D1716383

THE HISTORY OF
NATUROPATHIC MEDICINE
A CANADIAN PERSPECTIVE

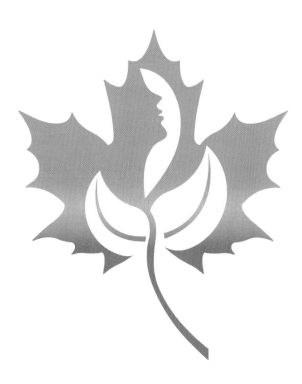

IVA LLOYD ND

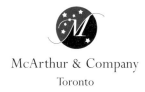

McArthur & Company
Toronto

First published in 2009 by
McArthur & Company
322 King St. West, Suite 402
Toronto, Ontario
M5V 1J2
www.mcarthur-co.com

Library and Archives Canada Cataloguing in Publication

    Lloyd, Iva
    History of naturopathic medicine : a Canadian perspective / Iva Lloyd.

ISBN 978-1-55278-778-6

    1. Naturopathy--History. I. Title.

RZ440.L585 2009   615.5'35   C2009-902733-X

Design and Composition by SZOL DESIGN
Printed and bound in Canada by Transcontinental

The publisher would like to acknowledge the financial support of the Government
of Canada through the Book Publishing Industry Development Program, The Canada
Council for the Arts, and the Ontario Arts Council for our publishing activities.
We also acknowledge the Government of Ontario through the Ontario Media
Development Corporation Ontario Book Initiative.

10 9 8 7 6 5 4 3 2 1

TABLE OF CONTENTS

ACKNOWLEDGEMENTS

THE COMPILING OF THE HISTORY of naturopathic medicine in Canada has been attempted, with limited success, in the past. The idea to pursue this task came about during a conversation between me and Dr. Verna Hunt ND as she talked about the tremendous change and growth in the profession over the years. The purpose of this book is to acknowledge the pioneers whose vision and devotion to the profession has paved the way for the future of naturopathic medicine, to inform the membership of the past achievements of those who have gone before them, to encourage the present members to zealously perverse the heritage they have been left and to provide a document that can be used to educate the public and the government on the strength, value and history of naturopathic medicine.

The first thing I did, once I agreed to the project, was to call my mother, Sherron Madeleine Lloyd. My mom has done genealogy most of her adult life. Madeleine is also my clinic office manager and over the years she has become a strong supporter of naturopathic medicine. She spent the next 26 months collecting boxes of information, contacting all the associations and schools and finding and compiling the names of all naturopathic doctors that had practiced in Canada, had graduated from a Canadian school or that were born in Canada and practiced elsewhere. She is a historian at heart, especially as it applies to family history, and she approached this project with the goal of ensuring that everyone was included. She has assisted with every aspect of the book, especially the collection of information. Without her gentle persistence and dedication this book would have never materialized.

With boxes and boxes of information the task of organizing the information began. Many people were skeptical as this project had been started a few times in the past. And thank goodness it had. A number of summaries and historic references served as a foundation for this book, such as documents written by Dr. Chris Turner ND, George Cody JD, Dr. Gerry Farnsworth ND, Dr. Sandesh Singh Khalsa ND and David Schleich PhD. Members of the provincial associations, regulatory boards and colleges were helpful in providing access to documentation, letters and journals. Many practitioners rifled through old files and provided needed information along the way. Books such as Nature Doctors, which was published by NCNM Press, have also served as a valuable reference.

The importance of collecting and writing about the history of Naturopathic Medicine had been recorded many times. The records of the naturopathic profession have encountered fire, floods, break-ins and have been lost in transport or mistakenly disposed of throughout time. Inconsistency in information and gaps in time frames have also added to the challenges. It is for this reason that the writing and retention of the history is so imperative. I am very thankful that National College of Natural Medicine and the Canadian College of Naturopathic Medicine have archives that include many of the initial books, journals and articles for the profession.

There have been many that have aided in this book including NDs Gerry Farnsworth, Mona Zarei, Chris Turner, Joe Pizzorno, Dugald Seely, David Lescheid, Gord Smith, Anton Ingard, Ken Dunk, Daria Love, Angela Moore, Ted Sleigh, Jim Farquharson, Lorne Swetlikoff, Mike Nowazek, Stephanie Ogura, Sinnoi Skaken and Elvis Ali. I also thank all those that wrote sections for the book, including Dr. Jim Wilson ND, Dr. Eric Shrubb ND, Dr. Pat Wolfe and Shawn O'Reilly. A special thanks to Dr. Verna Hunt ND who was a wonderful sounding board throughout the process; Dr. Pat Wales ND was a tremendous resource due to her years of being actively involved in the profession and Dr. Paul Saunders ND who was always available to clarify information and provide feedback. Glenn Cassie was instrumental in capturing the history from British Columbia and in reviewing many sections of the document.

I would like to thank the staff of CAND, Alex McKenna, Stuart Watson, Lisa Westlake and Heather Fleck and Lyle Clark from the BDDT-N. Every project like this requires people that are good at editing and proofing. There were many that assisted with this task, especially Madeleine Lloyd, Beth Riches, Hector D'Souza and Dr. Jodi Meacher ND. Kim McArthur and Company quickly grasped the essence of the book and provided guidance along the way.

Throughout the book the doctors listed are naturopathic doctors, unless stated otherwise. The book lists many individuals that have been involved in the profession, but my fear is that despite my best efforts, some who should be recognized have been left out. Please forgive any such omissions. You are welcome to send your thoughts to me or to the CAND to correct any oversights.

The Canadian Naturopathic Foundation (CNF), the Canadian Association of Naturopathic Doctors (CAND) NaturPharm Inc., Cyto Matrix and have financially supported the production of this book. All proceeds from this book will support CAND public awareness initiatives.

Iva Lloyd, ND

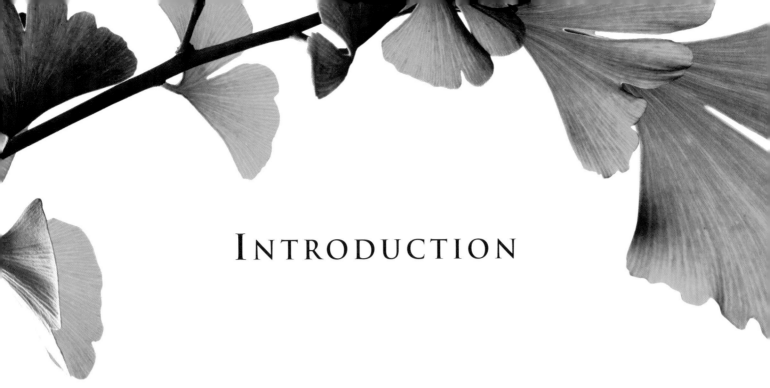

INTRODUCTION

THE YEAR WAS 1892. The first escalator was patented, the telephone switchboard went in to operation and X-ray machines were about to be invented. The "germ theory" of disease was receiving tremendous attention and gave great impetus to the pharmaceutical industry and shifted the focus away from hygiene, healthy living and individual responsibility for healthcare. Antibiotics were introduced a short-time later and with them the promise of "miracle cures." Over the next 30 years, more than 22 million people would pack their bags and their families and travel across the ocean in search of a better life, many of them bringing new concepts of healthcare to America. But it was the circumstances and actions of a twenty year old man from Germany that changed the face of natural medicine to this day.

Benedict Lust was an immigrant to America. In 1892 he came to New York to seek fortune. Instead, he found himself gravely ill. Lust had contracted tuberculosis. Given up on by medical doctors who advised him he would die from the disease, Lust decided he would return to his homeland. While in Germany, Lust heard about Sebastian Kneipp, a priest in a remote settlement west of Munich. Kneipp practiced hydrotherapy, a water cure that had worked wonders for many. Lust soon found his health improved dramatically and he not only became a firm believer in natural medicine, he become known as the 'Father of Naturopathy' in America.

In 1901 the term "Naturopathy" was used to describe all forms of natural healing that embraced health and disease from a vitalistic and holistic perspective. Although these terms are not commonly used today, they were in the 1800s and early 1900s. The concepts of vitalism and holism were the original philosophies for all forms of medicine. Over the years conventional medicine moved further and further away from its roots with every new discovery in chemistry and physics. The view of health and disease became reductionistic and dualist as medicine began to treat the body as a machine with individual parts and the body and mind as separate entities. Naturopathic medicine is a distinct system of medicine based on the philosophies of vitalism and holism. Naturopathic doctors are eclectic in their approach and, by staying true to the roots; they have become the leaders of natural medicine.

The history of naturopathic medicine in Canada is closely tied to that in the United States. Between 1896 and the 1920s, naturopathic medicine steadily developed: the number of colleges increased; regulation was achieved in four provinces and twenty-three states; and there were thousands of naturopathic physicians in America. This period was followed by fifty years of struggle and decline. Like all forms of medicine, naturopathic medicine is affected by the socio-economic environment and by politics and external factors. The decline in naturopathic medicine is attributed to the impact of wars and the Great Depression, the shifting of funding and support to allopathic-based medical schools; the birth of pharmaceutical medicine and the promise of 'miracle cures'; and the constant lobbying of the conventional medical associations. The interest in natural medicine diminished considerably between 1940 and 1970; enrolment at the colleges declined and the regulatory success that had been achieved was rescinded in many States. By 1950 there were less than a handful of naturopathic colleges remaining and many of the naturopathic programs were offered in chiropractic colleges.

Naturopathic medicine was developing as a profession one hundred years after conventional medicine which held the monopoly. There was tremendous pressure for naturopathic medicine, and other 'alternative' forms of medicine, to conform to the standards and rules that were being set based on allopathic principles. Even the governmental guidelines for medicine were, and continue to be, primarily allopathic in their approach to health and disease. Naturopathic medicine was faced with continual legal and regulatory battles that threatened the scope of practice and the ability of naturopathic doctors to practice.

Throughout it all, there were those practitioners - the champions of naturopathic medicine - that held true to their philosophies and principles. They dedicated their lives, volunteered their time, funded the schools, and continually put the profession ahead of their personal interests. There is great satisfaction in being a pioneer, but it comes with tremendous personal sacrifice.

Naturopathic medical institutions started the same way as most medical schools in the late 1800s - as apprenticeship-based institutions each spearheaded by a charismatic practitioner. During the first two decades, there were over twenty powerfully vitalistic naturopathic schools engrained in the philosophy of naturopathic medicine, yet lacking consistency in educational curriculum. Naturopathic education evolved as new standards of education were established for all systems of medical education in the early 1900s. By the mid 1950s naturopathic institutions were almost extinct due to the lack of funding, opposition and struggles with other systems of medicine, and because the profession was young and naïve. National College of Naturopathic Medicine was established in 1956 in Portland Oregon; naturopathic doctors from British Columbia played a significant role in the college with the intention of ensuring the survival of naturopathic medicine in Canada. It wasn't until twenty-two years later, in 1978, that the first naturopathic college opened in Canada. The Ontario College of Naturopathic Medicine, later renamed the Canadian College of Naturopathic Medicine, was established in Toronto and marked the time when the profession in Canada started to grow again. In 2001, the Boucher Institute of Naturopathic Medicine opened in Vancouver; now there are a total of seven colleges in the United States and Canada that meet accreditation requirements.

Health care in Canada is handled primarily at a provincial level. As such, provincial regulation is essential to ensure that Canadians can be guaranteed that practitioners have the education and standards to ensure patient safety. Every system of medicine is defined, to some degree, by the recognition and status that it achieves politically. Ontario naturopathic practitioners first received regulation in 1925 under the *Drugless Practitioners Act*. British Columbia followed in 1936 under the *Naturopathy Act*. Within five years, there were five provinces that regulated naturopathic doctors. Over the years, the major focus of the provincial associations has been to maintain or aquire regulatory status. In 2008, Nova Scotia gained title protection. This was the first 'new' province to achieve provincial recognition in over fifty years.

One thing that the naturopathic profession has not been able to do well is explain the research behind naturopathic medicine. This book will explore the different forms of research, the importance of choosing research designs that match the philosophy and criteria measured and the factors that determine and influence research. It is often reported that there are three criteria needed to establish a medical profession: quality education institutions, government recognition and provincial formation. It could be argued that there are others. The establishment of a profession requires ongoing support from and for members, continual research initiatives, building relationships with other professional associations and continual funding. To accomplish all of this requires dedicated individuals that have the vision, knowledge, patience and commitment to see it all happen and who are committed to moving the profession forward in one direction.

The return to naturopathic medicine in the 1970s was in direct response to a reawakening to the values of personal responsibility for health. The realization that a healthy environment and healthy individuals go hand-in-hand and that individuals have to be responsible for their health by living a healthy lifestyle, that emotions and thoughts affect health and that health promotion is a life-long journey. Consumers are choosing naturopathic doctors as their primary care doctors as the philosophies and treatments of naturopathic medicine are in line with these beliefs.

What has always been unique for naturopathic medicine is its broad scope of practice. For many, especially government and other health care professionals, the broad scope was viewed negatively. There have been many attempts to restrict the practice of naturopathic physicians. Yet, a strength of naturopathic medicine is its broad scope. It is the recognition that naturopathic medicine is not defined by the therapies that a practitioner uses; but by why and how they choose to use those therapies. There are many different ways to establish health and treat disease. A system of medicine that intends to grow and change can not be restricted in its scope. It is important to have a philosophy that guides and defines the path for the profession, but it is equally important to allow that profession to develop and expand over time. The aim of naturopathic medicine is to maintain the foundation for health and to embrace new discoveries as they arise. Naturopathic doctors have always been on the leading edge of natural health care and are true leaders in that field. This field of medicine is composed of practitioners who value subjectivity, intuition and spirituality, as well as those who value objectivity, reproducibility and practicality. Naturopathic medicine has truly bridged the art and science of natural health care.

Naturopathic medicine has established itself as a strong, viable primary health care system. Practitioners continue to interface with all levels of government stressing the importance of prevention, the focus on a healthy lifestyle and the value of treating the whole person.

PART ONE

THE ROOTS OF
NATUROPATHIC MEDICINE

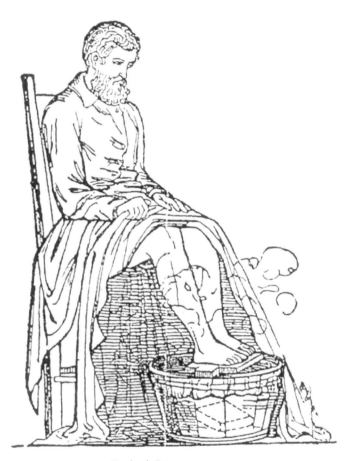

Kneipp's Foot vapor

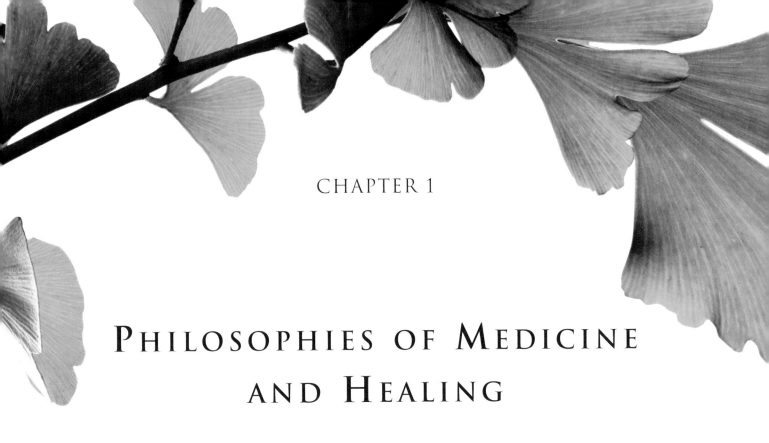

CHAPTER 1

PHILOSOPHIES OF MEDICINE AND HEALING

Vitalism and Holism: *the origins of medicine*

IN THE EARLIEST KNOWN CIVILIZATIONS people lived in a harmonious relationship with their surroundings and the understanding of disease was accomplished by observing nature and how it interplayed with human life. Traditional medical systems, such as Ayurvedic and Chinese medicine have been practiced for over 5,000 years. What these traditional forms of medicine have in common is the understanding that the body has an innate ability to heal – referred to as vitalism - and that life, health and disease follow certain laws and principles that are logical. They recognize that in order to achieve health, you must treat all aspects of an individual and that health is dependent on a healthy lifestyle and on the health of the environment – referred to as holism.

Hippocrates (460 – 377 BC), traditionally considered the father of western medicine, including naturopathic, acknowledged the concepts of vitalism and holism. Treatment was based on the fundamental assumption that nature had a strong healing force and tendency of its own, and that the main role of the physician was to assist nature in this healing process, rather than to direct it arbitrarily. Health was viewed as a state of the harmonic mixture of the body humors or fluids and disease was a result

"Let your food be your medicine and your medicine be your food."

HIPPOCRATES (460 – 377 BC)

of a faulty mixture. There was the understanding that nature itself would maintain balance and restore health through a number of internal processes. Hippocratic physicians based their treatments on each individual, not a disease; and the body was treated as an integrated whole, not as individual parts. The main allies of the physician in assisting nature in this process were food, exercise, hot baths and herbs which promoted the elimination of internal wastes.

The vitalistic concept was first articulated by the Greek philosophers Socrates and Aristotle around 300 BC. They used the term '*logos*' or 'will to live' to describe this vital principle. Aristotle was a great philosopher who sought to explain the human body's position in the universe, how it came into being and the meaning of its life. He believed that a "soul" animated and directed the body and that it contributed to one's state of health.

These concepts continued as a basis for the study of health and disease for centuries. The philosopher Moses Maimonides (1135 – 1204) was a court physician to the royal family in Cairo, Egypt. In contrast to other medical practitioners (viewed as philosophers in those days), who were embracing the use of drugs and surgery, he emphasized the use of diet, exercise and a positive mental outlook as the way to achieve health. Maimonides wrote a book, *Preservation of Youth,* which was based completely on natural methods and it documented how to live in harmony with the environment.

Scientific Methods: *a change in focus*

The Renaissance period (1300 – 1650) changed everything. The invention of the printing press resulted in the mass production of books and the ability for information to be compiled and shared more readily. Travel was easier and resulted in a sharing of medical practices and remedies from distant lands. With advances in technology and science, the functioning of the body started to be understood using the concepts of chemistry and physics.

During this time period the understanding of anatomy and physiology was greatly enhanced. Once dissections became common practice and physicians were able to understand what was happening under the skin, the focus of medicine changed and expanded. In contrast to the ancient tradition, which placed the origin of disease within the body (as a disturbance of the humors), the physician, Paracelsus (1493 – 1541), postulated that materials in food and drink and abnormalities in organs were primarily responsible for diseases. He was also one of the first to explain disease as a highly specific chemical process. This period of time provided tremendous insight into the biochemical and physiology processes in the body. Vitalistic and holistic concepts were downplayed and often completely dismissed, as the physical and scientific aspects became the focus of medicine.

Isaac Newton (1643 – 1727) was an English physicist, mathematician, natural philosopher and theologian. He provided the theories behind gravitation, the laws of motion and the ground work for classical mechanics that dominated scientific thought for the next three centuries.

The philosopher René Descartes (1596 – 1650) widened the gap between science and vitalism. Descartes was responsible for introducing the concept that the mind and body were split and that all elements of the universe were isolated from each other, divisible and wholly self-contained. Descartes saw the human body as a machine that could be studied and understood in terms of a mechanical model with little regard for the influence of environment on health, the acknowledgement of an innate ability of the body to heal itself or the presence of a vital essence.

"The art of healing comes from nature, not from the physician. Therefore, the physician must come from nature, with an open mind."

PARACELSUS (1493 – 1541)

This mechanistic approach shaped research and science for hundreds of years, and contributed to humans becoming more detached not only from their environment, but from their own mind and soul. It replaced the vitalistic and holistic perspective that had been held for centuries. The book, *What the Bleep Do We Know,* states, "The separation of mind and body that Descartes made into a fundamental rule of science, and which scientific discovery believed for hundreds of years, has caused endless problems. By viewing the world outside our minds as nothing but lifeless matter, operating according to predictable, mechanical laws and devoid of any spiritual or animate quality, it divided us from the living nature that sustains us. And it provided humanity with a perfect excuse to exploit all 'natural resources' for our own selfish and immediate purposes, with no concern for other living beings or for the future of the planet."

Two centuries later the Darwinian theories supported the idea of the separateness between mind and body. Charles Darwin (1809 – 1882) saw life as random, predatory, purposeless and solitary. He denied the concept that humans and their environment depended on each other and the need for them to live together cooperatively. He promoted the belief that life was about winning, getting there first; those that are first are on the top of the evolutionary tree. His theories influenced medicine and many other aspects of civilization for centuries.

The "germ theory" of disease had been proposed as early as 36 BC and, in the 1st century, the concept of quarantine was introduced due to the realization that diseases, such as tuberculosis, had an infectious nature. Yet, Louis Pasteur (1822 – 1895), a French microbiologist and chemist, is often credited with the germ theory discovery. Between the years of 1860 and 1864 he demonstrated that specific microorganisms were responsible for particular types of infection. He was also responsible for introducing the concept of pasteurization. The germ theory was beneficial in improving hygienic conditions in hospitals and surgeries and in improving awareness of everyday hygiene. It

The microscope was invented in 1590 by two Dutch spectacle makers, Zacharias Janssen and his son Hans. Anton van Leeuwenhoek (1632 – 1723) of Holland, expanded on their discoveries and built the first microscope.

influenced the field of microbiology and immunology and contributed greatly to furthering our understanding of disease processes within the body. It also gave rise to the "magic bullet" concept where the pharmaceutical industry creates a drug to kill a specific bug. For many scientists, medical practitioners and the pharmaceutical industry the germ theory became a primary focus of conventional medicine. It placed the emphasis of healing on drugs and caused an even greater separation between disease and lifestyle.

The reductionist and mechanistic schools view the body as an intricate machine which can be dissected and analyzed into its various parts. According to this theory, life and health can be explained as the product of complex reactions of chemical, electrical and mechanical interactions. Mechanistic medicine indentifies disease and its accompanying signs and symptoms as simply the result of a disruption of normal chemical reactions and hence uses drugs which function in the same way. This view is helpful in explaining biochemical processes, but it is inadequate in many ways, especially related to chronic degenerative disease and when explaining the overall impact of stressful situations on one's health.

Prior to the invention of microscopes, stethoscopes, x-ray machines and other diagnostic tools, the primary means of assessing illness was listening to a patient, how they recalled their symptoms and how they were impacted by lifestyle and environment. The emphasis was on observing the patient and on listening to the patient's story. As medicine became more focused on science and technology less attention was paid to the patient. Names and concepts of diseases changed from relating to the subjective symptoms and the causal factors to being associated with anatomical and pathological functions within the body.

Rene Laennec, a French physician invented the stethoscope in 1816

Vitalism and Holism Returns: *alternative medicine begins*

Prior to the 18th century, a number of practitioners still embraced vitalistic and holistic concepts and treatment facilities that utilized diet, exercise, water therapy and herbs started to appear. The following are a few of the significant practitioners and researchers that kept the concepts of vitalism and holism alive. Thomas Sydenham (1624 – 1689) who is recognized as the founder of European clinical medicine, believed it was the task of the physician to assist the body's natural processes while searching for the causes of disease, which were often due to lifestyle factors. George Ernst Stahl (1660 – 1734) believed that even though the organs of the body were subject to the laws of chemistry and physics, there was a soul that regulated and harmonized their functions. Jean-Jacques Rousseau (1712 – 1778) advocated a strong emotional attitude towards nature, a theory of health, disease treatment and cure, and a preference for treatments considered natural.

Christoph Wilhelm Hufeland (1762 – 1836) used treatments based on hydrotherapy, air and light baths, vegetarian diet and herbal remedies. He served as a royal physician to the King of Prussia and was a prolific author. He is viewed as one of the founders of holistic medicine. His book *The Art of Prolonging Human Life* (1796) was the first book written on preventive medicine and natural health care that became a best-seller.

By the end of the 18th century the field of medicine which became known as alternative medicine began to take root and the "old" ways of medicine started to reappear.

Modern Day Medicine: *blending together*

Early in the 19th century, new discoveries in the fields of quantum physics, energy medicine, systems theory and ecology started to question mechanistic, reductionist and dualist concepts. The pioneers of quantum physics, Erwin Schrödinger, Werner Heisenberg, Niels Bohr and Wolfgang Pauli recognized that many aspects of life could not be explained by the restraints of these concepts.

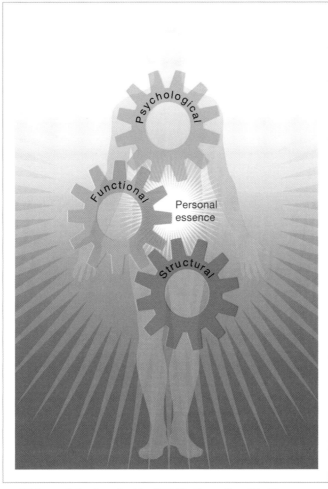

Every aspect of an individual works as a unit with a personal essence (vitality) that guides life and provides innate healing.

With permission from Iva Lloyd ND. The Energetics of Health, a naturopathic assessment, Elsevier 2009

The basis of quantum physics was the recognition that particles had no meaning in isolation, only in relationship to everything else. Also, at its most elemental state, matter couldn't be chopped up into self-contained little units, but was completely indivisible and part of the greater web of life. It describes how all living beings, including humans, are simply beings of light energy. Every cell of the body has it own energetic field and complex wave pattern, and all energetic fields 'talk' to each other and interact, both internally and with their external environment. It goes on to explain how the energy of a person can be affected by others, even when they are at a distance. It explains how thoughts and emotions impact health, the healing power of intention and prayer, the impact of colour and sound on health, and many other concepts that before were unexplainable. Quantum theories have impacted all aspects of medicine and continue to influence how doctors view and treat individual patients.

Systems theory illustrates how aspects of life are interconnected and how human beings are dependent on and a part of their environment. It explains the complexity and inner workings of the body as a complex system with each part able to impact every other part. Research shows that human beings are discovered to be self-organizing systems that had the ability to renew, grow and heal based on an inner wisdom or vital force. Human beings are able to influence and be influenced by factors outside their physical bodies. It illustrates how the mind is able to impact physiological functions and how a person's posture and physical structure is able to alter the mind. According to system theory, the body operates as a single unit, not as individual parts.

Modern day science recognizes that the concepts of vitalism and holism are as integral to understanding health and disease as the concepts of reductionism and mechanism. The true picture, and hence the answer to health promotion and disease prevention, lies in the blending of all the knowledge.

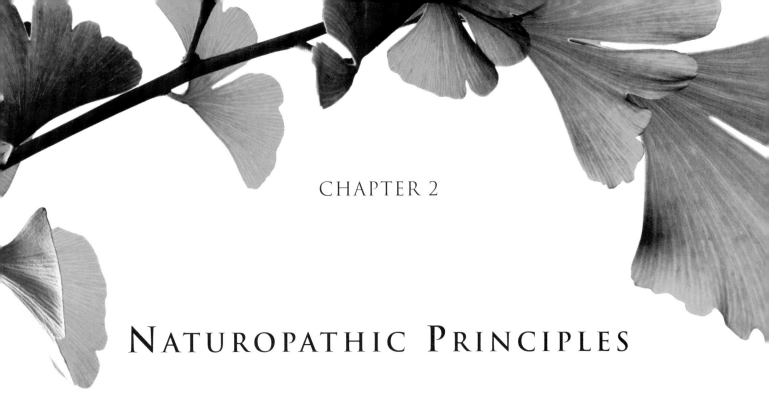

CHAPTER 2

NATUROPATHIC PRINCIPLES

VITALISM AND HOLISM REPRESENT the philosophy of naturopathic medicine. The principles represent how these philosophies are applied in practice. Before naturopathic medicine was described as six principles it was often written about and discussed according to its philosophy, science, art and practice. Over the years, as the educational standards of the naturopathic colleges became more rigorous and standardized and as the class sizes became larger, it was felt that the principles and philosophy of naturopathic medicine needed to be conveyed in a structured fashion in order to ensure consistency of the information and to ease communication both within the profession and between the profession and others. In 1986 the American Association of Naturopathic Practitioners (AANP) formed a committee that consisted of naturopathic doctors Andre Saine, Pam Snider, Jared Zeff and others. These practitioners spent over three years reviewing the historic data and documents and interviewing over 1,000 people. In 1989 there was a three day meeting on Dr. Saine's farm in Ontario that resulted in a unified definition of naturopathic medicine and the description of the six naturopathic principles. Later that year, at the AANP conference and at a Canadian Naturopathic Association board meeting both national organizations agreed on six defining principles of naturopathic medicine.

First, Do No Harm (*Primum non nocere*)

"First, do no harm" has been a principle of medicine since the time of Hippocrates. From a naturopathic perspective, it refers not only to the patient but to the patient's vital force. It refers to choosing treatments that support the innate healing ability of the body and that honour the laws of nature. To *"do no harm"*, a practitioner chooses the diagnostic techniques and therapies, and fashions the most gentle and non-invasive strategy necessary for each individual patient. By respecting the integrity and vitality of the patient, the healing process is supported versus overridden or suppressed. *"Do no harm"* involves practitioners teaching their patients insight and awareness of how their lifestyle choices affect their health.

It is important to address lifestyle factors in the initial part of treatment if they are the root cause of disease or a contributing factor. Often when these factors are appropriately addressed, minimal other treatment is required. Naturopathic doctors work on the basis that there is a hierarchy to treatment choices starting with lifestyle changes and then proceeding from the least invasive and forceful to the most.

In situations, especially when the progression of disease is advanced or the current state is critical, it is necessary to chose more aggressive treatments or treatments that pose the risk of adverse effects. An aggressive treatment may require referral for drugs or surgery, but at times it can be accomplished by changing many lifestyle, environment or external factors at once and supporting the body with the use of naturopathic therapies.

The Healing Power of Nature (*Vis medicatrix naturae*)

The followers of Hippocrates used the term *vis medicatrix naturae*, the healing power of nature, to denote the body's ability to heal itself. Naturopathic medicine recognizes that each person has an inherent healing ability which is organized, orderly and intelligent. The body automatically knows what to do to stimulate the healing process, for example when we cut our finger the wound automatically starts to close. A fever is a common advantageous reaction to the flu. Vomiting or diarrhea are the body's way of responding to the ingestion of spoiled food. There is no mistaking this innate healing ability. The aim of naturopathic physicians is to treat the patient, not the disease, by directing the vital force and encouraging it with naturopathic therapeutics to stimulate the body's own defences.

Medical therapy takes two forms: practitioners can attempt to strengthen the body so that it can heal, organize and defend itself; or it can attack the agents and mechanisms of disease directly. A naturopathic doctor addresses foreign agents of disease, but the focus is on strengthening the body thus decreasing its susceptibility to disease.

Symptoms often are the manifestation of the organism's attempt to defend and heal itself. For example take a patient who complains of hip pain and numbness down his leg. If the patient has poor posture and continually sits on a thick wallet, the treatment involves correcting the misalignment, educating the patient on proper posture, and informing him not to sit on his wallet. Once that is done, the remaining symptoms resolve on their own. Simply recommending an anti-inflammatory (whether drug, botanical or homeopathic) does not address the root cause and even if the symptoms diminish temporarily they will likely return.

"During the healthy condition of man the spirit-like force which animates the material body rules supreme as "dynamis". All parts are wonderfully maintained by it as a harmonious vital process, both in feelings and functions, in order that our intelligent mind may be free to make the living, healthy, bodily medium subservient to the higher purpose of our being."
SAMUEL HAHNEMANN, M.D.
(1755 – 1843)

Identify and Treat the Causes *(Tolle causam)*

Health and disease are logical outcomes of a person's genetics, vitality, lifestyle, environment and external factors. The primary goal of a naturopathic physician is to identify, address and/or remove the underlying causes of disease. The body naturally compensates whenever the internal functioning is overwhelmed. This compensation shows up as symptoms and as a disruption to health. The aim of the practitioner is to determine the specific trigger, event, or behaviour that initiated the disruption and that needs to be addressed.

Health and disease are complex and logical and they occur for specific reasons. The manifestation of symptoms or disease is never the root cause of the problem. To understand the root cause a practitioner starts at when and why the disruption of health was initiated. To elicit a cure, the factors that initiated the imbalance - the root cause - need to be addressed, especially if they are still occurring. For example, if someone is angry because of the way they are being treated at work and they hold in their anger, this suppression of emotion might result in digestive discomfort, headaches, changes in hormones or mood or in a red rash. If the treatment involves taking something to mask the digestive discomfort, relieve the headache, and a cream to minimize the redness of the rash, but does not address the anger, the suppressed anger continues to signal the body, resulting in the same or deeper, more severe symptoms.

Recognizing a relationship between lifestyle and health is a concept that has been around for centuries. Yet over the years, most people have moved further away from a lifestyle that is supportive of health. Fast food, stimulants, sedentary jobs, fast-paced lifestyles and less time resting and sleeping are all contributing factors. The invention of pesticides, plastics, paints, cell phones, video games, etc. have all had a negative impact on health. Human beings are complex, living multi-dimensional energetic systems that have a limited capacity to handle the onslaught of a toxic lifestyle and environment. Identifying the root cause of disease and the aggravating factors is an essential aspect of health care; now-a-days there are just more considerations and doctors need to be more thorough. As part of the therapeutic encounter, a naturopathic doctor explores a large number of variables. They understand that health is improved by reducing the number of factors that strain the body and interfere with its normal functioning and ability to heal. Naturopathic treatment involves teaching each patient that a return to a more simple and health promoting lifestyle often is the best medicine.

Treat the Whole Person

Disease affects the entire person, not just a specific organ or system. Health and disease are a result of a complex interaction of all aspects of a person, their life and environment. A naturopathic assessment includes addressing the nutritional status, lifestyle, family history, physical, mental, emotional, genetic, environmental, social, spiritual, external and other factors. The mind, body and spirit aspects of an individual are an inseparable whole that is interconnected and interdependent with family, community and environment.

"Treat the whole person" is a holistic concept that recognizes that the whole is greater than the sum of the parts. Each individual is unique with their own specific susceptibilities and way of manifesting disharmony and disease. It is the harmonious functioning of all aspects of the individual, within themselves and within their environment, that is essential to health.

"A careful physician. . . before he attempts to administer a remedy to his patient, must investigate not only the malady of the man, he wishes to cure, but also his habits when in health, and his physical constitution."
CICERO (106-43 B.C.)

Doctor as Teacher (*Docere*)

Docere, which means "doctor", comes from the latin word "to teach" and a naturopathic physician's role is to educate patients so that they are able to take responsibility for their own health. Each person has a choice whether to choose a healthy or a diseased way to live. Choices about food and eating regimen, occupational and environmental situations, exercise, spiritual well-being, posture, hygiene, rest and recreation and state of mind all impact health and healing. The role of the naturopathic doctor is

"Those that know, do. Those that understand, teach."
ARISTOTLE (384 – 1322 BC)

to ensure that choices are based on sound advice, specific to the health needs of each individual.

Teaching takes time and hence the time spent with a naturopathic doctor is typically longer than with other medical practitioners. In order for a person to have an understanding of why they are sick, what they can do to improve the situation and what they have to change for the future, it is important that each sessions allow time for the patient to talk and the doctor to listen. It is this awareness and understanding by the patient that determines long-term wellness, not just the knowledge level of the doctor.

Disease Prevention and Health Promotion

"People are beginning to realize that it is cheaper and more advantageous to prevent disease rather than to cure it."

Henry Lindlahr ND (1862 - 1924)

Naturopathic physicians encourage and emphasize disease prevention, promoting a healthy lifestyle, assessing risk factors, determining suscep-tibility to disease and making appropriate interventions. This approach prevents minor illnesses from developing into more serious or chronic degenerative disease.

Prevention of disease is a continual process that starts at conception and continues throughout all of life. It involves every aspect of a person – their lifestyle, emotional health, family and community and the envi-ronment in which they live. It is difficult for individuals to be healthy in an unhealthy environment. The role of the practitioner is to facilitate increased awareness, as well as to educate each patient on the changes required to address their health concerns and to ensure prevention. Maintaining health and preventing disease is an ongoing process, not a short-term project.

There is no magic bullet. You cannot eat a poor diet and have an unhealthy lifestyle and correct it by taking supplements or relying on vaccines and drugs to prevent disease. The basis of prevention is about lifestyle and about living in harmony with the environment.

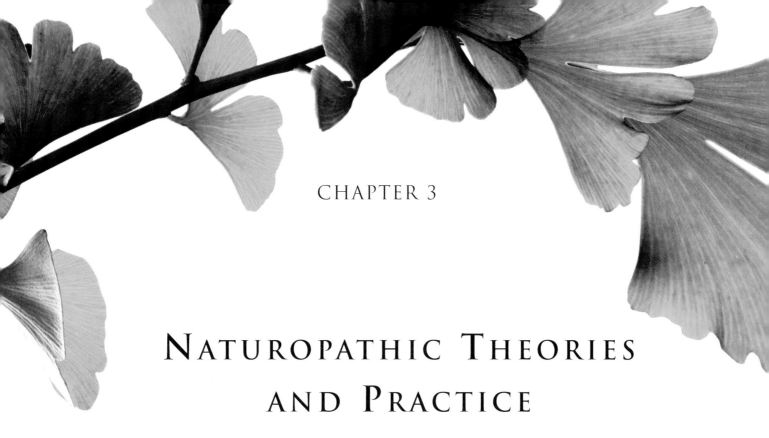

CHAPTER 3

NATUROPATHIC THEORIES AND PRACTICE

THE THEORIES AND PRACTICE of each system of medicine is determined by how the practitioners define health and disease and their expectations and beliefs about wellness. The theories influence every aspect of assessment, diagnosis, and treatment. They dictate what information is sought and how it is interpreted. They determine whether the emphasis of the patient-practitioner relationship is on addressing the factors that cause disease or just treating the symptoms. Whether health and disease are viewed as logical or random, and whether a practitioner is trained to integrate all aspects of a patient or just address specific pathological conditions, impacts the meaning that is assigned to symptoms and diseases and the approach used.

From a naturopathic perspective, health and ill-health are not two separate states of being. It is a continuum. This continuum allows a patient to move from a state of health to ill-health or from ill-health to health. At any point in time, if vitality, willingness, and the building blocks to health are present, a patient's innate healing power works to sustain life and restore health. The naturopathic definition of health and ill-health (or disease) is based on the concepts of vitalism and holism. It recognizes the uniqueness of each person and the logic of health and disease. It understands that there are essential building blocks to health and that each person is an individual. The naturopathic physician's role is to listen to each person and guide them back to health, with the recognition that true healing is an inherent ability and right.

What is Health?

"Health is more than just the absence of disease; it is a vital dynamic state which enables a person to adapt to, and thrive in a wide range of environments."

Iva Lloyd ND 2008

"And in the end, it's not the years in our life that count. It's the life in your years."

Abraham Lincoln (1809 – 1865)

The natural or desirable state of existence is health. A patient's view of health and disease changes as they mature and age and as a result of life experiences. People are affected by culture, religion, economics, race, class, gender, and other social and biological factors. Health is an attitude, and the desirability of the outcome depends on one's beliefs, expectations, and upbringing. For some this means the absence of signs or symptoms; for others it represents an awakening on a psychological or spiritual level. For others health is the absence of any symptoms that impact daily life; with the tolerance for symptoms varying greatly among patients. Some people perceive themselves as healthy, even when they have a disease or disability.

The body is continuously responding to, compensating for, and balancing the various internal and external stimuli that it encounters. There are periods of development, growth, and maturation as the body continually replaces, heals, and nourishes every aspect of it self. There is continual change and movement. Throughout all of this, the aim is to maintain health.

Every component of a patient functions autonomously to some degree, yet they are also interdependent on every other part. If one component is in a state of deficiency or excess, it impacts other components. For example, if the digestive system is not functioning appropriately the other cells, tissues and organs will not receive the nutrients that they require. As a result, other aspects compensate to ensure that vital organs and functions are preserved. Symptoms are initially subtle and arise whenever imbalances in lifestyle or environment exceed a person's ability to compensate or adapt appropriately. What shifts and how it shifts relates to a person's constitution, the disruptive factors, and how a person attempted to compensate. Likewise, as lifestyle and environmental factors improve, there is a return towards health.

Building Blocks to Health

There are eight basic building blocks to health. These are the components that provide the fuel and structure for the body to function. They ensure that the terrain of the body, that is the internal environment, has the nutrients and ingredients to sustain health and to aid in healing and repair. The building blocks are the aspects of health promotion, the healthy lifestyle habits, which influence all stages of life and all stages of health and disease. The building blocks are: posture, rest and sleep, movement, food, water, expression of emotions, breathing and positive mental outlook.

Posture represents the ability of the body to maintain structure and form. An aligned posture provides open and straight pathways for the flow of energy, nutrients and fluid. When posture is not aligned it is like having a kink in the hose. Poor posture causes stress on organs and tissues and can result in pain or stiffness and it is a contributing factor to many diseases.

Rest and *sleep* represents the body's ability to slow down, to heal and to grow. It can be disrupted by many factors, such as: poor dietary habits, ingestion of stimulants, like caffeine and sugar; excessive mental activity, too much physical activity right before bedtime, musculoskeletal pain, poor sleep environment, stress, excessive television or computer usage, too much noise or light, shift work or a sense of discontentment at one's core. It can also be affected by different diseases. Adequate rest and sleep are essential to health.

Movement is about flexibility, range of motion and internal and external motion. Many physical symptoms are triggered by the lack of internal movement of blood, lymphatics, nutrients or water. Physical movement is an important factor in maintaining internal movement and hence the body needs to move. It requires horizontal movement like walking and vertical movement like rebounding or bouncing on a daily basis to maintain health.

Food is more than protein, carbohydrates and fats. It is the primary way that we nurture ourselves and it supplies the basic fuel for the body. Food assists in healing, influences health, mood and energy on a daily basis and

"If a patient complains of one or more trivial symptoms that have been only observed a short time previously, the physician should not regard this as a fully developed disease that requires serious medical aid. A slight alteration in the diet and regimen will usually suffice to dispel such an indisposition."

SAMUEL HAHNEMANN, MD (1755-1843)

can contribute to disease. There is a difference between good food and food that is good for you. The first step is to get a sense of how you feel after a meal. A meal that includes foods that are suited to you and that is nutritious increases your energy and does not cause any symptoms. Addressing food intolerances and eating regimen are often the first step to achieving better health.

Water comprises over 70% of the body and is one of the most essential components. It is a life-sustaining and life-giving substance that is required for every living function and structure. Without sufficient water on a regular basis the body soon becomes dehydrated. This affects energy, health and longevity. A general rule of thumb for calculating how much water you need is to consume half your body weight (in pounds) in ounces each day. Keep in mind that the best source of water is plain water. Coffee, soft drinks and many fruit juices are actually dehydrating due to the high caffeine and sugar content in these drinks.

Breathing represents the ability to take in air to every cell of the body. It is the only activity that you do throughout our whole life both consciously and unconsciously. Many people do not breathe properly. Try this exercise. Put one hand on your upper chest and one on your low abdomen while sitting in a chair with both feet on the ground and your back straight. Take a deep breath. Your top hand should stay still and the hand on your low abdomen should move outward. Proper breathing is about taking deep slow breaths into your low abdomen. It is one of the most effective ways of calming the nervous system and is an essential skill.

Expression of Emotions Health is most easily maintained when a person feels safe and is able to express their emotions. Chaos is created when there is a difference between what a person feels inside and what they express. This chaos contributes to disease. For example, if a person is unhappy with their marriage or job they often feel sad. This sadness is a true reflection of their life. Health is restored by addressing the situation or changing one's beliefs or expectations; not by suppressing the feelings.

The mental outlook that a person has influences every aspect of health and disease. It can restore health on its own, it can intensify the impact of subtle interventions and it can nullify the impact of a treatment. Over the next few generations the focus of the mind in healing will become one of the greatest areas of research and study. A person's mind chatter, mental state, outlook on life, beliefs and their ability to work with their mind is an important component of health.

For some, health is achieved by addressing a few building blocks that currently aren't part of their lifestyle. For others, it involves a dramatic shift. What you'll find is that when the basic building blocks are part of your lifestyle, there is a greater chance of preventing disease, healing from any injury and promoting ongoing health.

Individual Constitution

Each person is unique, with different builds, body compositions, and attitudes. Much of western medicine has been based on the principle that because each patient has similar parts, they can be treated the same. Naturopathic medicine, as well as the eastern medicines, recognizes that it is the uniqueness of patients and the integration of all the parts that holds the key to achieving and maintaining health.

A person's constitution is their baseline. It represents their natural tendencies, their primary makeup, their appearance, and their disposition. It represents their inherent strengths and their weaknesses. It is determined at conception, but is influenced throughout life due to learned behaviour and experiences. It is also affected by a person's lifestyle and environment. A person's constitution indicates their healing potential, their resistance to disease and their susceptibilities.

Susceptibility is affected by past injuries, beliefs and thoughts. If a person believes that disease and a lower level of health comes with age, a decrease in healing potential might be more a reflection of this belief than their actual health status. If a person believes that they are likely to suffer the same symptoms and diseases as their parents, it is more likely to happen. The aim of maintaining health is supporting and maintaining areas of strength, and adjusting and balancing for areas of weakness.

"Health is linked to emotional responsiveness in the face of changing life circumstances and social interactions. The word "e-motion" tells it all — we need to keep our feelings and energy in motion, rather than locking them in our tissues."

SAT DHARAM KAUR ND

Transformation between Health and Disease

"Chronic disease never develops suddenly in the human body. Nature always tries to prevent its gradual development by acute and sub-acute healing efforts. If these, by any means whatever, are checked and suppressed, then they are followed either by fatal complications or chronic after effects, the mysterious "sequelae" of medical science."

HENRY LINDLAHR ND (1862-1924)

Some people are able to define a point in time that their health shifted. For others, it is a more gradual progression over a longer period of time. For everyone the balance between health and disease oscillates over a lifetime. The concept of disease, like health, depends on a person's expectations and beliefs. For example, some people view disease as the onset of symptoms, and others view themselves as having a disease when informed by a doctor or when their health concerns disrupt their life or their sense of well being.

Disease is a process and it often starts with subtle changes in health. A person's energy may decrease; sleep or appetite maybe disrupted or digestion and elimination show signs of stress. Prevention involves paying attention to subtle changes and becoming aware of what caused them. Naturopathic doctors have a number of theories about the process of disease. These theories influence how they approach the assessment process; diagnose diseases and the treatment strategies that they employ.

Acute Healing Response

Acute states come on suddenly and are usually initiated by an exposure to an external pathogen or a minor injury, such as flus and colds, a fall, food poisoning or coming in contact with poison ivy. The innate response is for the body to heal, balance and compensate for whatever factor has disrupted health. Usually acute conditions result in inflammatory symptoms as the body attempts to release "toxins" through one of the routes of elimination – bowels, urine, nasal passages, lungs, or skin.

"Every acute disease is the result of a purifying, healing effort of nature."

HENRY LINDLAHR ND (1862-1924)

During an acute healing response, it is best to support the body, not to override it or suppress it. For example, a natural response to the flu is a fever and it is important to support this response, even to encourage it. Doing so supports the ability of the body to heal. Suppressing the fever, which is done all-too-often, weakens the immune system; making a person more susceptible over time to infection.

The body returns to health when acute conditions are properly handled. If the response is suppressed or does not completely restore, the area of the body affected becomes weakened and more susceptible to injury or attack in the future. The continual suppression or lack of resolve of acute conditions contributes to chronic disease.

A Healing Crisis

The path from disease to health involves symptoms or signs of healing referred to as a healing crisis. These signs and symptoms come on suddenly and tend to resolve on their own. A 'healing crisis' is often a necessary part of the process of recovery. The symptoms that arise relate to those symptoms that were suppressed or unresolved. For example, if a patient has a history of respiratory infections that had been suppressed, it would be common, and often desirable, for that person to get an infection, as the respiratory and immune functions are strengthened. In a situation such as this, the practitioner would have most likely discovered during the intake that as a child they had several ear infections that had been suppressed with antibiotics or other treatments.

The suppressed symptoms typically arise in reverse order, i.e., the symptoms that a patient experienced last manifest first in the healing process; ending with the symptoms that caused the initial episode. The presence of a healing crisis is a positive sign, as it indicates the strength of the body's healing potential. It is common for a naturopathic doctor to intentionally stimulate a healing crisis, such as using hydrotherapy to stimulate a fever. Those new to naturopathic medicine, may interpret a healing crisis as a sign that a previous disease state is returning.

Progression to Chronic Disease

A worsening of the symptoms occurs when mild symptoms are not addressed or resolved. Chronic disease and destruction of tissues and function is a multi-factorial process and involves the prolonged and continual disruption in the needed resources for health. The timing and progression depends on a number of factors that are continuously at play, such as a patient's constitution, their susceptibilities, their adherence to the building blocks of health, and their exposure to external and environment disrupting factors. The onset of disease is influenced by the manner in which a patient addresses and handles signs and symptoms throughout their life, and it depends on the severity and impact of any particular disrupting factor.

Disease is a progressive process that has the ability to move in both directions. The initial symptoms often involve an excretory reaction – similar to an acute healing response - and results in symptoms such as irritation or inflammation, rash, sweating, fever, diarrhea, acute muscle pain, tiredness or psychological disturbances such as mild anxiety, frustration. Symptoms become more intense and more constant as the excesses build at a greater degree than they are excreted or balanced. When one specific organ or part of the body reaches its threshold, it creates an internal aggravation which spills over into other parts and the signs of disease begin to affect multiple organs and functions. If the appropriate steps are not taken, symptoms become more engrained in the body and overtime become more internal. Eventually the tissues start to deteriorate and break-down and there is destruction in overall function and structure. The progression eventually results in diseases such as cancer and autoimmune disease or in death.

Naturopathic Assessment

During an assessment, a naturopathic doctor conducts a detailed history, including information relating to diet, emotional state, exercise, lifestyle, past and current stressors, and exposure to environmental toxins. A naturopathic doctor inquires about a patient's family history, accidents and injuries, past and present medical history, procedures and treatments, as well as current medications, supplements, and all other forms of treatment.

The time frame of a patient's history is relevant in determining whether the symptoms are a result of an event or situation or as a result of lifestyle, stresses or environmental factors that have affected health over a long period of time. A naturopathic physician takes the time to listen to the patient's story and to

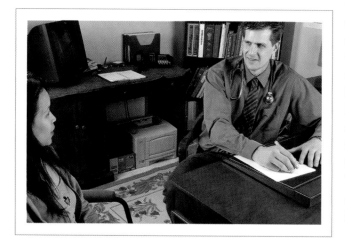

understand how their health concerns are impacting their life. Symptoms are a warning sign that something is wrong or something needs to be changed. A part of assessments includes learning how to listen to the body and how to understand what it is doing and why. It involves awareness and understanding of how the body responds to life. Together, the patient's and the physician's aim is to identify the underlying causative factors.

The detailed history is followed by a standard physical examination. Naturopathic doctors are also trained in additional examination procedures such as tongue and pulse assessment as these tools provide information on internal functioning often prior to any abnormalities showing up on other tests. Laboratory tests are done, or requested, as needed, including X-ray examinations and/or scans, gynaecological exams, blood tests, urine analysis, allergy testing, etc. It is common for naturopathic doctors to embrace other forms of diagnostic testing such as hair mineral analysis for heavy metals, saliva testing for hormone levels, stool analysis for an assessment of metabolic activity, basal body temperature readings to assess thyroid function, etc. There are many tools that provide a window into the inner functioning of the body, each with its own specialization. As naturopathic doctors often assess a wide range of causal factors it stands to reason that they would utilize a wide range of assessment tools.

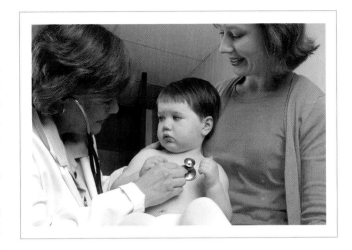

"Naturopathic doctors make sense of the complexity of health."

Iva Lloyd ND

The purpose of the physical examination and additional testing is to link the patient's subjective experiences and symptoms to what is happening on a physiological level. Patients often experience symptoms long before standard laboratory tests show any abnormalities. In cases like this, the lack of positive laboratory findings often indicates that the disease pattern has not progressed far enough to disrupt internal function or structure. The naturopathic doctor would still recommend treatments based on the subjective experiences of the patient, as a way of ensuring that the pattern of ill-health does not progress. In other words, the subjective experience, in many cases, overrides and carries more weight than the objective findings.

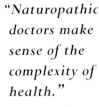

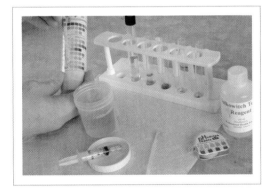

Naturopathic Diagnosis

Conventional medical diagnosis is categorical that is it explains "what" is happening within the body based on anatomical and patho-physiological terminology; naturopathic diagnosis uses the conventional medical diagnosis but it includes an explanatory diagnosis that is one that indicates "why" something is happening. It is the why that relates back to the root cause.

Most conventional diagnoses are labeled in such a way as to aid in the communication between medical practitioners. They provide little, if any, information as to the root cause. Naturopathic doctors aim to communicate diagnoses so that it provides information to the patient that is relevant and informative to them.

The effectiveness of any treatment plan depends on the correctness and thoroughness of the diagnosis. A diagnosis that informs a patient what needs to be changed and why has the greatest chance of achieving a positive outcome. The achievement of health is dependant on what the patient does; not the doctor.

Naturopathic Treatment

Naturopathic physicians recognize that many illnesses are self-limiting, that is they will heal on their own provided that the body has what it requires. The aim of all treatments is to stimulate the healing power of nature and starts with a practitioner determining where a patient is on the continuum between health and ill-health. Naturopathic treatments often involve a patient addressing any obstacles to cure, that is lifestyle, environmental, or external factors that are causing the symptoms and it involves a patient changing something in their life, not just taking something.

Healing is a process, not a project. A naturopathic doctor has often been referred to as a gardener. The role of the gardener is to ensure that each individual has the essential nutrients that they require, that they can eliminate wastes, and that they have the room and space to grow. Naturopathic doctors recognize that healing and health takes time and patience. A quick fix, especially for health issues that developed over time, is not the correct path to choose.

"Whereas an allopathic approach seeks cure (based on some objective criteria), a naturopathic approach aims for healing which will be based in large part on subjective (the patient's) criteria. Consequently there will not be a single measure of outcome, but a pattern of healing that includes physical, emotional, and social functioning."

Christa Louise, PhD 2008

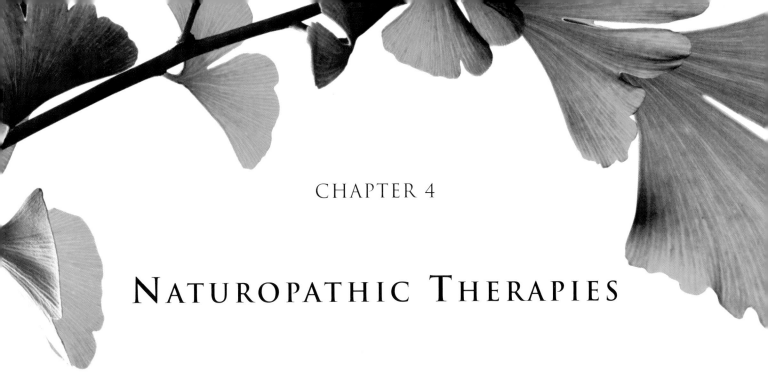

CHAPTER 4

NATUROPATHIC THERAPIES

NATUROPATHIC MEDICINE HAS ALWAYS been an eclectic and diverse field of medicine. It encompasses many different forms of treatment. What unites the treatment options is that they are all based on the same principles and philosophy. Naturopathic medicine encompassed the therapeutic methods of hydrotherapy, nature cure, hygiene, nutrition, mind-body therapies and herbalism when it was introduced to America in 1896. Within a few years, homeopathy, physical medicine, acupuncture and forms of therapies, such as environmental medicine were added. The therapies used by naturopathic doctors continue to change and expand as new ways to stimulate the healing power of the body are discovered.

Hydrotherapy – *Water Cure*

The ideas held by Hippocrates and other European philosophers and practitioners received new impetus in the hydrotherapy – nature cure movement in the 19th century. Vincent Priessnitz (1799-1851), a Silesian famer is considered the founder of the hydrotherapy movement. He developed a system of water cure based on the keen observation of animals in their natural surroundings. Priessnitz began a simple therapy of using water to initiate and augment the cleansing or detoxification processes of the body. Using cold water packs and immersions, he was able to stimulate circulatory changes by causing a strong vasoconstriction (narrowing)

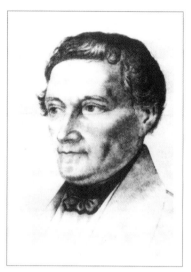

Vincent Priessnitz (1799 – 1852)

"Our task is not to treat the disease, but the patient."

VINCENT PRIESSNITZ

(1799 – 1851)

of the surface blood vessels followed by a strong external vasodilation (expansion) response that increased perspiration. The result was that toxic metabolic wastes from the body were eliminated via the skin and other routes. He relied on nothing except cold water, air, a simple diet, and physical activity to heal his patients. At age twenty-six he established the first water-cure institute in Graefenberg, Austria. "Our task", he would say, "is not to treat the disease, but the patient." Wilhelm Winternitz, MD carried on this practice and did much to popularize hydrotherapy in Vienna.

J.H. Rausse was the first person to lay down the scientific principles of water cure. In 1837 he spend ten weeks receiving treatment from Priessnitz and he began to ponder the principles underlying water cure that Priessnitz followed by intuition. He wrote *The Spirit of the Graefenburg Water Cure* in 1838. His writing increased Priessnitz's fame. His cousin, Theodor Hahn (1824 – 1883), a chemist and a contemporary of Vincent Priessnitz, advocated using water cure along with a vegetarian diet. Hahn promoted the belief that the nature doctor should educate people on how to live a healthy life, how to use natural treatments, and to realize personal responsibility for their own health. He wrote a system of water cure known as "Enforced water cure" and he wrote the book *Hahn's Water Doctor.* Of greatest and lasting influence in the hydrotherapy movement was the work of Father Sebastian Kneipp (1821 – 1894). A physician and priest, Kneipp was cured of a chronic lung disease by Preissnitz through the liberal use of ice-cold water. He was also influenced by the writings of Theodor Hahn. His approach to healing was holistic, advocating "the balance between work and leisure, stress and relaxation and the harmony between the mental, emotional, physical, social and ecological planes." In short, "he asked for a different life, not for better pills; he asked for the active patient and rejected the passive one." Using an eclectic and integrated approach, Kneipp combined hydrotherapeutic baths with heliotherapy (sun therapy), exercise, vegetarian and fruit diets and indigenous herbs. His fame spread throughout Europe and his small town of Woerishoften grew from a hamlet of 500 to a permanent population of 15,000. His establishment received some 20,000 people per year, including the crowned heads of Europe. He was very successful in curing many human illnesses using his holistic approach. Father Kneipp provided the link between the European nature cure and American naturopathy. He mentored and commissioned specific practitioners, such as Benedict Lust, to take hydrotherapy to America.

Johann Schroth (1798 – 1856) smashed his knee in an accident with a horse and was advised to use the Preissnitz method of cure. In order to avoid the frequent changing of the packs, as prescribed by the Preissnitz method, he placed several packs on top of one other and wrapped his whole knee with a woollen cloth which he left on for several hours. The moist heat worked and he was cured. What he theorized was that the moist heat caused the poisonous toxins to dissolve and be swept away. Over time he developed the famous Schroth cure in which he used damp packs in conjunction with the consumption of only dry grain products and the gradual reintroduction of fluids. The Schroth cure was renamed by F. E. Bilz to "the regenerative treatment" which was used quite successfully in treating chronic diseases. Bilz established a Nature Cure sanitarium in Germany and authored the first naturopathic encyclopedia, *The Natural Method of Healing*. It has been translated into a dozen languages, and in German alone there have been over 150 editions.

In the early 1900s Dr. Otis G. Carroll, a naturopathic doctor from Illinois, modernized hydrotherapy techniques by introducing constitutional hydrotherapy, a series of hot and cold compresses applied to the chest, abdomen and back during which the patient is wrapped snugly in wool blankets. Constitutional hydrotherapy was kept alive after his death by naturopathic doctors Leo Scott and Harold Dick. In the 1980s constitutional hydrotherapy was brought back into the mainstream of naturopathic medicine by Dr. Andre Saine ND who was practicing in Ontario at the time.

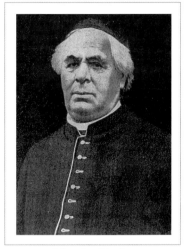

Sebastian Kneipp

"Those who do not find time every day for health must sacrifice a lot of time one day for illness."

FATHER SEBASTIAN KNEIPP (1821 – 1894)

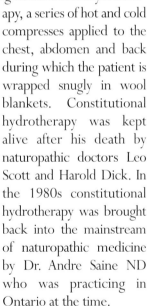

THE ONLY AUTHORIZED AND ORIGINAL
EDITION

POPULAR EDITION FOR AMERICA

MY WATER-CURE

TESTED FOR MORE THAN 40 YEARS

AND PUBLISHED FOR THE CURE OF DISEASES

AND THE PRESERVATION OF HEALTH

BY

SEBASTIAN KNEIPP

SECRET CHAMBERLAIN OF THE POPE, PARISH PRIEST OF WÖRISHOFEN (BAVARIA)

TRANSLATED FROM THE 118 GERMAN EDITION

With 100 Illustrations

JOS. KOESEL, PUBLISHER
KEMPTEN (BAVARIA).

My Water-Cure

THE

Kneipp Water Cure Monthly

Subscription
$1.00
a year.

SINGLE
COPIES
10 Cents.

A Magazine devoted to the late Rev. Father Kneipp's Method and kindred Natural Systems.

PUBLISHED BY THE KNEIPP MAGAZINES PUBLISHING COMPANY.

B. LUST, *Editor and Manager.*   *Office : 111 East 59th St., bet. Park and Lexington Aves., New York.*

Vol. I.   JANUARY 1900.   No. 1.

TO OUR READERS!

A new year has commenced and with its beginning our new publication the "Kneipp Water Cure Monthly" presents itself to our friends, followers and the public in general. It is an old custom to wish a happy New Year to one's friends. We follow this custom with good cheer and will endeavor to make our "Kneipp Water Cure Monthly" a messenger of glad tidings of good health to all (all year round). Good health is most undoubtedly the foundation for real happiness.

There also is no doubt that it is the wish of every human being to be the happy owner of sound brains in a sound body. Unfortunately only very few people know. how to attain this end, only very few people think it worth while to study the laws of nature. They wait until they find themselves at death's door, they wait until it is too late to effect a cure, they wait until their system is poisoned by drugs, they sin against the laws of nature for years; until nature takes matters in its own hands and punishes the sinner mercilessly. The laws of nature are supreme. Every crime against them is severely and vigorously punished. Therefore it is men's duty to study the laws of nature and to learn how to obey them. An obedience to its laws will produce that what we all long for, to wit: Sound brains in a sound body.

What shall men do to attain this end?
Where is the road to health and happiness?
Where is the guide who knows this road?
Where is the mentor who will guide us?

The "Kneipp Water Cure Monthly" will be mentor and guide to all those who need and want health and happiness. The "Kneipp Water Cure Monthly" will give advice in regard to all branches of natural healing and will tell its readers the best way of living according to the laws of nature. The "Kneipp Water Cure Monthly" will not be onesided, it will treat all systems alike and show to its readers where their best points are.

The "Kneipp Water Cure Monthly" will also show to its readers the ways and means which the different branches of natural healing possess to prevent sickness. It will prove that a great deal of suffering is only due to the obstinacy of a class of men who are more business-men than healers of ailments. Mankind is only a part of nature, and nature provides for everything needed by its parts, but these parts have to obey nature's laws and must

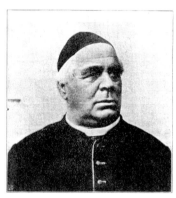

Seb. Kneipp

only use such means of healing disorders which are provided by nature for this purpose, to wit: air, light, sun-heat, water, exercise, rest, massage, gymnastics, diet, magnetism, electricity and in connection with the different herbs of healing power. Men's artificial means are nothing but poisons. The "Kneipp Water Cure Monthly" will further show, that by means of these simple remedies the science of natural healing is able to produce good and lasting results, surer and quicker than any physician of the old school would be able to do.

The time is not far off, when people will look at to-day's so-called medical science as the curse of our times and bless the moment in which men like Sebastian Kneipp showed to the world the errors of the old way and pointed out to this same world the only natural road to real happiness and health.

The "Kneipp Water Cure Monthly" will always be an advocate of the principles of this great master of natural healing. "Return to nature" will be our war-cry.

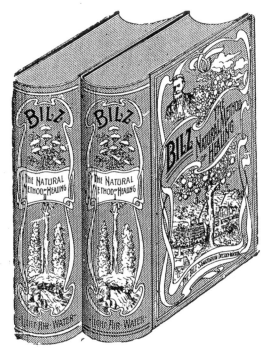

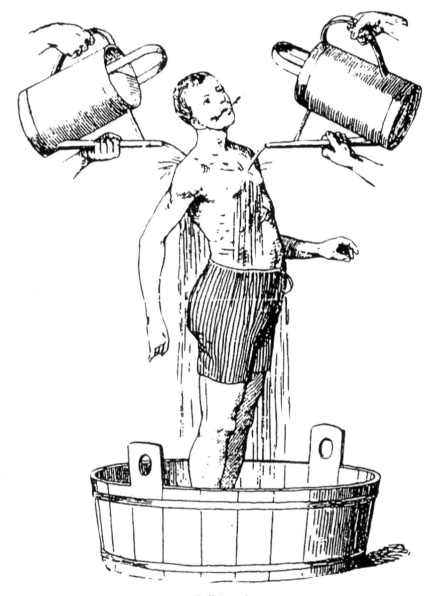

Full Douche

Nature Cure

One of the early contributors to natural living and healing was Arnold Rikli (1823 – 1906) who practiced in Germany and Switzerland. He is considered the founder of light and air cures. He stated "water is good, air is better, but light is best of all." This seemingly obvious remark was startling to his European countrymen at a time when hygiene was still unknown and it was customary not to expose any area of the flesh to public view, nor to the air and sun! He introduced the concept of contrast water baths, used steam for treating colds and other diseases and was famous for his sun baths which consisted of simply exposing the body to the sun. He also emphasized the importance of walking barefoot on the grass, especially when there was dew on the ground to aid in the drainage ability of the body. In 1869 he taught that it was "extremely injurious to harden the head by keeping it bare, and on the other hand to keep the feet covered all the time, as people suffering from headache are prone to do . . . The balance of circulation between the head and the feet and between the intestines and the skin is the most important principle for the preservation and restoration of health."

In 1891 Louis Kuhne (1835 – 1907), a European nature curist, wrote *The New Science of Healing* which was one of the greatest works written on the basic principles of natural healing and his books were used in the initial naturopathic schools. Kuhne advocated sun, steam baths, a vegetarian diet, and whole-wheat bread. He considered raw food to be the most digestible and nutritious. He believed that excess intake of food created toxins, which if not

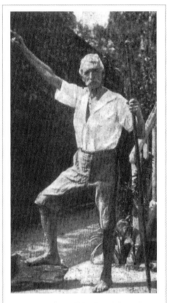

Arnold Rikli in his air bathing suit (Archive of the Eden Foundation, Bad Suden)

"The light and airbath cure leads to a faster more efficient restoration of a human being than any method of water cure no matter how refined it might be. A human being is not a fish. Water is not our highest element of life . . . Light and Air are our highest, most delicately organized life-vessels. All organic life would degrade and die in the shortest time without them."

Arnold Rikli (1823 – 1906)

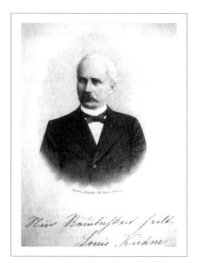

Louis Kuhne
(Kuhne ND, fr ontspiece)

"Food precisely in the form nature gives it to us is always best for the digestion."

LOUIS KUHNE (1835 – 1907)

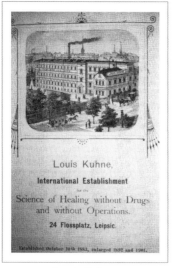

Louis Kuhne.
International Establishment
Science of Healing without Drugs and without Operations.
24 Flossplatz, Leipsic.

Louis Kuhne
(International Establishment)

excreted, would be subject to fermentation. This fermentation would cause disruptions in health and typically occurred when the routes of elimination - the bowels, urinary tract, skin and lungs - were deficient and not working optimally. Kuhne's concept was similar to Hippocrates' idea of "cocotion" - the body's ability and intent to isolate and discharge morbid or toxic wastes via skin, mucous membranes, bowels, kidneys, etc. He emphasized the "unit of disease" theory stating that "disease is the presence of foreign (morbid) matter in the body . . . cleanliness only cures." Kuhne's book "*Neo-Naturopathy*" was one of the first textbooks that looked at pathology of disease from a naturopathic perspective.

The clinical observation of the "healing crisis" in which the body throws off its toxic accumulation with an acute episode was also emphasized by Adolph Just (1859 - 1939) in his book *Return to Nature*. Just utilized primarily moist heat and promoted self-care and responsibility, stating "Nature does not err". He also advanced the theory that acute diseases are the most favourable healing crisis and should be greeted with joy.

Heinrich Lahman (1860 – 1905) was trained as a medical doctor, but did not ascribe to many of the beliefs and practices of conventional medicine and he became known as one of the first scientific nature doctors. He became a staunch advocate of natural healing and spent much of his time refuting the practice and ideas of medical science. He was a strong believer in the light and air cure and constructed the first appliances for the administration of electric light treatment and baths. He emphasized raw food, stressed the concept of no salt on foods, no water with meals, and he promoted the steaming of vegetables as well as the use of vegetable extracts and soy and almond milk. He authored many books on diet, heliotherapy (sun therapy) and nature cure, including the first scientific treatise on nature cure written in 1891.

Hygiene

The hygienic school of thought is considered a forerunner of American naturopathy. It originated as a lay movement and followed the popular teachings of Isaac Jennings (1789 – 1875), Sylvester Graham (1794 – 1851) and William Alcott (1798 – 1859), all American practitioners who taught that the body was governed by natural laws. Sylvester Graham began preaching the doctrines of temperance and hygiene in 1830, and in 1839 published *Lectures on the Science of Human Life*, two hefty volumes that prescribed healthy dietary habits. He also published a journal called *The Graham Journal and Longevity* that was later known as the *Water-Cure Journal*. He emphasized a moderate lifestyle, recommending an anti-flesh diet and bran bread as an alternative to white bread. The introduction of hygiene gained popularity after 1834 when William Kelly, a physician introduced the idea of preventing the spread of disease via sanitation following epidemics of cholera.

Early hygienic practitioners used a mixture of hygiene and hydrotherapy (also called hydropathy). In 1856, the phrase *Hygiene System* came into use. The physician Russell Thacker Trall, MD (1812-1877), influenced by the writings of Graham and Jennings, was instrumental in promoting the hydropathic and hygienic movement. He was also a leading advocate of vegetarianism. His combining of many different hygienic agents and systems into one holistic system caused him to be considered an activist and a health reformer. He was opposed to 'drug therapist', a term used to classify many of the allopathic physicians in those days. His contribution had a significant impact on the later growth of naturopathy.

Trall contended that when the laws of nature were broken, sickness and death could result. The role of the doctor was to remove the cause of any illness, rather than suppressing symptoms. Once the causes were removed, the body tended to heal itself. Trall maintained that drugs harmed the body; they did not act upon the body but the body acted upon the drugs. Trained as an allopathic physician, Trall had observed patients who had become well without drug intervention and those who had been made sicker by drugs. He noticed that the body was helped when patients were prescribed rest, vegetarian diet,

"If the people can be thoroughly indoctrinated in the general principels of Hydropathy, they will not err much, certainly not fatally, in their home-application of the Water-Cure appliances to the common diseases of the day. If they can go a step further, and make themselves acquainted with the laws of life and health, they will well-nigh emancipate themselves from all need of doctors of any sort."

RUSSELL THACKER TRALL

(1812 – 1877)

treatments such as massage and hydrotherapy, and when a patient's mind was filled with positive thoughts.

Trall opened the second water cure establishment in America, in New York City in 1844. The first Kneipp Sanitarium was opened in New Jersey by Chas. Lauterwasser, a hydropathic physician and natural scientist. In Trall's sanitarium he combined the full Preissnitzian range of water-baths with regulation of food, air, heat, exercise and sleep. He opened and directed a number of other hydropathic institutions around the country. In 1852 Trall founded a school of natural healing arts in North America, the "New York Hygieo-Therapeutic College". This school was the first to have a 4-year curriculum with the authorization to confer the degree of MD and it was chartered by the New York State Legislature in 1857. It also was the first medical school to admit women on equal terms with men. In 1862 Trall presented a famous lecture on *The True Healing Art or Hygienic vs. Drug Medication* at the Smithsonian Institute in Washington.

For more than 15 years, Trall was editor of the *Water Cure Journal*, the *Hydropathic Review*, and a temperance journal. During this period, the *Water-Cure Journal* went through several name changes including the *Hygienic Teacher* and *The Herald of Health*. He also authored over 25 books on the subject of physiology, hydropathy, hygiene, vegetarianism, and temperance, among many others. The most valuable and enduring of these was his *Hydropathic Encyclopedia*, a volume of nearly 10,000 pages that covered the theory and practice of hydropathy and the philosophy and treatment of disease advanced by other schools of medicine.

In the late 1800s and early 1900s there was much focus and education on the need for proper sanitation and hygiene by both practitioners and the governments in Canada and the United States. In the mid 1880s, natural hygiene was so enthusiastically received and popularized that its practitioners outnumbered those of allopathic, homeopathic, and all other forms of medicine. This period saw important advances which included the provision of safe drinking water, public baths, beaches, municipal garbage services and government introduced sanitation standards.

Nutrition

Food has always been associated with the maintenance of health. Whether practitioners were using hydrotherapy, nature cure, or hygiene, specialized diets were employed in some fashion. The focus on nutrition as a stand-alone therapeutic tool developed gradually over time. In traditional systems of medicine food was often looked at based on its properties, such as hot or cold and dry or moist. Specific foods were chosen based on their ability to balance the body.

In the 1920s Ragnar Berg, a Swedish nutritional scientist, was one of the first to analyze the mineral content of food. He correlated the mineral content of what was eaten with the excretion of minerals in the body. He drew conclusions about metabolic disorders and faulty nutrition based on the mineral balances. His work became known as the acid/alkaline effects of food on pH balance of the body, a concept still used effectively by many naturopathic physicians.

In the 1930s naturopathic doctor Otis G. Carroll discovered eight major food intolerances: dairy, fruit, meat, eggs, sugar, potatoes and grain, as well as salt. He later determined that most people had a combination intolerance between cereal or grain products and other foods. He was an advocate of fasting and in identifying and removing food intolerances in order to promote healing.

Macrobiotic diet, from the Greek "macro" (large, long) and "bios" (life), is a dietary regiment that includes grains as a stable in the diet with other foods such as vegetables and beans. It advocates the avoidance of highly processed and refined foods. Macrobiotics also address the manner of eating, by recommending against overeating and requiring that food be chewed thoroughly before swallowing. The term macrobiotics is found in the writing of Hippocrates, Aristotle, Galen and other classical writers. It was used to describe a lifestyle, including a simple balanced diet, that would promote health and longevity. George Ohsawa (1893 – 1966) was born in a Japanese

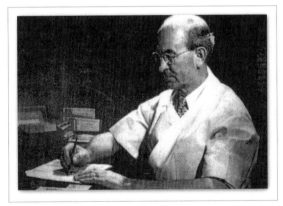

Otis G. Carroll (1879 – 1962) Courtesy of William J. Carroll ND, DC Used with permission, *Nature Doctors*, NCNM Press

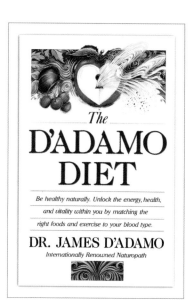

The
D'ADAMO DIET

Be healthy naturally. Unlock the energy, health, and vitality within you by matching the right foods and exercise to your blood type.

DR. JAMES D'ADAMO
Internationally Renowned Naturopath

"The cornerstone of any method of healing is the individualized diet ... nutrition will bring you health, energy and well-being."

DR. JAMES D'ADAMO ND

family whose father was descended directly from Samurai. He is considered the founder of macrobiotics and he brought this concept to North America in the late 1950s. Michio Kushi and his wife Aveline were students of Ohsawa and they have continued to advance the field of macrobiotics.

Naturopathic doctor James D'Adamo introduced the concept of blood type diets in 1950 while working in New York. His theory is based on the concept that there is a correlation between the foods tolerated and the four different blood types – 'O', 'A', 'B' and 'AB'. His son, Peter D'Adamo ND continues to further this theory by researching the link between different blood groups and disease.

There are many different therapeutic ways to use nutrition and food. Naturopathic practitioners over time have embraced many of these different theories. What is common with naturopathic practitioners is the understanding and the belief that diet and digestion are an integral component of healing, promo health and preventing disease.

Mind-Body

Mind-Body medicine is a current term for what was originally referred to as psychotherapeutics. Psychotherapeutics or 'psychotherapeia' was a term coined in 1853 to describe the treatment of mental and emotional symptoms and disorders via "talk therapy". In current day language it is considered psychotherapy or mind-body medicine, depending on what system of medicine is being employed and the designation of the practitioner. In an informal sense, talk therapy can be said to have been practiced through the ages, as individuals received counsel and reassurance from family and friends.

Mental illness has a history of being poorly understood in most cultures. In some, mental illness was interpreted as a sign that the supernatural or gods were upset with an individual and, as a result, torture and rituals were performed to rid "mentally ill" patients of demons. Paracelsus (1493 – 1541), a Greek philosopher, was one of the first to advocate talk therapy for the treatment of mental illness. Hundreds of years later mental illness still remained a mystery, especially when the mind and body were viewed as separate. Systems of medicine, such as Chinese and Ayurvedic medicine emphasize the important link between the mind and the body.

They also recognize that different emotions and mental states have specific patterns and that each emotion "sits" or is correlated with a specific organ of the body. Emotional or mental disturbances are assessed and treated according to the overall pattern of disharmony in the body.

Due to Darwinian theories, the germ theory and the focus on biochemical processes, the connection between the mind and body over time was dramatically downplayed in conventional medicine. Re-igniting the focus on the mind-body connection is occurring with new discoveries and research methods. For example, the relationship between worsening of symptoms and mental state can be observed in many diseases. The impact of relaxation and meditation has been shown to be effective in treating and managing symptoms and diseases. It has been shown that mental and emotional states affect digestive function, immunity, reproductive function, etc. There is research to show that every emotion releases different hormones and that the physical body contracts or relaxes depending on one's thoughts and emotions. Certain emotions have also been linked to disease and it is generally accepted that holding in emotions is detrimental to health.

Over the years, the practice of psychotherapy has been influenced by many psychologists and practitioners. Sigmund Freud, near the end of the 19th century, developed the "talking cure" which was one of the first scientifically based applications of psychotherapies. In the 1920s, behaviourism became the dominant paradigm, and remained so until the 1950s when the focus switched to cognitive therapy and therapies which promoted positive, holistic change through the development of a supportive, genuine and empathic therapeutic relationship. In the 1970s the strengths of cognitive and behavioural approaches were combined and the emphasis became on symptom-relief and modifying core beliefs. Cognitive behavioural therapy has gained widespread acceptance as a primary treatment for numerous disorders. Family and group dynamics, and transpersonal psychology, which emphasizes the spiritual facet of human experience, are being adopted and integrated within the field of psychotherapy.

Psychotherapeutics or mind-body medicine, as it applies to naturopathic medicine, emphasizes three points: firstly, that the state of the mind influences health and disease; secondly, that the mind and body are one and that changes in one aspect will always result in changes in the

"Mind-Body Medicine (MBM) is basically the study of how our thought, emotions and experience of life affect our health. Mostly, MBM is about stress reduction and living in the moment, to fully experience all moments of life, thereby enriching our experience of life, allowing us to feel more fullfilled and having a greater sense of purpose."

DENIS T. MARIER ND

others; thirdly, that a positive mind and thoughts are an integral part of healing. In naturopathic medicine, psychotherapeutics focuses on identifying the natural tendencies of the mind and training the mind how to be positive and support healing and health. It also involves listening intently to patients and on understanding the impact that symptoms and their concerns are having on their health. An integral part of any naturopathic treatment is the recognition of the mind-body connection and acknowledging the role of the mind in health and healing. Many naturopathic doctors offer a form of counselling and lifestyle modification. They also work with and refer to other therapists as required.

Herbalism

Herbalism or botanical medicine is the traditional medicinal practice based on the use of plants and plant extracts. Plants with their therapeutic properties have been used as healing agents since prehistoric times by people all over the world. Hippocrates (460 – 370 BC) and Galen (129 – 200 BC) advocated the use of herbs – along with fresh air, rest and proper diet – as the basis of achieving and maintaining health. The medicinal properties of plants have been documented from the first century AD and since the 1700s there have been many practitioners who have written books on the therapeutic properties of plants. The therapeutic use of herbs continues to be the most common therapy as about 80% of the world's population use them as therapeutic agents.

THE

AMERICAN FLORA,

OR

HISTORY OF PLANTS AND WILD FLOWERS:

CONTAINING

THEIR SCIENTIFIC AND GENERAL DESCRIPTION,

NATURAL HISTORY,

Chemical and Medical Properties, Mode of Culture, Propagation, &c.

DESIGNED

AS A BOOK OF REFERENCE FOR BOTANISTS, PHYSICIANS, FLORISTS, GARDENERS, STUDENTS, ETC.

BY A. B. STRONG, M. D.

VOL. I.

IS ILLUSTRATED WITH

SEVENTY BEAUTIFUL COLORED ENGRAVINGS, TAKEN FROM NATURE.

NEW-YORK:
PUBLISHED BY GREEN & SPENCER,
67 *Bowery*.

1851.

Every area in the world has its own unique plants. One premise is that the plants that grow in a certain area cure the diseases of that region. Each part of the world has been provided with its own medicines. Early explorers presumed that a careful cataloguing of the region's botanicals and the identification of herbs, barks and roots used by native peoples would measurably add to the range of therapeutic tools that they had at their disposal.

Although the therapeutic effects of many herbs have been studied and verified by scientific research, traditional use over thousands of years is the primary basis for our understanding the therapeutic properties of many herbs. Herbs are prescribed therapeutically in many different forms: as food, tea, tinctures, extracts, capsules, tablets, syrups as well as topically in oils, salves, creams, lotions, poultices, and compresses. The method chosen depends on the specific herb and the therapeutic effect desired.

Western medicine has its roots in the use of herbs. Until the 1950s, herbs were the basis of all pharmaceutical drugs. Even today, about 25% of pharmaceuticals are derived from herbs - opium, aspirin, digitalis, quinine. Others are extracted from plants such as corticosteroids and oral contraceptives. The difference between herbs and drugs is that botanical medicine tends to use whole plant extracts, such as the roots or leaves, whereas drugs isolate individual chemicals. Pharmaceutical medicines prefer single ingredients on the grounds that the dose can be more easily quantified. Herbs are holistic by nature. Hence, practitioners using them often reject the notion of single active ingredients, arguing that the various chemicals present in herbs interact to enhance the therapeutic effects of the herb and to minimize or eliminate adverse effects and toxicity.

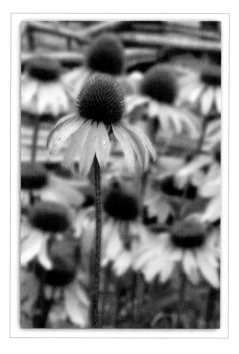

Herbs can be classified based on the type of compounds present or on their actions. These include warming or cooling, adaptogens that help to regulate hormones and homeostatic function, calming and nerve effects, cardio-tonic effects and so forth. The classification used varies with indigenous culture (e.g. Chinese, Ayurvedic, Native American, etc) but are effective means for each medical tradition to understand, use and evaluate the herb's actions. Naturopathic doctors learn over 250 botanical medicines. This education includes both the traditional and modern scientific knowledge.

Homeopathy

In the early 1800s, Samuel Hahnemann (1755 – 1843), a German physician who was disenchanted with the medical system of his day, believed that there were better and safer ways of restoring health. Through observation and experimentation, he founded homeopathy which means 'like cures like'. Homeopathy was based on the belief that the curative power of medicines stemmed from their ability to induce in healthy persons symptoms analogous to the diseases for which they were administered. He and his followers subscribed to the vitalistic approach to medicine, believing that a spirit-like force was present in every organism and that sickness was due to an alternation of the vital force.

Hahnemann used the word "homeopathy" to distinguish his use of infinitesimally small doses of substances to treat the spiritual causes of illness. Homeopathic remedies are made from plants, animals and minerals. They are created by diluting these substances many times until what remains is the energetic blueprint or essence, not actual chemical components. Homeopathy is known for three central doctrines:

• The "law of similar" (that like cures like).

• The effect of a medication can be heightened by its adminstration in minute doses (the more diluted the dose, the greater the "dynamic" effect).

• Nearly all diseases are the result of a suppression.

Most homeopathic consults consist of a practitioner

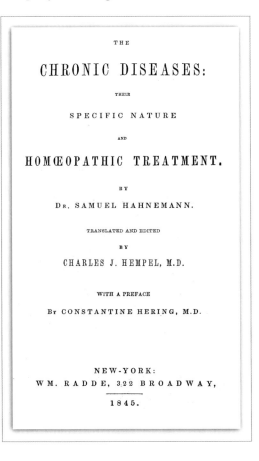

THE

CHRONIC DISEASES:

THEIR

SPECIFIC NATURE

AND

HOMŒOPATHIC TREATMENT.

BY

DR. SAMUEL HAHNEMANN.

TRANSLATED AND EDITED

BY

CHARLES J. HEMPEL, M.D.

WITH A PREFACE

BY CONSTANTINE HERING, M.D.

NEW-YORK:
WM. RADDE, 322 BROADWAY,
1845.

listening intently to not only what a patient says, but observing a patient's body language and mannerisms. It is the uniqueness of individual symptoms (i.e., what makes a symptom better or worse, or what emotions are linked with a specific symptom) that determines the correct remedy. A practitioner then chooses the correct remedy by matching the symptoms of a person to the characteristics of a remedy.

In 1825 homeopathy was brought to the US by Dr. Hans Burch Gram (1787 – 1840). In 1833 Dr. Constantine Hering (1800 – 1880) immigrated to America and later became known as the father of American homeopathy.

Physical Medicine

Physical medicine is the term used to describe all forms of manual therapy, such as those involving the use of the hands or machines on the body to address structural misalignment, neuromuscular concerns or functional imbalances in the body.

Physical medicine has always been a component of naturopathic medicine. In fact, physical medicine has been part of most healing systems since the beginning of time. The introduction of naturopathic medicine to America coincided with the founding of osteopathic and chiropractic medicine. Many of the early naturopathic doctors held degrees and licenses in many of the different facets of natural medicine. The early physical medicine techniques used by naturopathic practitioners included: Ling massage, mechanotherapy, zone therapy and reflexology, vibrational and membraneous massage, spondylotherapy, neurotherapy, manual therapy techniques, neuromuscular techniques, high velocity with low amplitude mobilization, graded mobilization, lymphatic drainage, exercise therapy, or the more modern approaches of visceral manipulation, hydrotherapy and electrotherapy. Some of the initial physical medicine terms are not currently used and over time techniques have been lost due to a lack of documentation and integration into the naturopathic curriculum.

Bernarr Macfadden (1868 – 1955) was the founder of the physical culture movement in the early 1900s. He embraced diet, lifestyle and exercise. He was very influential in pioneering today's exercise industry and initiating the still popular fitness movement.

The central concept that distinguishes naturopathic physical medi-

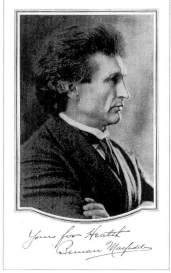

Bernarr Macfadden (1868 – 1955)

"Lack of activity destroys the good condition of every human being, while movement and methodical physical exercise save it and preserve it."

PLATO (428 – 348 BC)

cine from other forms of manual medicine is the perception of human beings as vitalistic and holistic organisms. It is the recognition that the physical structure shifts and adapts to internal and external stressors. This adaptation can result in changes in internal functioning, psychological well-being as well as physical misalignment. There is the realization that every aspect of the body is connected and that imbalances on the structural level often affect other aspects of health. The early schools of naturopathic medicine placed a tremendous focus on the importance of physical structure and the use of physical medicine as an integral part of all treatments.

Acupuncture and Traditional Chinese Medicine

Chinese Medicine is a holistic system of medicine that has been part of the Chinese culture for over 5,000 years. The ancient Chinese perceived human beings as a microcosm of the universe that surrounded them and believed that they were motivated and driven by the same primeval forces of the macrocosm. Chinese Medicine is based on vitalistic concepts and recognizes that health is based on the accumulation and balance of the attributes within an individual (Yin-Yang, hot-cold, blood-chi. Optimizing human life by preserving the conditions within which it thrives is the purpose of Chinese Medicine.

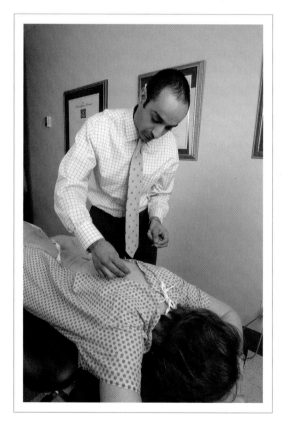

Acupuncture is a part of Chinese Medicine, as well as other forms of healing. It involves inserting fine needles into specific parts of the body in order to relieve symtoms and to establish health. The ancient Chinese hypothesized that energy circulated in the body via specific channels, called meridians. On each meridian there are acupuncture points which are stimulated by these needles, thus influencing the appropriate body organs, nervous systems or affected areas allowing the healing life force to flow uninhibited.

The Chinese believed that in addition to being in balance, the energy or life force (which they called *"chi"*) had to be able to circulate freely around the meridians. If a break or congestion occurred anywhere in the movement of the energy, symptoms or illness would result. An example is backache, viewed by the Chinese as a blockage in the "chi". The remedy is to insert a needle at the point of discomfort, thus encouraging flow to re-establish itself. Acupuncture treatment regulates the flow of chi and blood - tonifying where there is deficiency, draining where there is excess and promoting free flow where there is stagnation.

Most of the acupuncture points are found on the twelve main meridians and two of the eight extra meridians. Each meridian channel refers to a particular organ, and the energy flowing through that meridian can be taken as indicating the functional state of that organ. The concept of organ and organ function is different in Chinese Medicine compared to Western Medicine. The liver, for example, relates not only to the actual liver, but to the concepts of frustration, irritation, motivation, internal heat and other "fiery" qualities (eg red rash or burning pain). Inserting a needle into a point on the liver meridian could be expected to affect the function of the liver, to dissipate anger and frustration, to clear internal heat or a rash – all depending on the actual point used and the state of the patient at the time of treatment.

Any practitioner in Canada that practices acupuncture must use disposable stainless steel needles. The needles are very fine in diameter (0.18 mm to 0.51 mm) as they are not hollow. Most people experience acupuncture as relaxing and calming. Some patients experience a sensation known as *"de qi"* which means that the qi has been stimulated. This is similar to a mild electric sensation and is viewed as a positive sign in acupuncture. Acupuncture is a safe, effective form of treatment when done by a properly trained practitioner.

Other Therapies

Naturopathic medicine is eclectic and it has always encompassed many different forms of natural therapeutics. In addition to what is listed above, it has included therapies such as iridology and colour and sound therapy. In the early 1900s when the many of the new therapies were being introduced, the lack of scientific understanding of how they worked impacted their acceptance and they were removed from most naturopathic programs. Science is now catching up to the mysteries that nature has to offer. The way that these energetic therapies stimulate healing is not only witnessed, but understood.

Over time, as new therapies or techniques are discovered, the breadth of naturopathic medicine changes and grows. Therapies such as colon therapy, energetic therapies, Chelation, intra-venous therapy, and others serve a valuable role in naturopathic treatments. There will also be new ways discovered that can stimulate the innate healing of the body, and as they are, many will be embraced by naturopathic medicine.

PART TWO

THE HISTORY
OF THE PROFESSION

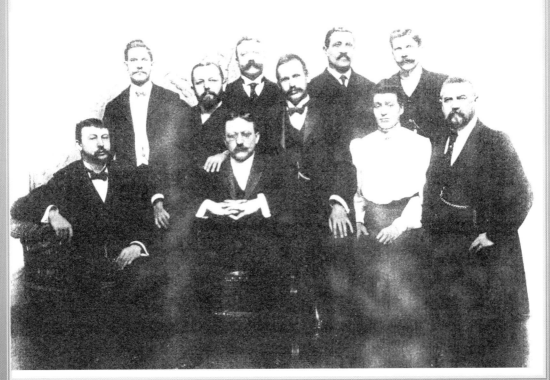

The charter members of the American Naturopathic Society

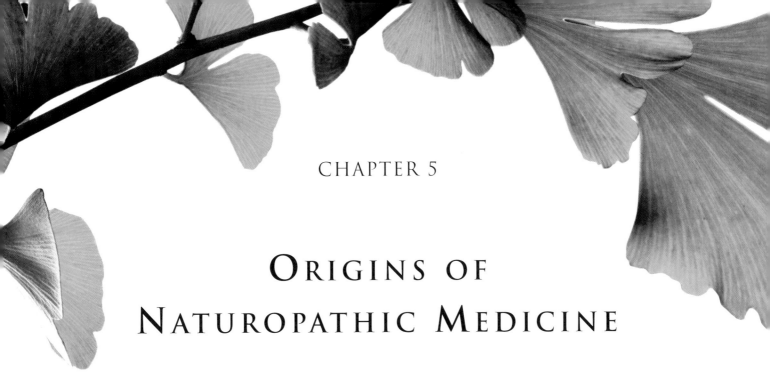

CHAPTER 5

ORIGINS OF
NATUROPATHIC MEDICINE

Naturopathy, as it was originally called, was brought to America in 1896. To appreciate the origins of naturopathic medicine, it is help-ful to understand the early medical climate in Canada and the United States and to be introduced to the early pioneers.

Medical Climate in the 1800s

Prior to the 1800s the practice of medicine and healing was done at home where family and friends nursed an ill person to health. The skills and tech-niques were passed on verbally from generation to generation. After the invention of the printing press in the mid 15th century, medical techniques started to be written down. Those who were so inclined became self-taught physicians often referencing written works such as John Wesley's *Primitive Physic* (1747), William Buchan's *Domestic Medicine* (1769) or John Gunn's *Domestic Medicine* (1830). In the 1800s, the practice of medicine started to become more formalized, yet the "house-call" was still the norm. It wasn't until the 1900s that the practice of medicine became office and hospital ori-ented.

Before the Civil War (1861 to 1865), hygiene was the form of medicine most commonly practiced. All forms of medicine at the time – hygiene, conventional, eclectic and homeopathy were accepted and practiced. In the mid 1800's the Canadian Medical Association and the American

Medical Associations were formed. During the Civil War the germ theory gained new momentum, and as a result of these and other factors, the conventional (also referred to as allopathic) model of healthcare became the system held by the majority. Other natural forms of healing, such as naturopathy, osteopathy and chiropractic, were established thirty or forty years later. The number of natural healers in the late 1800s was small, yet they were visible and respected in their own communities for their abilities and expertise.

As of the early 1900s conventional medicine moved away from it roots and embraced science as the foundation of medicine. The natural healing systems of medicine, such as naturopathic medicine, were not as eager to give up their roots. The debate between the science and art of medicine and the struggle between conventional and alternative began. The struggle with homeopathy was because it resulted in the conversion of a substantial number of medical doctors and because homeopaths generally also made a better income. The rejection of the eclectic and hygienic schools was more fundamental as many of these practitioners had limited education and this challenged the validity of the practice of medicine being one for a select, privileged, professional group of men. Natural healers were forced into the role of "alternative" practitioners, fighting for their right to treat patients, as the allopathic medical profession gained power and acceptance.

The first schools of conventional medicine required little or no college education and were largely apprenticeship based. The first medical school in the United States opened in Philadelphia in 1765; the first one in Canada, founded in Montreal in 1824, later became of the Faculty of Medicine of McGill University.

The establishment of large sanitariums or medical institutions were common practice for natural healers in the 1800s and early 1900s. These sanitariums offered the full range of natural therapeutics and focused on both acute and chronic illnesses. In the early twentieth century conventional medical institutions cared for the poor, those with mental illness or those suffering from tuberculosis. The institutions initially were not-for-profit and were run by municipal governments, charitable organizations and religious denominations. Conventional medical institutions and hospitals grew in numbers as Canada and the United States developed as nations and the influence of government continued to increase. Sanitariums and asylums were replaced by hospitals and additional subsidies were paid to encourage admission and treatment of all patients, regardless of their ability to pay.

The tremendous social impact of the Great Depression and the devastation of World War II contributed greatly to the increasing desire for a public health system and in decreasing the initial opposition of medical doctors. After the early 1900's, the ability to establish natural therapy institutions became impossible due largely to government regulations.

By 1920, medical care in a hospital setting became increasingly accepted and hospitals became major training and clinical research facilities. Initially naturopathic doctors were granted hospital privileges in a number of institutions both in Canada and the United States. The privilege that naturopathic doctors once enjoyed was removed as greater regulations were put into place and as the domination of hospitals fell under the conventional framework.

Benedict Lust, the Father of American Naturopathy

Dr. Benedict Lust (1872 – 1945) is considered the father of American naturopathy. Born in Baden, Germany he, like many of the founders of naturopathy, had been introduced to natural forms of healing due to personal health concerns. Dr. Lust had originally immigrated to the United States in 1892 to seek his fortune, yet when he contracted a severe case of tuberculosis that was not getting any better with conventional treatments, he returned to his homeland to undergo the water-cure treatments of Father Kneipp. During his time in Europe, Dr. Lust visited and studied with many of the nature-curists of his day including Kuhne, Lahmann, Just and others.

Once Dr. Lust was cured, he was asked by Kneipp to spread hydrotherapy to America. He returned to the United States in 1896 with his colleague Dr. Robert Foster and established two Sanitariums and Kneipp Water Cure Institutes, one in Butler, New Jersey in 1902 and another in Tangerine, Florida in 1914. In 1901 Dr. Lust opened the American School of Naturopathy in New York, which was the first naturopathic college in America. He also opened what could be considered the first health food store or Kneipp store as they were initially known. From the onset, Dr. Lust integrated the Kneipp water-cure methods with the many other therapies that he had encountered.

Over the years, Dr. Lust undertook further training in a number of other natural therapies. He graduated from the Universal Osteopathic College of New York in 1898, received his medical degree in 1902 from the New York Homeopathic

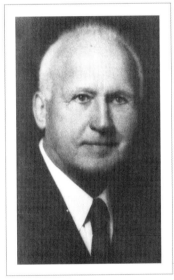

Benedict Lust ND (1872 – 1925)
Used with permission, *Nature Doctors*, NCNM Press – Gift of John B. Lust

Medical College and received an eclectic medical degree from the Eclectic Medical College in New York in 1913. He was editor of the professional journal *Father Kneipp Blatter* — which came to be called *Naturopathy and Herald of Health*. As well, for over thirty years he edited the public journal, the *Nature's Path*. The early naturopathic journals provided valuable insights into the prevention of disease and the promotion of health.

The Kneipp convention held in New York in 1901 marked the birth of naturopathy. "Naturopathy" was a term first coined in 1895 by Dr. John Scheel, a German homeopath practising the methods of Kneipp and Kuhn at his Badekur Sanitarium in New York. Lust purchased the name in 1901 to describe the eclectic practice of 'nature doctors'. The word "naturopathy" was viewed as a word that would not be seen to be competing with conventional medical doctors. Many early naturopaths objected to the name because, in its literal translation, it means *natural disease*. However, Lust credited it with helping to end his own persecution and that of the profession at large. In 1921 Lust remarked that "The persecution became so intense that we could not use the words cure, healing, therapy, therapist, physician, doctor, or any similar title. We were all in despair. Finally we decided to use the word 'naturopath' as being the only safe term by which we could designate ourselves as having to do with 'the nature cure' and disease."

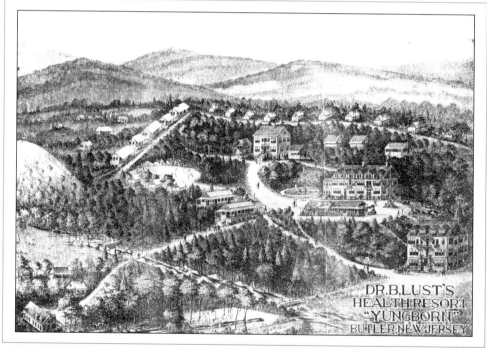

This is an artist's rendition of the buildings and facilities of Dr. Benedict Lust's Health Resort in Butler, New Jersey at the turn of the century.

Lust stated that the term naturopathy was well suited to the profession as it "stood for the reconciling, harmonizing and unifying of nature, humanity and God." Lust went on to explain that the term "Naturopathy" is a hybrid word and "it is purposely so. No single tongue could distinguish a system whose origin, scope and purpose is universal – broad as the world, deep as love, and high as heaven. Fundamentally therapeutic because men need healing; elementally educational because men need teaching; ultimately inspirational because men need empowering, it encompasses the realm of human progress and destiny. Dietetics, physical culture and hydrotherapy are the measures upon which Naturopathy is to build; mental culture is the means and soul-selfhood is the motive."

"The human body possesses an inherent ability to heal itself through the mechanisms of homeostasis – restoring balance in structure and function and adapting to environmental changes."

BENEDICT LUST ND

(1872 – 1945)

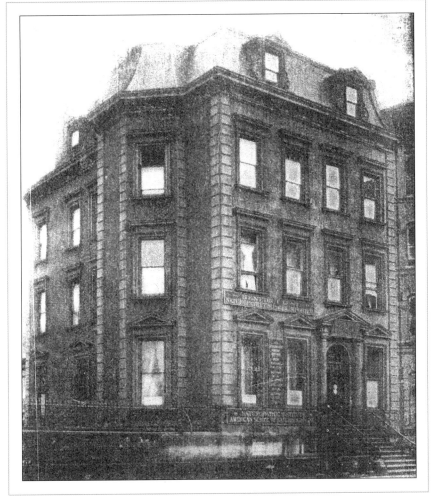

This entire building of 55 rooms was used by Dr. B. Lust's Naturopathic Institute, Clinic and Hospital and the American School of Naturopathy in New York City from 1907 to 1913.

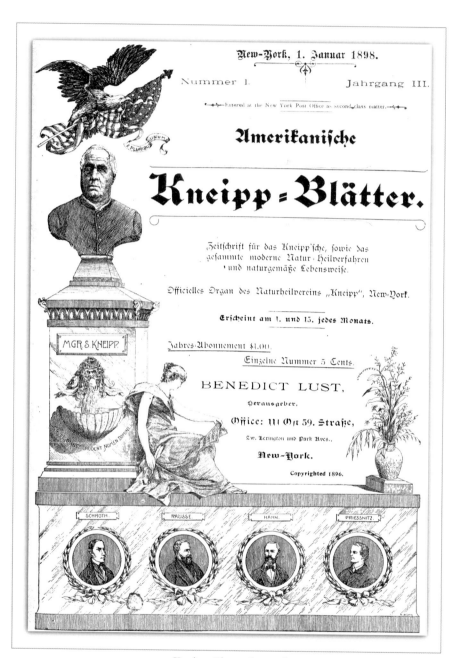

Kneipp-Blatter journal

Edited by
Benedict Lust,
N.D., D.O., M.D.

Herald of Health
and
Naturopath

Price, 20c copy
Subscription,
$2.00 a year

THIS magazine, which is the professional organ of the American Naturopathic Association, first appeared in 1896 as **The Kneipp Water Cure Monthly**; then in 1902 it became known as **The Naturopath and Herald of Health**; and finally, in January, 1916, it became **The Herald of Health and Naturopath**. As the name indicates, this publication is the exponent of every phase of drugless healing. It is many years older than the Naturopathic Society, the name by which the American Naturopathic Association was first known, and which was founded December 2nd, 1902, in the city of New York.

The **Herald of Health and Naturopath** is the only journal published in the United States that espouses the healing of disease by the simple and natural methods, as opposed to the vile nostrums and superstitions of Allopathy, otherwise known as official medicine.

The Natural System of Healing alone has the courage to assert that Nature cures, that the only healing force is the vis naturae medicatrix, and not the potions, pills and powders of the empirics. It had its inception in Germany. Priessnitz of Gräfenberg, Kuhne of Leipzig, Schroth of Lindewiese, Bilz of Dresden, and Kneipp of Woerishofen, established sanatoria, and proved to a world sick unto death with swallowing paralyzing palliatives, of annihilating fermenting substances with chemicals, of suppressing fevers with poison, of relieving constipation with purgatives, causing the muscular system of the intestines to lose tone and elasticity, all practices antagonizing nature in her benign efforts to get rid of the offending materies morbi that is the cause of the specific disease, that the benign forces of sunshine, air, light, exercise, simple foods, earth cure, water cure, mental science, etc., are a thousand times more curative of the ills of mankind than the poisons of the allopaths.

The epoch-making work done by these great pioneers in Natural Healing is fully described in the pages of our magazine. The twentieth century will be known as the Century of Naturopathy. The long slavery of mankind to the bag of bones and feathers of the primitive medicine man, the Witches Brodth of the Middle Ages, the vacuous "megrims" and "vapors" of le docteur a la mode, the bleeding craze of our immediate forefathers, the drugging craze, and the present craze for serums, inoculations, and vaccines, has been broken at last, and many allopaths are now turning naturopaths, thus fleeing from the wrath to come.

The specialties in Natural Healing, no matter by whom introduced, receive most elaborate exposition. These include the German Water Cure; the Nature Cure or Naturopathy, which includes Diet, Hydrotherapy, Thermotherapy, Phototherapy, Heliotherapy, Chromotherapy, Electrotherapy, Psychotherapy or Mental Healing, including suggestive therapeutics, Mechanotherapy, or Massage, and Physical Culture, Osteopathy, Ophthalmology, Chiropractic and Spondylotherapy.

All these various drugless methods, and others not specifically mentioned, are parts of an immense whole that forms a body of medical principles and practice that are the very antithesis of allopathic medicine, which is but a system of ignoring the cause of disease, thus leaving it intact to break forth again. The system is an attempt to enable man to violate the laws of nature, and yet secure immunity from punishment for so doing by the vicarious virtues of drugs, serums and vaccines. This false system of finding "cures" for disease, by treating the effect, even if successful, would only result in our seeing a new series of ailments springing from the unextirpated roots thereof, each requiring a new artificial "remedy," produced in most cases with the infinite suffering of animals in the shambles of the medical laboratory.

The Natural Method of Healing, on the contrary, seeks to change the very habits of the individual by urging a return to nature in eating, drinking, breathing, bathing, working, resting, dressing, thinking, by making use of elementary remedies of nature, by correct physiological principles.

THE HERALD OF HEALTH AND NATUROPATH contains biographical sketches of all the prominent pioneers of Naturopathy, not only those of foreign countries, but also those of the United States. Biographies of Dr. Trall, Graham, Jackson, Kellogg, Walters, Page, Still, the originator of Osteopathy, Weltmer, who enlarged suggestive therapeutics, Palmer, originator of Chiropractic, B. Lust of New York and Butler, N. J., the Naturopath, Drs. Lahn, Strueh, Lindlahr, Carl Schultz, Collins, Deininger, Davis, Havard, professors of Neuropathy, Dr. McCormick, the Ophthalmologist, etc., etc.

These apostles of Natural Healing and their disciples are doing a wonderful work in the prevention and cure of disease, having reduced the death rate of over fifty per cent. under the old and false drug treatment to less than five per cent. by the drugless method.

THE HERALD OF HEALTH AND NATUROPATH is a magazine for the people at large, as well as for the Drugless profession. Each issue is full of ideas that will emancipate the reader from the tyranny of the drug superstition. It is the most desirable factor in the regeneration of the race.

Back volumes from the year 1900 on up to now, each volume, $2.00, postpaid. Single back numbers, except current year, cannot be supplied.

THE NATURE CURE PUBLISHING CO., BUTLER, N. J.

Herald of Health and Naturopath journal

NATURE'S PATH

TO HEALTH AND POWER

A monthly journal of approved methods for gaining, renewing and maintaining superb health and power of body and mind. A frank but clear exponent of the attainment of what human beings want most, through better ways of living, healing, thinking, planning, working, saving, hoping, loving, conquering and achieving.

A supplementary periodical to *Naturopath and Herald of Health,* published by Dr. Benedict Lust since 1896, the original naturopathic magazine, of national and international scope.

This magazine is devoted to the proper care, use, knowledge, development and enjoyment of life. It covers, in particular, all rational, safe and effective methods of healing. And it opposes all irrational, unsafe and ineffective methods. It offers a means of proper health education and acquisition for everybody, and is the only authorized naturopathic journal of a popular character in the United States.

Official Journal of the Lay Department of the American Naturopathic Association, the American School of Naturopathy and Chiropractic and several other Societies and Movements devoted to Natural Life, Nature Cure and Medical Freedom.

| Volume I | JULY, 1925 | No. 1 |

CONTENTS

Edited and Published by Dr. Benedict Lust, 110 East 41st Street, New York, N. Y.

Articles, letters, and personal experiences of general interest are welcomed by the Editor. Please write on one side of paper only; have your manuscript typewritten if possible; and in case you wish manuscript that proves unavailable returned, enclose self-addressed stamped envelope. No compensation can be paid for contributions.

The Editor does not assume responsibility for signed articles. He may not always agree with statements or opinions expressed, but he approves full and fair discussion of all vital topics, and urges readers to form their own conclusions.

Outside of a few special articles labeled "copyrighted," the text of the magazine is not thus protected, and may be reprinted as desired. Please give credit, however, to both magazine and author, and mail us copies of all reprints.

SUBSCRIPTIONS per year to United States, Mexico, Cuba and Insular Possessions, $3.00; Foreign Countries, $3.50, invariably payable in advance. Single copy, 25c. Back issues or back volumes supplied at regular rates. All new subscriptions start with July or January. Back numbers will be mailed to new subscribers.

Application for entry as second-class matter is pending.

Nature's Path to Health and Power journal

Naturopathy embraced all known means of natural therapeutics, including diet, herbs, hydrotherapy, homeopathy, exercise, manipulative therapies, electrotherapy, psychological and spiritual counselling. Dr. Lust believed that the human body possessed an inherent ability to heal itself, that it was able to restore its own balance and function and that it was able to adapt to environmental changes. He was a man of strongly held opinions. For example, he was: *"Opposed to the processing of foods because such 'manufacture' tends to destroy their true nutritional values . . . Opposed to the administrations of all drugs and narcotics because they are unnatural elements which the human body is not capable of assimilating . . . Opposed to the regimentation of the American people under medically controlled elements because such legislation will wipe out other methods of treatment and bring inestimable damage to the health of every man, woman, and child affected . . . Opposed to any legislation which in practice would prevent a family from attending to its own ills or the choosing, by such family, of any type of treatment it might desire because such legislation restricts personal liberty and tends to take from the American people the right to use the beneficial homespun efficient remedies which have been handed down from generation to generation."*

In his efforts to promote the growth and understanding of the science and art of naturopathic medicine, Dr. Lust's life was not without personal sacrifice. He

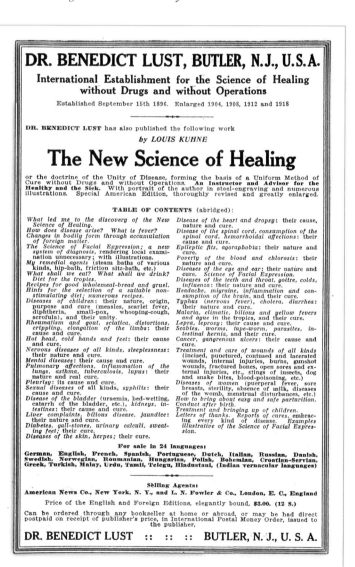

The New Science of Healing

was arrested some three dozen times for practicing medicine without a license, but attempts to suppress his efforts were thwarted, as all cases were dismissed from the courts. It was not as a practitioner, however, but as an educator, promoter and organizer of naturopathy that Lust had his greatest impact. He was the founder of the American Naturopathic Association, which was known as the Naturopathic Society of America from 1902 to 1919. One of Lust's greatest disappointments was the internal struggles that developed within the naturopathic profession just a few years before his death in 1945.

Louisa Lust, the First Matriarch of Naturopathy

Dr. Louisa Lust (1868 – 1925) is considered the matriarch of naturopathy. She studied the nature cure methods of Rikli and Kuhne in London prior to coming to America where she met and married Benedict Lust. She was a successful naturopathic physician specializing in the treatment of women. Dr. Louisa Lust was the leading financial partner in establishing the sanatoriums in New Jersey and in Florida and she provided the financial wherewithal for the establishment of the first naturopathic college. She was also instrumental in paying for most of the legal defences for her husband. Although Louisa studiously avoided the limelight, she was a powerful presence behind the scenes.

Dr. Louisa Lust was an accomplished writer, especially with respect to living a healthy vegetarian lifestyle. She believed firmly in the life force within as the great healing agent of the body. For her the successful practice of naturopathy rested on three factors: freedom from fear, mastery of hygiene and never forgetting to treat the individual by modifying and adjusting to each person.

Dr. Louisa Lust was a strong believer in the healing power of food. "We can lengthen our life," she wrote, "or shorten it by eating."

In sickness she recommended the lightest possible diet. "One of the greatest evils to be avoided by those who are nursing the sick," she wrote, "it is that of over eating." Dr. Lust was also a staunch advocate of hydrotherapy. "If all people understood how to use water," she wrote, "one half of all the afflictions from disease would be removed."

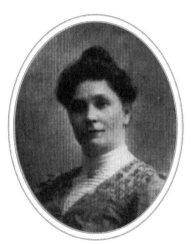

Louisa Lust ND (1868 – 1925)

Used with permission, *Nature Doctors*, NCNM Press

"Do not under any circumstances; shut the air and sunshine from your home. Do not mind if the furniture, curtains, draperies, etc. will fade. It is better to let them fade than you should."

LOUISA LUST (1868 - 1925)

Lindlahr's Influence

Another significant figure in the history of American naturopathy was Dr. Henry Lindlahr (1862 – 1924). He was mayor of a town in Montana and a thriving businessman. In his thirties he was over weight and diabetic. When he was unable to find appropriate treatment for his diabetes in America, he travelled to Europe and found curative results under the guidance of Father Kneipp.

On returning to America in early 1900 he enrolled in the Homeopathic and Eclectic College of Illinois. After graduating in 1904, he opened the Lindlahr Sanitarium in Chicago, and shortly thereafter, he founded the Lindlahr College of Natural Therapeutics which included hospital internships at sanitariums. It became the leading naturopathic colleges of the day.

In 1908, Dr. Lindlahr began to publish the *Nature Cure* magazine and began publishing a series of books titled, *Philosophy of Natural Therapeutics*. His therapeutic regimen combined the use of breathing, fasting and specialized diet, fever therapy, exercise and rest, sun and light, as well as counselling to address mental and emotional concerns. He utilized various detoxifying or cleansing foods, in particular - orange juice, lemon, grapefruit, garlic, bean sprouts, fiber and laxatives. Besides these items, he pioneered the use of vitamin and mineral supplementation, forming what may have been the first company that produced Thiamine (Vitamin B1) commercially. It was written that Henry Lindlahr ". . . is remembered for his conviction that disease did not represent an invasion of molecules, but the body's way of healing something. In other words, he viewed symptoms as a positive physiological response and proof that the body was fighting whatever was wrong."

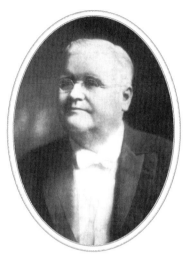

Henry Lindlahr ND (1862 – 1924)
Used with permission, *Nature Doctors*, NCNM Press

"Every acute disease is the result of a purifying, healing effort of nature."
HENRY LINDLAHR ND (1862 - 1924)

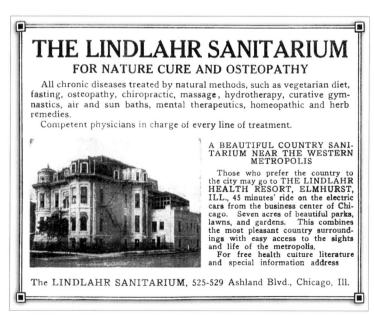

THE LINDLAHR SANITARIUM
FOR NATURE CURE AND OSTEOPATHY

All chronic diseases treated by natural methods, such as vegetarian diet, fasting, osteopathy, chiropractic, massage, hydrotherapy, curative gymnastics, air and sun baths, mental therapeutics, homeopathic and herb remedies.
Competent physicians in charge of every line of treatment.

A BEAUTIFUL COUNTRY SANITARIUM NEAR THE WESTERN METROPOLIS

Those who prefer the country to the city may go to THE LINDLAHR HEALTH RESORT, ELMHURST, ILL., 45 minutes' ride on the electric cars from the business center of Chicago. Seven acres of beautiful parks, lawns, and gardens. This combines the most pleasant country surroundings with easy access to the sights and life of the metropolis.
For free health culture literature and special information address

The LINDLAHR SANITARIUM, 525-529 Ashland Blvd., Chicago, Ill.

The Lindlahr Sanitarium

Nature Cure, philosophy and practice

Other Significant Contributors

Dr. John H Tilden (1852 – 1942) was an eclectic medical doctor who believed that disease was due to the build up of toxins in the body. He was a strong supporter of preventive medicine and addressing the cause of disease, not just treating it with drugs. Dr. Frederick W. Collins (1873 – 1948) and Dr. Joe Shelby Riley (1889 – 1946) were naturopathic practitioners who embraced the eclectic aspect of naturopathic medicine. Dr. Riley introduced the field of acupuncture into naturopathy and was also an advocator of zone therapies such as reflexology. The National University of Therapeutics was founded by Dr. Riley, Dr. Hallan Parker and Dr. Collins in 1911 for the teaching of all types of medical and alternative therepies. Dr. Collins was one of the early students of Dr. Benedict Lust. Over time he became known as the "consulting drugless physician of America." He was a true Renaissance man, with doctorates in medicine, naturopathy, osteopathy and chiropractic. Dr. Collins founded the New Jersey College of Chiropractic and Naturopathy in 1910 and was the first physician in America to establish a free clinic treating polio victims. A prolific author and speaker, he helped to form, advance and define the new profession of naturopathic medicine. At the Golden Jubilee Convention of the American Naturopathic Association, held in New York City in 1947, Dr. Collins received the award of "Dean of Naturopathy" as he was the last of the five great Naturopaths of America – Drs. Lust, Lindlahr, Collins, Riley, and Tilden.

Dr. John Harvey Kellogg (1852-1943) studied at the Hygieo-Therapeutic College and at the Michigan Medical School. He became the editor of *Health Reformer* in 1874, and in 1879 he changed the magazine's name to *Health*. He published over 50 books on various aspects of healthy living and advocated vegetarianism, regular exercise, plenty of fresh air and sunshine, drinking eight to ten glasses of water a day, and abstinence from alcohol, tobacco, tea and coffee. He became famous for the cereals that he patented and introduced, including Granola and Corn Flakes. His younger brother then built a successful company to market his cereal creations. Dr. Kellogg also invented peanut butter, artificial milk made from soybeans and other foods.

Otis G. Carroll (1879 – 1962) suffered from rheumatic fever and severe juvenile arthritis. He found help from Dr. Alex LeDoux, a medical doctor who had studied with Father Kneipp. After his cure, he studied herbalism, then later studied with Dr. LeDoux. It was only after years of informal education that he enrolled at the Cleveland College of Chiropractic, while continuing his

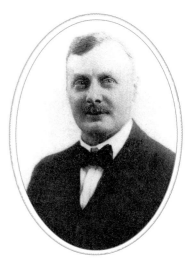

Fredrick.W. Collins ND
(1873 – 1948)

"Health and disease are related in that they are two phases of one state, and neither can be known without contrasting it with the other."
J. H. TILDEN (1852-1942)

informal education with Dr. Lindlahr. Dr. Carroll became a naturopathic doctor and the focus of his practice was on improving his patients' abilities to digest foods and absorb nutrients. To do this, he relied on hydrotherapy, herbs, and diet. Dr. Carroll is remembered for originating constitutional hydrotherapy and developing one of the first means for discerning food sensitivities. The clinic that he started in the early 1900s is still in operation today. After Dr. Carroll's death in 1962, his practice was taken over by Dr. Harold Dick, one of his preceptors. After Dr. Dick's death, the practice still focuses on hydrotherapy and diet and is run by his daughter, Dr. Letitia Dick-Watrous ND in Washington.

Alternative Medicine Flourishes

During the early 1900s, naturopathic medicine flourished in America. There were many reasons for its acceptance and growth. The Canadian and American landscapes were untamed with respect to the practice of medicine. Both countries were experiencing a high amount of immigration, especially from European countries which were already familiar with nature cure therapies. There was also growing dissatisfaction with the blood-letting, mercury purges, drugs and potions of the allopathic practitioners. From this beginning, the ideas and philosophies of naturopathic medicine spread until it was on the leading edge of the nature cure movement of the early and middle 20th century.

It was a time of expansive thinking and many additions to the methods of the natural healing arts were made. Osteopathy, chiropractic and treatment by all kinds of artificial lights, electricity, colour, etc., were discovered and many were integrated into the practice of naturopathy. Homeopathy had been introduced in 1825 and flourished in the United States into the early 1900s. In 1874 osteopathy was founded by Dr. Andrew Taylor Still (1828 – 1917), a medical doctor who felt that the current medical system was inadequate and that many drugs could be avoided if practitioners were properly trained to treat the physical structure. In 1895 chiropractic care was founded by Dr. Daniel David Palmer. Chiropractic was built on the foundation that the body is a self-healing organism, that structure determines function, the nervous system controls and coordinates every organ and tissue of the body, there is a relationship between the spine and the health of the nervous system and that the role of the practitioner is to find and eliminate the blockage so that the body will move back toward health. Homeopathy, chiropractic, osteopathic, and naturopathic became known as the four major practices of natural medicine and in the 1900s there was much mixing and cooperation between them.

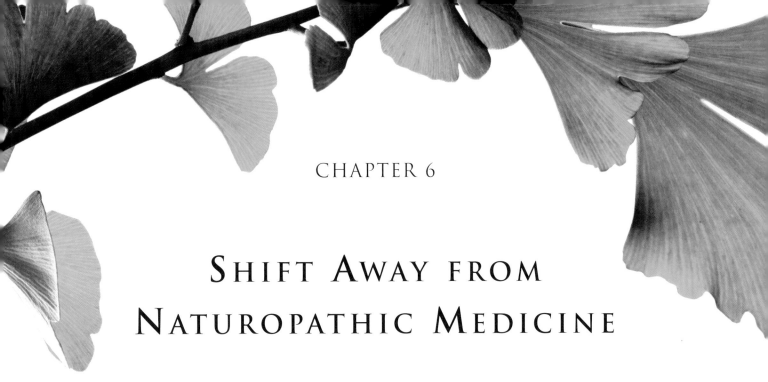

CHAPTER 6

SHIFT AWAY FROM NATUROPATHIC MEDICINE

Naturopathic medicine enjoyed wide acceptance and growth for its first thirty years. The period of 1930 to 1970 marked its legal and economic suppression. Factors that contributed included the social-economic impact of the Civil War, the Great Depression and World War II; the Flexner report resulting in a shift of funding and support to only scientifically based conventional medical schools; the birth of pharmaceutical medicine with its promise of 'miracle cures'; and struggles within the naturopathic profession itself.

Socio-Economic Factors

The Civil War (1861 – 1865) impoverished the nation and resulted in a shift away from hygiene as a major focus of health and ill-health. The Great Depression of the 1930s and World War II which subsequently followed, resulted in further economic impact. It was during the second World War that antibiotics were introduced and the War is credited with the advancement of surgery. Despite the devastation of these events, there was a sense of a new future that would support longer, healthier and richer lives. This was something that many believed would come from drugs and surgery and from a government run health care system, rather than the old tradition of each individual taking responsibility for their own health and living lifestyles that promoted well-being. America was entering the post-war period with a strong sense of individual entitlement at the expense of personal responsibility. The focus on hygiene, lifestyle and good eating was left in the shadows and with it the practice of naturopathic medicine.

Flexner Report

A focus of the American Medical Association (AMA) in the late 1800s was to establish medical educational standards, licensing laws and to ensure that scientific medicine was integrated into medical educational institutions. In 1871 Harvard University created the first four-year medical curriculum in America, John's Hopkins University and others schools followed suit twenty years later. In 1904, the AMA established a Council on Medical Education that was made up of members from the faculties of schools modeled on the John Hopkin's prototype.

Shortly after, an educator was hired by the Council and the Rockefeller and Carnegie Foundation to do a report on the medical schools of America. The purpose of this report was to establish standards and a certifying body as the current medical schools and the health care system were viewed as disorganized with diverse standards. The educator chosen was Abraham Flexner. In a matter of months he reviewed 186 allopathic medical schools, assigning them an A, B or C rating. In 1910 the Flexner Report was released and the emphasis on medical education in America changed significantly. Although the report was aimed at the quality of allopathic medical education, it also included sections that discredited botanical, hydrotherapy and homeopathic treatments. The report made many recommendations including the banning of midwives, female doctors and non-white doctors, and set up a committee to investigate and accredit only those schools and hospitals that met certain standards.

Federal, public, and private funds were channelled to select institutions as a result of the Flexner report recommendations. Those institutions that emphasized science-based medicine, drug therapy and surgery received funding; those schools which found themselves philosophically opposed to this emerging paradigm did not. Notably, many millions of dollars were poured into the allopathic schools and hospitals, while the homeopathic, naturopathic, chiropractic, osteopathic, and few surviving eclectic colleges and hospitals were not certified and were left to fend for themselves. The Canadian medical system and schools soon followed suit.

Fewer schools meant that there were fewer opportunities to attend and the process became more selective. For the next forty to fifty years, the allopathic medical doctor population consisted primarily of white male Protestants from higher income and influential families, a combination that quickly led to the MDs rise in power and prestige in the United States and Canada. Additionally, the growing political sophistication and intense lobbying by the emerging AMA helped to provide a favourable regulatory climate for conventional medical schools and for their own political agenda.

In the early 1900 there were 186 allopathic, 22 homeopathic, about 20 naturopathic, and at least 30 other chiropractic and osteopathic institutes of higher learning. By 1927 there were only a dozen naturopathic schools. Many of the naturopathic and chiropractic colleges merged in order to survive. By the mid 1950s over half of the allopathic schools, all of the homeopathic, most of the chiropractic and osteopathic schools and all of the original naturopathic schools had been closed.

The Rise of Pharmaceutical Medicine

The first half of the twentieth century saw many advances in pharmaceuticals to replace the crude, poisonous, and often ineffective medicines that were previously used by allopathic physicians. The development of penicillin and other antibiotics, diuretics, insulin, hormones, anti-inflammatory and psychoactive drugs helped to bring about an expectation of quick and effective relief from a wide variety of ailments. While many of these drugs save lives and improve the quality of life, they were and are not without toxicity themselves. They also foster a dependence on passive care and are often used to alleviate symptoms without addressing the underlying causes of disease.

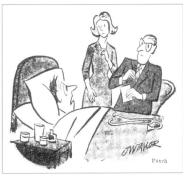

"Drugs, side-effects, more drugs, more side-effects – couldn't I go back to the original cold?"

The emphasis of scientific research and of health care became increasingly focused on technology and the use of pharmaceuticals. With the promise of miracle drugs such as antibiotics and vaccinations, there became a decreased focus on self-responsibility and on the relationship that human beings had to their environment. There became a greater separation between the physician and the patient, and the patient to the cause of their disease.

The separation between allopathic and the non-allopathic physicians also widened. The marketing campaigns of the medical associations and the pharmaceutical industries were focused on the idea that drugs could eliminate disease. Naturopathic medicine, as well as chiropractic and osteopathic medicine, encountered strong opposition in the public and political arenas.

Intra-Professional Struggles

There were many external factors that contributed to the decline in naturopathic medicine and there were internal factors. When Benedict Lust died in 1945 the profession was disorganized and the eclectic nature of the profession resulted in internal struggles. There were some practitioners that desired the scientific path of allopathic medicine and wanted to pull away from the naturopathic philosophies; others insisted that the profession maintain its roots.

The profession, already small, became split into even smaller groups. As well, since many naturopathic doctors held dual licences a number of doctors gave up their naturopathic practice in search of a more secure future.

The naturopathic profession has had established educational standards since the 1920s and had tried repeatedly to ensure that only those schools that adhered to these standards were recognized or supported. Yet, the profession has been hampered by schools that offer inferior programs, some nothing more than diploma mills. The challenge has been that practitioners working in unregulated states or provinces are not required to meet the high standards of education that have been set by the profession. Only by regulation can the profession enforce and ensure that all practitioners are qualified and properly trained.

Over the years there have been many discussions about the direction and focus of the profession. The outcome was the realization that, in order for the profession to survive, it must remain a distinct healing profession based on the roots of nature cure and the original principles of healing. The years of internal and external struggle would have resulted in the demise of the profession if it had not been for a small group of practitioners, such as naturopathic doctors Joe Boucher, Otis Carroll, Joe Pizzorno, Arno Koegler, Fred Loffler, Gerald Farnsworth and others - many from Canada - who dedicated their lives to ensuring that the profession survived.

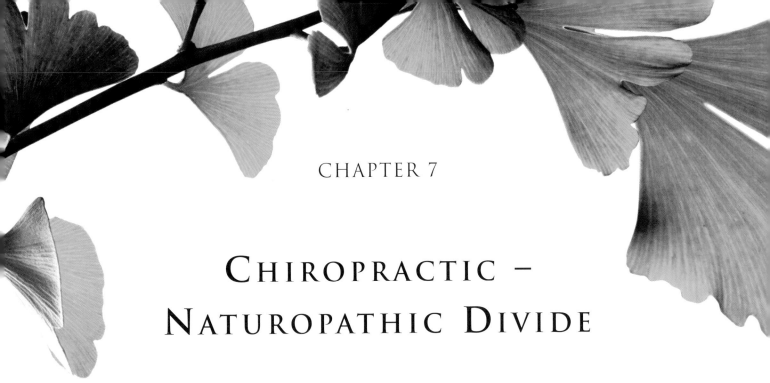

CHAPTER 7

CHIROPRACTIC –
NATUROPATHIC DIVIDE

The chiropractic and naturopathic professions have both had their successes and their challenges. For many years the two professions walked a common path and were cooperative in their educational and legislative initiatives. They started going their separate ways as each profession struggled for survival and recognition. Today, both professions are established and the relationship is supportive and professional.

Origins of Chiropractic

Dr. Daniel David Palmer is the founder of chiropractic medicine. He was born in Port Perry, Ontario in 1845 and moved to the United States when he was twenty years old. In 1885 Dr. Palmer became familiar with the work of Paul Caster, a magnetic healer, and in 1887 he opened the Palmer Cure and Infirmary.

In 1895 Dr. Palmer was communicating with a janitor in his office who was deaf. The janitor told Dr. Palmer that he became deaf all of a sudden when he was bent over and something in his back "popped". Dr. Palmer deduced that the two events – the popping in the man's back and the deafness – had to be connected. After conducting a spinal assessment he realized that one of the vertebrae in the man's back was not in its normal position. The man's hearing returned once his vertebrae was realigned.

Over the succeeding months, other patients came to Dr. Palmer with every conceivable problem, including sciatica, migraine headaches, stomach complaints, epilepsy, and heart trouble. Dr. Palmer found that the conditions responded well to the adjustments which he was calling "hand treatments." Later he coined the term *"chiropractic"* – from the Greek words, '*chiro*' meaning hand and '*practic*' meaning practice or operation.   Dr. Palmer started teaching his techniques and the practice of chiropractic quickly grew.

Working Together

In the early 1900s naturopathy, chiropractic, homeopathy and osteopathy were the main "natural" health-care systems that existed in America and each one was in its infancy. Each profession was striving for recognition and acceptance as a legitimate form of healing. Many of the "natural" healers were trained in more than one system of healing; as such, the relationships were mostly co-operative and strong. The chiropractic and naturopathic professions became quite close, often combining their efforts for regulation against the constant lobbying of conventional medical associations. In the 1920s and 1930s naturopathic medicine and chiropractic were both successful in achieving legislation with naturopathic medicine being regulated in twenty-three states and in four provinces. Over the years, chiropractic medicine was more politically savvy in their lobbying efforts and achieved greater government acceptance. As such, the number of chiropractors increased faster than naturopathic doctors. In the late 1940s it was estimated that there were about 8,000 naturopathic practitioners in North America; by comparison, there were about 17,000 chiropractors.

To address the impact of the Flexner report, attacks from the medical profession and the limited resources that each profession had its disposal the two professions combined their educational programs. Institutions which offered combined programs included Western States College of Portland, Oregon and the National College of Drugless Physicians located near Chicago, Illinois. In these colleges, the chiropractic programs were dominant. Those individuals looking to receive a degree in naturopathic medicine did extra courses, over six to twelve months, in topics such as nutrition, naturopathic philosophy and botanical medicine. The combining of the naturopathic and chiropractic programs resulted in the naturopathic profession being inextricably tied to that of chiropractic.

Growing Apart

Dual degree programs caused friction both within and between each profession. There were concerns that those practitioners with dual licenses would have split loyalty. There was also a concern that many programs within the dual degree schools did not teach enough naturopathic medicine. Adding to this friction was an inconsistency in the standards in different licensing jurisdictions and in the colleges that were recognized by the associations in the United States and Canada. For example, British Columbia did not approve colleges that did not meet certain requirements for basic science education. Even many of the straight naturopathic colleges did not have programs that met the standards of the regulated provinces. These differing standards did not serve either profession well.

By the 1950s the legislative rights won earlier by both professions were rapidly being eroded and challenged especially in the United States. Each profession was struggling to stay alive. The chiropractic profession in the United States wanted to be recognized by the Department of Health, Education, and Welfare as this would allow them access to federally insured student loans and federal research money. One of the conditions of obtaining recognition was the removal of all naturopathic programs from their colleges. At the same time, there was growing discord within the chiropractic profession. Some chiropractors embraced a broad range of treatments; others wanted to limit the scope - primarily to aid in legislative acceptance. The International Chiropractic Association was committed to the view that chiropractors should limit their practice to manipulation of bone. Those adhering to this point of view were called "straights". Those who believed chiropractic should have a greater scope of practice and use multiple modalities were represented by the National Chiropractic Association and were known as "mixers". The "straight" practitioners practiced primarily in the West; the "mixers" in the East. The Canadian Chiropractic Association and the provincial chiropractic associations soon followed in the footsteps of those set in the United States.

Schools that refused to discontinue their naturopathic programs were threatened with loss of accreditation. This was a threat that could not be ignored. This shift in focus to "straights" aided in the growth of the chiropractic profession. The National College of Drugless Physicians in Illinois graduated its last class of naturopathic physicians in 1952 and Western States College of Chiropractic in Portland, Oregon closed its program in 1955. The Canadian Memorial Chiropractic College in Toronto dropped the naturopathic aspect of its program in 1977.

Separation

The long time ally the naturopathic profession had found among chiropractors virtually evaporated as the chiropractic profession chose to disassociate itself from the naturopathic profession. The gap between chiropractors and naturopathic doctors widened due to the difference in the number of practitioners, the resources that each group had available, the closure of the ND programs and the difference in level of social and government acceptance. From the 1940s to the 1980s the chiropractic profession was rising while naturopathic was declining. Although the initial naturopathic practitioners, such as Lust and Lindlahr, were charismatic leaders, during the difficult years, naturopathic medicine did not have a central charismatic figure and lacked a strong organizational structure.

Over the years, there have also been 'territorial struggles' with reports of chiropractors instituting legal proceedings against naturopathic physicians for practicing chiropractic; all of which were decided in favour of naturopathic medicine. There have also been legislative battles between the two professions with respect to scope of practice and the use of terms 'chiropractic' and 'manipulation'.

The division between the chiropractors and naturopathic practitioners in Canada widened in December of 1964 when the Ontario Chiropractic Association (OCA) published a very explicit directive urging chiropractors who held dual licenses to:
- Not renew their naturopathic license;
- Discontinue using the letters "ND" after their name;
- Discontinue using 'naturopath' or 'naturopathy' on their business card, stationery, door, window, and/or sign; and
- Discontinue using a naturopathy listing in the telephone book.

The OCA took this stand as they believed that a more complete government recognition would only come when their profession was clearly defined with no confusing boundaries; and that it was a continual source of embarrassment to chiropractic delegates when asked by government representatives why so many of their members also hold naturopathic licenses. The perception was that chiropractors were not satisfied with their own present system of treatment.

The chiropractic profession was rewarded for abdicating the philosophy of their founder by receiving increased legitimacy in the eyes of the government. The naturopathic profession, on the other hand, endured more struggle with government and the medical establishment as they never conformed to the external demands of conventional medicine. They saw the breadth of their scope, their principles and philosophy, and the fact that they lacked a single distinctive focus, as their strength, not as a weakness.

Mending Fences

The strength of chiropractic medicine reached a plateau in the late 1980s and since then, the chiropractic profession has found that its decision to relinquish the breadth of its scope is again causing discord within the profession. The benefits that the chiropractic profession enjoyed, such as medicare coverage, has been withdrawn over time as the Canadian health care system encounters continual financial challenges.

The relationship between the chiropractors and naturopathic practitioners has enjoyed new strength and cooperation since the 1990s. Part of this is due to the increasing organization structure, demand and acceptance of naturopathic medicine and partially to the realization that the naturopathic philosophies and principles, which they once shared, are an integral part of healing and health care.

Today it is common for naturopathic doctors and chiropractors to work together in integrated clinics. There is also renewed effoorts in the two professions supporting each other in legislative and political arenas.

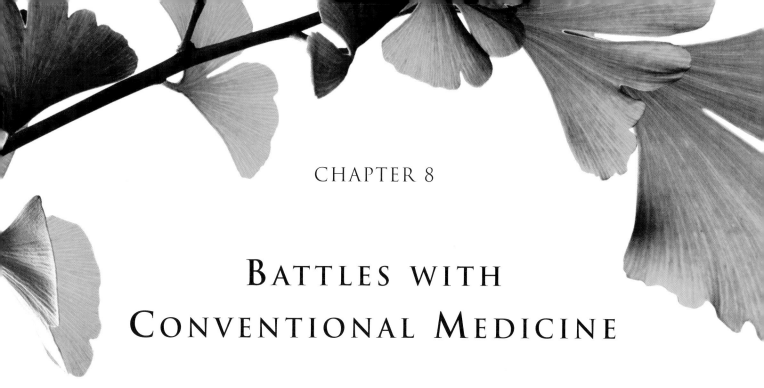

CHAPTER 8

BATTLES WITH CONVENTIONAL MEDICINE

THE BASIS FOR A LOT of the territorial struggles in the health-care industry, both in Canada and in the United States, has been driven by the conventional medical associations and the pharmaceutical companies desire to create a monopoly in healthcare. Until the late 1970s, Canada relied on the United States for the education of naturopathic practitioners. Hence, the political environment in the United States, especially as it related to health care, greatly impacted the practice of naturopathic medicine in Canada.

The conventional medical system was on lead. They had the in with government and political officials and they created a framework that defined the practice of medicine. They then measured all other practitioners and systems of healing by this framework. If you did not fit the conventional paradigm, you were an outcast and the overt intentions and actions of the American Medical Association (AMA) and Canadian Medical Association (CMA) were to limit the practice of all other forms of medicine. Natural systems of healing, such as naturopathic medicine, had four options - they could be absorbed by medicine, as osteopathy in the United States had; they could become a speciality within the field of medicine, as chiropractic had chosen to become by sacrificing all aspects of its scope other than manipulation; they could disappear, which is what happened to homeopathy after they united with conventional medicine; or they could hold their principles strong, grow slowly and steadily and wait for the time when they could emerge with their principles and full scope still intact. The latter is the path that naturopathic medicine chose. Not fitting in with the conventional medical standards was a cause for struggle, but it was also confirmation that naturopathic medicine was a distinct and unique system of healing.

In the 1956 Annual Report of the Canadian Naturopathic Association, the President Fred Parsons ND commented,

> *"We no longer live in a world of unorganized individuals, or a world where unorganized individuality can prosper or compete with organized society. We must conform to society's requirements, but that does not mean that we must practice as medicine, chiropractors or others do. It does mean though, that we must conform to our own predetermined and scientifically proven scope of practice, which will fit in and enhance other forms of practice rather than be antagonistic and destructive to other established professions. We must demonstrate that we respect the laws and the opinions of others if we in turn wish to be respected."*

Early Regulation of Medicine in America

In the 1850s there was limited acceptance for the government regulation of medicine due to the existence of different professional medical groups – the allopathic practitioners, the homeopaths and the eclectic practitioners and due to the fact that they were all enjoying strong social acceptance. In the late 1870s and into the 1880s all medical practitioners agreed to work cooperatively to obtain common professional goals, including the enactment of new licensing laws and the creation of respectable medical educational systems. Once the cooperation between the different medical systems started, the allopathic view of medicine came fully into power due to their numbers, their professional infrastructure and the political astuteness of many of their members. Ironically, even though the homeopaths and the other eclectic practitioners wanted to share in the legal privileges of the medical profession, it was only after they started working cooperatively with them that they started to lose their popularity. The non-allopathic doctors thrived when they were shunned and denounced by the allopaths (conventional doctors), but the more they gained access to the privileges of allopathic physicians, the more their numbers and scope of practice declined. For example, in the 1920s there were over 11,000 homeopathic practitioners, many of them were converted conventional doctors. Within a few years of the homeopathic curriculum becoming part of medical training, their curriculum was thrown out and medical practitioners were discouraged or banned by the AMA from practicing homeopathy. The practice of homeopathy in America had, for the most part, disappeared over a span of less than 20 years. Even today, over 75 years later, there is reported to be fewer homeopathic practitioners in American than there were in 1920.

"All along the history of medicine, the really great physicians were peculiarly free from the bondage of drugs."
SIR WILLIAM OSLER, MD
(1849 – 1919)

The history of medicine in Canada follows a similar trend as that in the United States. For example, in 1869 in Ontario all medical professions – allopathic doctors, homeopathic practitioners and the eclectics - were regulated and governed by the same council, the College of Physicians and Surgeons in Ontario (CPSO). Five homeopaths, five eclectics and seventeen physicians comprised the CPSO at this time. This legislative arrangement led to some disagreement between the "regulars" (MDs) and the "irregulars" (homeopaths and eclectics) as the different groups attempted to stake out their own territory. The "regulars" were mainly concerned that the standards for medical education and licensure would be weakened by this infiltration of the "irregulars". In the late 1800s, the scientific view was becoming the dominant view in North America. Both the homeopaths and the eclectics offered an independent and alternative approach to medical care based on a healing paradigm that challenged the fundamental assumptions of allopathic medicine. The allopathic profession attempted to further its own interests by invoking exclusionary techniques against these groups.

Beginning in the early 1900s, the CPSO council started actively seeking routes to restrict the practice of all non-allopathic or drugless practitioners in Ontario. In response, the Drugless Physicians Association was established and recognized by the government in 1915. This association was successful in obtaining more specific protective legislation, partly due to the public support for alternative medicine and the working-class opposition to the monopoly of allopathic medicine. The Drugless Physicians Association was dissolved in 1952 as regulations were put in place for "non-allopathic" (also referred to as alternative or drugless) practitioners.

The introduction of osteopathy, chiropractic and naturopathic medicine in 1874, 1895 and 1896 respectively, happened within this political backdrop. There was already an established struggle between allopathic and all other medical practitioners.

American and Canadian Medical Associations Begin

In 1847 the American Medical Association (AMA) was formed. It took about 50 years for it to have a lot of clout but over time its influence, both politically and professionally, became quite strong. From the onset the AMA established restrictive guidelines with respect to the practice of medicine and with respect to the relationship between allopathic (conventional) medical practitioners and other practitioners. For example, their initial code encouraged the adoption of uniform rules for payment in geographical areas, condemned the practice of contract work, prohibited advertising and fee-sharing, eliminated blacks and women from practicing medicine and prohibited any consultation or contact with irregulars or sectarian practitioners. Irregular practitioners were classified as any practitioner who did not follow conventional medicine's dogma. Although the AMA initially rejected women in medicine, by the end of the 19th century, the number of women physicians in the United States had increased to more than 7,000 up from about 200 in 1860.

The Canadian Medical Association (CMA) started in Quebec City in 1844 but due to internal struggles, it did not become an official association until 1867, just three months after the birth of Canada. The CMA was created by 164 physicians who recognized the need for a national medical body to represent the views of their profession. Similar to the AMA, when the CMA was first formed it too had restrictive guidelines, for example it refused to allow membership to any medical doctor who was known to consult with homeopaths. In 1868 the CMA tried to get a bill passed with respect to medical education and registration. It took over forty years to become law due to internal struggles and opposition from the 'irregular' practitioners and those who supported them.

During the late 1800s and early 1900s, Canada was in the process of setting up an organized and functional judicial system. Conventional medical practitioners were very successful at ensuring that they occupied many seats in government, especially as it related to the regulation and overseeing of Canadian health care. For example, with the exception of a two-year period from 1969-1972, every Minister of Health in Ontario, as well as his deputy minister, until 1974 was a conventional medical physician. In fact, the first president of the CMA, Charles Tupper, later served as Canada's Prime Minister. With medical doctors in primary positions of power, the environment for conflict with all other health professions was ripe. Conventional medicine was in charge and they developed definitions, regulations and criteria that matched their philosophies and principles.

"Natural healing, that has drifted so long and, by reason of a lack of organization, has been made for so many years the football of official medicine, to be kicked by any one who thought fit to do so, has now arrived at such a pitch of power that it has shaken the old system of bureaucratic medicine in its foundations. The professors of the irrational theories of life, health and disease, that are looking for victims to be inoculated with dangerous drugs and animalized vaccines and serums, have begun to fear the growth of this young giant of medical healing that demands medical freedom, social justice and equal rights for the new healing system that exists alone for the betterment and uplifting of humanity."

1st UNIVERSAL NATUROPATHIC DIRECTORY PRINTED IN 1918, LUST PUBLICATIONS

Different Approaches to Health Care

The common ground between naturopathic and conventional medicine is the desire to improve the health of Canadians. The goal is the same; the approach very different. Conventional medicine is based on dualistic, reductionist assumptions; naturopathic medicine embraces vitalism and holism. Conventional medicine focuses on 'killing the bug'; naturopathic medicine focuses on 'strengthening the healing power of the body'. Conventional medicine is pharmaceutically based, naturopathic medicine is based on lifestyle and natural therapies.

The relationship between conventional medicine and naturopathic medicine, especially in the mid 1900s, was distant, antagonist and territorial as a result of their differences. The conventional medical establishment has always been much larger and more powerful. They have more practitioners, more money and more political power. Over the years, the naturopathic profession has spent endless hours and resources on responding to the overt attacks made upon them.

The different approaches have often been a disadvantage from a political and legislative point of view; but there are also advantages. The differences provide choice,

Co-operation Urged With Healers

Sun Victoria Bureau

VICTORIA — A Socred MLA Tuesday objected to a bill which he said prevents doctors from co-operating with naturopaths and chiropractors.

Bert Price, (Vancouver-Burrard), told the legislature it was wrong to limit such co-operation.

He protested a section of a bill amending the Medical Act, which strengthens regulations imposed on doctors by the College of Physicians and Surgeons of B.C.

The section prohibits doctors from practising in partnership, contract, or business association with any person not qualified to practise medicine, surgery, or midwifery.

Doctors who violate this are liable to a fine of from $100 to $250 and to lose their licences.

··I don't think this should be done," Price said. "If a doctor sees fit to co-operate with a chiropractor, naturopath or one of the other trained people in healing, he should be able to do it.

"It's an imposition on the members (of the college) and an imposition on the general public."

But Price had no answer to his plea to Health Minister Eric Martin to change the bill and it was approved on a voice vote, Price remaining silent.

With permission from the Vancouver Sun. Article appeared in the Vancouver Sun March 23rd, 1966.

they allow for a broader perspective of health and disease. Each perspective is valuable and necessary and in specific situations each one is superior.

The goal is not to come to a single view of health-care; the goal is to establish a framework that allows a wider acceptance of the differences.

Legal Challenges

Through lobbying efforts, newspaper reports, channelling of funds, the prosecution of naturopathic doctors and targeted regulatory efforts, the conventional medical system has tried to eliminate or, at least restrict the practice of naturopathic medicine in Canada. In fact, the medical leadership was instrumental on many occasions in arguing that naturopathic legislation should be withdrawn or the scope of naturopathic doctors restricted. Many analysts have commented that conventional medicine has hindered the development of other occupations while protecting its own dominant position.

Denoting alternative medicine as quackery was and continues to be, a common statement made by members of the conventional health care system. In 1961 in British Columbia, Dr. Fred Loffler stated that it had recently been noted in the press that the CMA plans a battle against quackery. They stated chiropractors, naturopaths and osteopaths were an avenue through which quackery was being practiced and suggested something be done about this. Many of the early naturopathic practitioners dedicated their life to defending the naturopathic profession against unwarranted claims such as this.

The differences in medical terminology has always been a reason for confusion and misunderstanding. Words such as 'health' and 'disease', 'preventive medicine', even 'doctor' and 'physician' are defined differently in the various systems of healing and in different jurisdictions. The term 'doctor' means 'to teach'; and 'physician' means 'to heal'. Throughout history, there has been much discussion and debate with regards to which practitioners have the right to use these terms. British Columbia, for example, has been allowed the right to use the term 'physician' since it was first regulated in 1936; whereas, in most other provinces it has not been allowed or has been removed from regulation. In 1951 the naturopathic profession started the process of incorporating the national association under the name of Canadian Association of Naturopathic Physicians. The incorporation was held up for over five years due to debate over the term physician. Members of the naturopathic association were unwill-

"History has proven that whenever any practice surrenders to medicine, it disappears. Medical tenant is that they will not tolerate co-operative branches of healing. Medicine depends upon creating conflict for the removal of disease, while Naturopathy attempts to remove the condition by external, physiological, psychological, nutritional and biochemical means."

ALBERT RUSSELL ND ANPBC

PRESIDENT 1951

"It's a travesty for a person to be judged solely and completely on the standards (if you can call them that – opinions) of a totally different profession... true justice can only come when one's profession can be judged on standards that that profession has."

Joseph Bucher ND, president of the CNA 1980-1985

ing to give up the name and the federal government was unwilling to grant the association its use. Eventually, the association agreed to accept the term, Canadian Naturopathic Association (CNA).

Naturopathic medicine has enjoyed a history of safe and effective treatments with few adverse reactions. In fact, naturopathic doctors have one of the lowest malpractice claims of all the primary health care professions. Yet in the past, the conventional medical establishment has taken the opportunity to exploit situations that arose. The most public example in Canadian naturopathic history was a trial in Alberta in 1984 that involved a prominent naturopathic doctor with over ten years of experience. One of the treatments that he used quite successfully was called the Stober procedure. This procedure consisted of inflating a balloon into the nasal cavity, with the aim of opening up the sinuses and relieving pressure on the brain. During the treatment of a 20-month old child with cerebral palsy and microcephaly, the equipment failed which resulted in the balloon bursting and being lodged in the child's throat. The child died of suffocation. At the time, the Alberta regulatory board did not have sufficient regulatory guidelines or the ability to take disciplinary action. Therefore, the practitioner was charged with negligence and manslaughter.

During the first trial the jurors could not agree on a verdict, but in the second trial the naturopathic doctor was found guilty. The case received tremendous publicity across Canada. The parents of the young girl testified that the treatments were relieving their daughter's condition and they did not hold the ND responsible. During the court case the crown prosecutors relied on expert testimony from medical doctors who were not familiar with naturopathic treatments. In doing so, the judge pronounced that it was acceptable for medical doctors to judge other health professions and to determine reasonable skill, care and knowledge in undertaking any procedure or therapy.

The sentence was not steep as many realized that the faulty equipment was to blame; not negligence. The judge ruled the Stober procedure could not be performed in Alberta. Hence, the technique was banned in Alberta and all other provinces, except British Columbia.

The impact on the profession and on the regulations in Alberta was tremendous because of the precedent set. The concern for the profession was that if any action, whether civil or criminal, was taken against naturopathic doctors in the future, medical doctors could be called as witnesses and be the sole judge of their performance.

Conventional Medicine's Monopoly

Conventional medicine has had a monopoly on the health care system in Canada and in the United States for over 100 years. The concern with a monopoly is that all decisions favour the provider rather than the consumer. In the past there were occasions for naturopathic medicine to expand and enjoy increased public access and acceptance, but those situations were inhibited due to the power and overriding regulations of conventional medicine. For example, in 1943 Sir Victor Sassoon, a British philanthropist, who had regained his health as a result of naturopathic treatments, offered to finance a Chair of naturopathic medicine at the University of B.C. He sent a cheque to the then Premier of British Columbia (B.C.). His cheque was returned and his offer refused. Also, in 1952, a group of private citizens offered to finance the building and operation of a 52 bed hospital in Vancouver for the use of naturopathic physicians. The offer could not be accepted owing to clauses in the B.C. Medical Act and the B.C. Hospital Act.

Practitioners and the public have argued that the marginalizing of naturopathic medicine is unconstitutional as The Charter of Rights and Freedoms provides for equality before and under the law and equal protection and benefit of the law. At the same time, such legislation, as the Canada Health Act, provides the mandate for a diversified health care system. The Canada Health Act is quite specific and its preamble reads as follows:

> *"Whereas the Parliament of Canada recognizes . . . that Canadians can achieve further improvements in their well-being through combining individual lifestyles that emphasize fitness, prevention and health promotion with collective action against the social, environmental and occupational causes of disease, and that they deserve a system of health services that will promote physical and mental health and protection against disease; - that further improvements in health will require the cooperative partnerships of governments, health professionals, voluntary organizations and individual Canadians. – that continued access to quality health care without financial or other barriers will be critical to maintaining and improving the health and well-being of Canadians."*

Although conventional medicine still holds the monopoly on health care, there is a growing acceptance and understanding of alternative medicine. The scientific model is still the overriding focus of conventional medicine, yet the holistic and natural therapeutic methods are being recognized as an integral part of disease prevention and health promotion. There is a sense of hope and trust that all systems of medicine will be valued for the unique services and insight they provide.

From a naturopathic perspective the goal is to remain a distinct medical profession with an expertise in natural medicine. There are increasing opportunities for naturopathic and other forms of medicine to work co-operatively and in an integrated fashion, yet it is essential for each profession to maintain their own identity in order for the whole paradigm of patient care to be realized and to ensure the survival of a fully functional and viable health-care system.

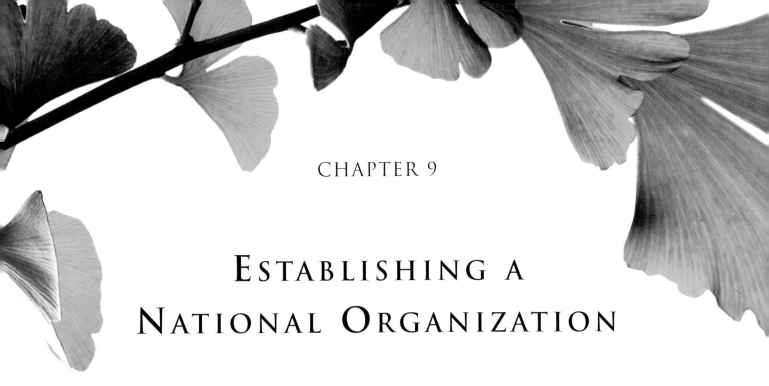

CHAPTER 9

ESTABLISHING A NATIONAL ORGANIZATION

Ɪɴ ᴛʜᴇ ᴍɪᴅ 1900s the majority of naturopathic doctors (NDs) in Canada were located in the western provinces. When it was decided that a national organization was required, Alberta took the lead in ensuring that it happened. In the 1990s the growth of the profession was centered in Ontario and the Canadian Naturopathic Association (CNA) was moved from Alberta to Ontario. In 2002, the name of the association was changed to the Canadian Association of Naturopathic Doctors (CAND) to better reflect the mission of the association. The CAND has become a strong and respected national voice for naturopathic doctors and naturopathic medicine.

Creation

In 1949 Alberta convention it was decided that a national association was necessary in order to present a unified national presence. The promise and concern of government-sponsored health insurance plans, the fact that naturopathic visits were not eligible for income tax deductions, and the inequality and confusion of legislation at the provincial level were a few of the reasons.

During 1950, due to the efforts of many naturopathic doctors, including Dr. Ross Skaken, president of the Alberta Association of Naturopathic Practitioners (AANP), considerable progress was made in formalizing the national association. The Alberta association's lawyer, Mr. Millard, was retained and instructed to draw up the by-laws and an application for incorporation. All provincial associations and naturopathic physicians in Canada were notified and invited to take part in annual association meetings. The Canadian Association of Naturopathic Physicians (CANP) was decided as the name for the national association.

At this point everything looked rather rosy so a membership drive was started in Alberta, British Columbia, Manitoba and Ontario. When the first application was made to the federal government for the CANP charter the first sign of difficulty arose. The federal government took exception to the use of the word "physician" in the title. Members from the provincial associations and individual members sent numerous letters and appeals, but to no avail. The whole matter was shelved pending the next meeting. Between 1951 and 1954 much time and effort was spent on this initiative, especially by the NDs who were part of the Alberta and British Columbia associations. The naturopathic profession was adamant that it would not relinquish the word 'physician' from the name; the government, on the other hand, absolutely refused.

In 1954 the situation seemed hopeless. With this in mind a discouraged and disappointed Dr. Ross Skaken ND attended the British Columbia annual convention in April and asked them to relinquish their stand and accept the name "Canadian Naturopathic Association" (CNA). The British Columbia members agreed, providing the word physician remained in various places throughout the text of the by-laws and the charter application. Later that year, four and a half days were spent in Ottawa with various Government officials and on April 1, 1955, after five years of concentrated effort, the CNA received its incorporation under the federal laws of Canada. The first official annual meeting and convention was held during the annual convention of the British Columbia Association of Naturopathic Physicians on April 13 – 15th 1955 at the Hotel Georgia in Vancouver.

Early Days

The initial annual membership dues were set at $30. British Columbia and Alberta automatically affiliated themselves with the national organization. In 1958, Ontario officially affiliated with the CNA, but each member was responsible for paying their CNA dues directly. In 1955 there were about 400 naturopathic practitioners in Canada, many of them residing in the western provinces and many of them already elders in the profession. This small number of NDs were spread far and wide across the country making membership efforts often tedious and difficult, especially as the primary means of communication was either face-to-face or by written letter.

From the onset, a primary focus of the CNA was to increase its membership. There were many initiatives taken to make this happen. For example, in the late 1950s arrangements were made with Dr. McGill ND who was travelling by car across the country. He was asked to look up as many naturopathic doctors and drugless therapists as possible along the route. He brought in seventeen new active members and eight new associate members.

Despite all the efforts, in 1960 the CNA had a membership of only 22. As an incentive to entice new members the annual dues were decreased to $15. Again the call for unity was sent out and, in a report by the CNA president, it stated, "It is a glaring reality that our profession is being placed under fire at every opportunity and unless we have a united front on a national basis the inevitable result will be disastrous." It was felt that the very life blood of the profession was dependent on a strong united national association, and there was growing concern that the most formidable opposition was not from other groups but rather from the lethargic indifference and non-supportive practitioners within the profession.

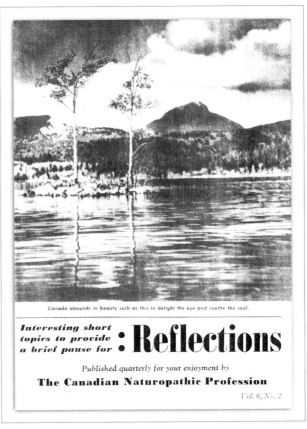

Canada abounds in beauty such as this to delight the eye and soothe the soul.

Interesting short topics to provide a brief pause for : **Reflections**

Published quarterly for your enjoyment by
The Canadian Naturopathic Profession

Vol. 6, No. 2

Reflections was the CNA journal from 1963-1972

The challenge with membership was that many of the older doctors were not in the mind-set to engage in something new especially as many were close to retirement. Adding to the challenge was that there were few new NDs entering the profession due to a lack of educational institutions. The feeling of solidarity across the naturopathic profession began in the 1970s and the membership started to grow. The profession was past its most difficult times and there were many exciting and positive changes. By 1990 only 30 percent of the eligible naturopathic practitioners in Canada were members of the CNA, but by 2008 that percentage had grown to over 90%. The membership was over 1200 and the national association was truly the national voice for the profession.

Working Together

The sustainability of the profession has been due to the cross-border cooperation, especially between the 1950s and 1980s. In fact, the feeling was that there was one naturopathic profession without any borders. Most major decisions, such as educational standards and defining the profession, have been decided jointly. There is also a history of support with respect to legislative and regulatory issues. Today the cooperation between the Canadian and US schools and between the two national associations - the CAND and the AANP - remains strong. The political climates and challenges are different, yet the desire is to advance the profession in a united way. The stakeholders from Canada and the United States continue to meet on a frequent basis to discuss the growth and development of the profession.

Over the years NDs from across Canada have met periodically to discuss the direction of the profession. Once

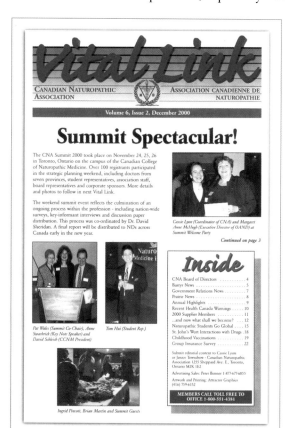

such occassion was in November of 2000 when the CNA hosted a two day strategic planning event at the Canadian College of Naturopathic Medicine (CCNM) to identify significant challenges impacting the naturopathic profession in Canada and to determine strategies to increase awareness, growth and acceptance of the profession. Over 100 participants attended, including naturopathic physicians, association staff, CCNM faculty and staff and other key stakeholders. The CNA Summit was part of a larger strategic planning process that involved extensive environmental scanning, a widely distributed discussion paper, and the subsequent identification of key issues for the profession. Areas of consensus were identified and collaborative strategies were established. In the following five years, many of the initiatives were addressed. Prior to the Summit, the CNA's influence and status with the profession was low. During the following years, the CNA (later named the CAND) has been positioned as a strong national leader for the profession.

Taking a Stand

Naturopathic doctors have a history of taking a stand on issues that affect health, such as the use of fluoride in the water supply, non-smoker's rights, the causes of obesity in children, the importance of detoxification before pregnancy, the harmful effects of toxic chemicals in personal care products, and the impact of heavy metals on health.

Naturopathic doctors have a role to play in medical emergencies, such as pandemics and epidemics and they continue to educate the public and government on the value of their involvement.

For example, in 1918, during the worst flu pandemic in history, homeopathic medicine was found to be extremely effective. The death rate of those treated using conventional treatments was reported to be about 28%, while that of patients treated with homeopathics was just over 1%.

Naturopathic doctors encourage patients to become aware of the factors that affect health, to understand what questions they need to ask and to recognize that they have options. The profession produces position papers to assit in making informed decisions. To access CAND position papers visit their website at www.cand.ca.

Fulfilling the Mandate

The roles and responsibilities of the national association have changed over time, in part due to the changes in the profession itself and also due to the development and growth of the provincial associations. The following highlights a few of its key initiatives.

Setting Standards of Education

Initially the setting of educational standards was done at the provincial and national level. Educational standards were an initiative that the CNA undertook even prior to being recognized as a national organization. On September 21st to 23rd, 1951 eight representatives from the CANP (later changed to CNA) met with the purpose of creating a committee whose duty it would be to approach the various naturopathic schools to establish standards of education and to keep records of schools that adhered to the standards. The representatives included naturopathic Drs. Fred Parsons, Ross Skaken, Albert Russell, Ronald Holtum, Ronald Grant, William Budnick, Fred Loffler and William Budden. At that time it was stated that *"Our naturopathic colleges must turn out graduates who are capable of standing beside the other professions as learned men. It was impressed upon the Committee that in order to be accepted by the powers that be and the public, Naturopathy must be put on a sound and scientific basis. The colleges must be supported and completely controlled by the naturopathic profession and become institutions of higher learning. . . ."* When the Council of Naturopathic Medical Education was established in 1979, it assumed the role of ensuring the standards of education for the profession.

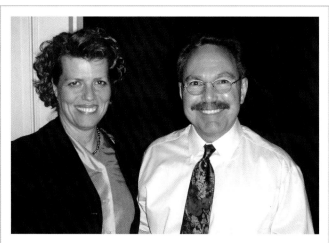

Pictured above are colleagues Dr. Ingrid Pincott ND and Dr. John Cosgrove, DC ND, both recipients of CAND awards for their outstanding work on behalf of the profession in Canada. Dr. Pincott ND was presented with the Verna Hunt award in 2005 and Dr. Cosgrove ND with the Lifetime Achievement Award in 2008.

Supporting the provincial regulatory efforts

Health care in Canada is a provincial mandate. It is up to each province to regulate its health practitioners and to determine the scope of practice of each profession. The CAND's role is to support the provincial regulatory efforts of the individual provinces. It provides both human resources and financial assistance when needed and continues to participate in legislation across Canada. The CAND also sets fee guidelines for the profession and provides many members benefits such as malpractice insurance.

In 1963, Drs. Douglas Kirkbride and Joe Boucher, prepared a CNA document titled, *A Brief Respecting National Health Services*. The brief was presented to the federal government with the request that naturopathic physicians receive the same recognition as other established practitioners, that the services of naturopathic physicians be available on an equal basis to Canadians, that the governments perspective on preventive medicine be broadened to allow for the process of referrals between health practitioners, to ensure the government would provide sponsorship for naturopathic students as they did for other medical students and to request that naturopathic services be included under Medicare. Similar documents were prepared and submitted during the 1970s and 1980s. Since that time the CAND has been recognized as a stakeholder with the federal government.

The CAND provides the national perspective and is often called upon to meet with provincial government officials to explain the status and scope of practice of naturopathic medicine in Canada. The CAND is also involved on issues that impact all the provinces, such as the Agreement on Internal Trade which was initiated in 1994 and became law in 2009. Part of the Internal Trade agreement is the Labour Mobility chapter which ensures that naturopathic doctors that are qualified and regulated in one province can move to another province or territory without barriers.

Working with the federal government

One of the main reasons that the national association was formed was to ensure that the naturopathic profession had a voice at the federal level. In 1995, after the CNA offices moved from Calgary, Alberta to Toronto, Ontario the work with the federal government substantially increased.

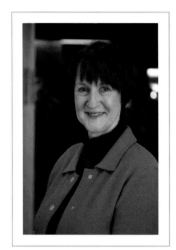

Shawn O'Reilly, Executive Director and Director of Government Relations for the CAND.

Heather MacFarland, executive director of the CNA was initially responsible for establishing these relationships with the federal government.

In 1995, naturopathic Drs Pam Snider, Pat Wales and Paul Saunders were involved in a grass roots push for regulation of natural health products. Dr. Paul Saunders ND was a member of the transition team that created the Office of Natural Health Products, which later became the Natural Health Products Directorate.

Since the late 1990s, the CAND has been very active at the federal level. In addition to its ongoing work with the Natural Health Products Directorate, the CAND participated in the revisions to *Canada's Food Guide*, the development of the *Adverse Reaction Training Module* which provides an avenue for NDs to report suspected and known adverse reactions of drugs, and drug-herb or other natural product interactions and was a member of the stakeholders committee on *Enhancing Interdisciplinary Collaboration in Primary Health Care* which was designed to encourage health professionals to work together in the most effective and efficient way to produce the best health outcomes for patients. The CAND continues to lobby for regulatory changes, participates in consultations, and provides participants for scientific panels and expert advisory committees on health issues.

The CAND is involved in international health issues and has participated with the World Health Organization (WHO) in the development of guidelines including the training and safety of the use of traditional medicines in naturopathic healthcare, quality for safety of homeopathic medicines and the selection of substances for quality control of herbal medicines. It has also made submissions to the

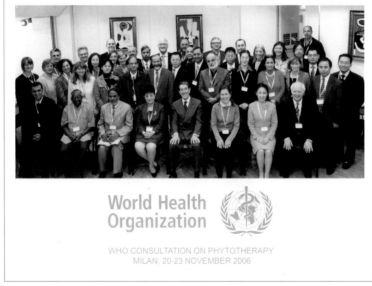

World Health Organization

WHO CONSULTATION ON PHYTOTHERAPY
MILAN, 20-23 NOVEMBER 2006

Attendees included Shawn O'Reilly and NDs Iva Lloyd and Dennis O'Hara

International Government Working Group (chaired by Health Canada) on the draft global strategy and plan of action on public health, innovations and intellectual property.

It is anticipated that the work of the CAND on an international level will continue to expand, especially as Canada is the country with the highest number of regulated naturopathic doctors per capita and the CAND, as a national association, represents the largest percentage of regulated NDs in any country.

Promoting the profession

The initial focus of the association was to assist provinces in their regulatory efforts and to support the internal organization and formation of the profession. There was little attention on external marketing or the image of the profession.

Promotion was done primarily through the production of professional and consumer journals and newsletters. Due to limited resources, some of the journals were done cooperatively with the American national association, such as the consumer booklet entitled, *Health for You*. From 1963 until 1972 the CNA produced *Reflections*, a magazine aimed at educating the public. In 1965 the CNA started to publish a professional journal, *Canadian Journal of Naturopathic Medicine*, which was later replaced with *The Vital Link* in 1995. The *Vital Link* is published three times a year and has become a professional peer-reviewed journal.

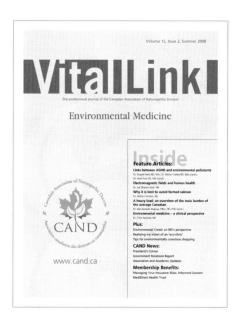

In 1966 the CNA published a booklet entitled, *Naturopathic Medicine in Canada*. Its aim was to increase awareness and understanding for the public and the government with respect to naturopathic medicine. A similar document, *Naturopathy: A Separate and Distinct Healing Profession* was published in 1972.

The CNA has had as many as five different logos and letterheads. This diversity in the CNA's image was a contributing factor in the association's struggles in establishing itself as the recognized leader in naturopathic medicine. As the profession became more developed and stable in the late 1990s, there was a shift from survival to growth mode. In 2003 the ability to expand the public awareness initiatives was realized, thanks to a generous donation from Eileen Gingrich, a grateful patient.

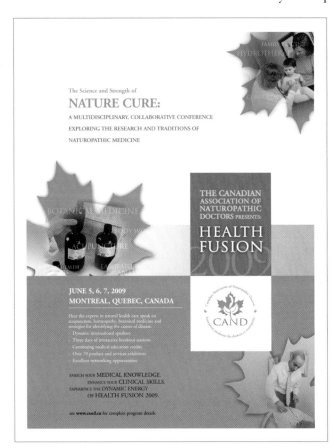

Improving the image of the national association started with the renaming of the association from the CNA to the CAND in 2004. This decision was made to more accurately reflect its aim of promoting naturopathic doctors as primary care providers and supporting the growth and development of naturopathic medicine. At the same time a logo was created to assist in the new branding of the CAND and to put a "professional face" to the profession. The bequest enabled the CAND to increase its promotional efforts: a national television campaign was created which has run for four consecutive years, the CAND website was professionally redone, CAND increased the marketing materials that were available to practitioners; and other forms of advertising, such as newspaper ads were initiated.

In 2005 the CAND decided to hold a national conference, the first one in over 15 years. The conference was called Health Fusion, to illustrate the aim of bringing together health professionals, from many different systems of medicine who were interested in natural healthcare. The conference was held in Alberta as that was where the CNA started. Health Fusion conferences continue to be held bi-annually.

For an updated listing of the CAND's mandate and current initiatives visit the website at www.cand.ca

CHAMPION:
DR. VERNA HUNT, DC ND
Written by Dr. Patricia Wales ND

VERNA WAS BORN IN BRANTFORD, ONTARIO in 1951 and was raised on a dairy farm in Troy. She always was very curious about nature and about human health, acquiring her first anatomy book in early childhood. She graduated from the University of Waterloo with a BSc Honors in Kinesiology in 1973 with an adjunctive specialty in dance and drama. Verna began her journey with natural medicines when she contracted mononucleosis during her time at Waterloo and realized that allopathic medicine did not have ways to promote healing.

Verna managed a dance and theatre company before entering the Canadian Memorial Chiropractic College (CMCC) in 1975, graduating in 1979. She was the first person with a kinesiology degree to attend CMCC and was one of only 12 women in a class of 150. Verna realized that, as much as she found chiropractic sciences a useful avenue to promote healing, she felt there had to be more. Upon graduating, she immediately broadened her scope with the Drugless Therapist license and began the three year accelerated program with the Ontario College of Naturopathic Medicine (OCNM), graduating in the second class in 1982.

From 1979–1994, Dr. Hunt had a solo practice at Yonge and Summerhill in Toronto. She then joined a new practice at the West End Holistic Health Centre and in 2005 opened the Centre for Health and Well

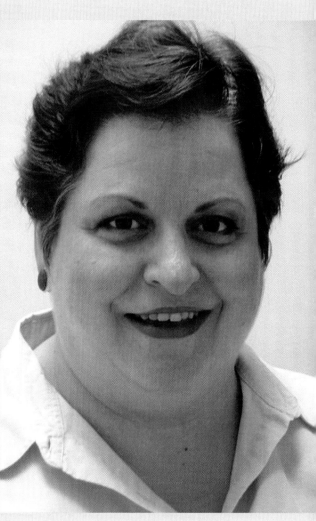

Being on Dundas St. W. in downtown Toronto. Throughout her practice and teaching to the public, students and professionals, she has been a pioneer in and proponent of Applied Kinesiology / Touch for Health, advanced physical modalities, practice management, healthy living, cleansing, proactive breast health, fertility, sound and colour therapy and many other topics of practical application.

From 1982-1996 she served on many boards and committees for the naturopathic profession at the college, provincial and national levels. Dr. Hunt was a key person involved in revitalizing the Ontario Naturopathic Association. She worked on many committees, served as Vice President and Secretary, and was awarded *Naturopathic Doctor of the Year*. During the 1980s and early 1990s, Dr. Hunt worked closely with Pat Wales ND and others in Ontario on resolving legal battles, maintaining regulation of the profession and the birthing of OCNM by contributing her time, extensive experience and finances to assure the continuation of the profession. In 1988 she and others were key in preserving the educational integrity of the OCNM, protecting it from those who would have decreased the credibility and the educational standards of the institution.

In the mid 90's she was the key player in restructuring the CNA (now CAND), moving the head office to Toronto and hiring full-time staff. Verna also served as a Board member and Vice Chair. In 1996 in recognition of her work and influence, the CNA established the Dr. Verna Hunt Award to be given to a Naturopathic Doctor who has made a significant contribution to the naturopathic association. Dr. Hunt was the first recipient.

Dr. Verna Hunt is an exceptional teacher and mentor, bringing an experiential focus and practical problem-solving to her work both as a clinician and as an ardent supporter of the naturopathic profession.

CHAMPION:
DR. PAUL SAUNDERS, PhD ND, DHANP
Interview by Shawn O'Reilly, written by Stuart Watson

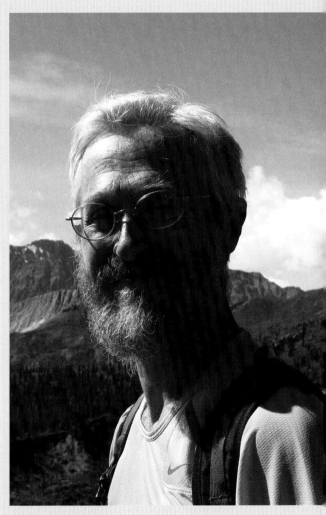

BORN IN INDIANAPOLIS INDIANA and raised not far away, in rural Kokomo, young Paul was an avid reader and spent plenty of time on his grandparent's farm where he enjoyed admiring and studying the local flora and fauna. He had, as a young man, aspirations in the medical and forestry fields. This in time brought him to Perdue University where he enrolled in their premedical course. Growing disillusioned with his original choice, Paul switched over to the forestry program in which he received his Bachelor's and Master's degrees.

It was shortly thereafter that Paul's number was called in the first Vietnam War draft lottery; his was lucky number sixty-six. A sense of self-preservation tied with the fact that a medical education was no longer applicable as a deferment for serving, Paul followed another field he was keenly interested in, philosophy. This saw him enrolled at Duke Divinity School. In his time spent at the seminary at Duke, he befriended a professor of botany who inspired him to leave the seminary and pursue his PhD in plant and forest ecology. During his PhD fieldwork he was employed as a teacher at Clemson University in 1977. In 1979 he received both his PhD and an assistant professorship at Washington State University (WSU). It was within his first year at WSU that Paul became an associate professor and was also granted tenure.

While at WSU, Paul was in charge of the recreation resource management program with their Department of Forestry and Range Management. This was a position involving a lot of travel and research in the field. It was during one of these research expeditions in the remote Wallowa Mountains of Oregon that he met his future wife Marilyn May. Shortly after this Paul found the time to make the trip to Portland to visit Marilyn at NCNM, at the same time he was introduced to naturopathic medicine. Recalling a thwarted education in medicine and realizing the correlation to his current field and expertise in plant life,

Paul started to research deeper into the naturopathic field.

Paul decided to apply to the three naturopathic colleges existing at that time. At OCNM Peter Cook and Tony Manolis interviewed Paul, and upon completion of the interview accepted him into the program. He began his new educational path at OCNM in August 1986.

As OCNM was not accredited at that time of Paul's graduation, he transferred his OCNM education to NCNM. He then embarked on completing all NCNM 3rd and 4th year course work, his clinic hours, a homeopathic residency shift one night a week under John Cullen who was teaching at Mayrl Mersis University, as well as being NCNM's interim research director. This amazing feat was accomplished in 9 months and Dr. Saunders graduated with his ND degree in 1991.

NCNM offered both Dr. Paul Saunders and Dr. Marilyn May positions. However, Dr. May was keen to return to Canada and they decided to return to set up a home base in Ontario. As luck would have it Dr. Saunder's old alma mater, OCNM, offered him a position as Clinic Director.

For the past 20 years Dr. Saunders has been heavily involved with the regulation and promotion of naturopathic medicine Canada wide and has been a major asset to the profession in those areas. He has championed the cause of naturopathic medicine before government hearing committees, participated in scientific review panels and expert advisory committees as well as appearing as an expert witness in court.

Dr. Saunders is a prolific researcher and writer with over 200 papers to his credit. He believes strongly in keeping pace with changes in medicine which motivates him to read as much as he does noting "we can't rest on what we learned yesterday, we must keep up."

The profession has recognized his commitment by presenting him with the OAND Naturopathic Doctor of the Year award twice, the Verna Hunt Award and the CAND Presidents Award. His students at CCNM have also expressed their gratitude by presenting him with the Instructor and Mentor of the Year Award. Dr. Saunders feels that promoting and supporting the profession is every ND's job and duty. In the good doctor's own words: "It's all for the patients and the profession."

Drs. Paul Saunders and Marilyn May own a farm and currently practice in their clinic located in Dundas, Ontario. Dr. Saunders continues his involvement with the naturopathic profession as a member of the CAND's Government Relations Committee; President of NPLEX, reviewer of grants for the Institute of Health Research and as Adjunct Professor at CCNM.

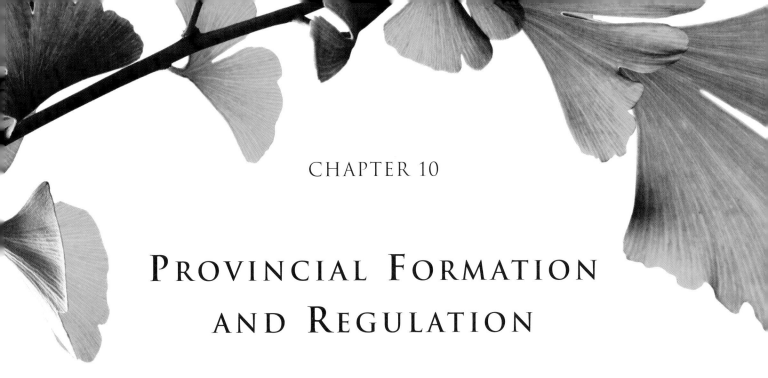

CHAPTER 10

PROVINCIAL FORMATION AND REGULATION

British Columbia

The following is a history prepared by Dr. Arthur William Dennis ND around 1940. Some sections have been shortened for the purpose of this book and subsequent entries have been added to bring the history up-to-date.

THE HISTORY OF NATUROPATHIC MEDICINE in Canada started primarily in British Columbia in the early 1900s when a handful of practitioners, graduates from various schools of healing in the United States, England and Europe, began their professional careers in natural healing. These dedicated men were rugged individualists and practical idealists who openly opposed the then-current doctrines of allopathic medicine.

In 1886, the practice of medicine and surgery became regulated in British Columbia under the Medical Act, creating a statutory monopoly of medicine by allopathic (and homeopathic) physicians. This marked the birth of the College of Physicians and Surgeons of British Columbia. As of this time, only allopathic (conventional) practitioners could be employed by any hospital or provincial public service.

This was the back-drop upon which these new naturopathic physicians decided to meet together for a common purpose, unite as an association and then work for social, political and legal recognition.

The first meeting of naturopathic doctors was held in March of 1920

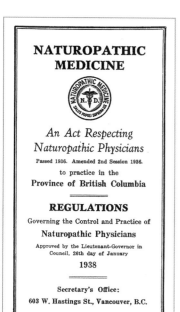

NATUROPATHIC MEDICINE

An Act Respecting Naturopathic Physicians

Passed 1936. Amended 2nd Session 1936.

to practice in the
Province of British Columbia

REGULATIONS

Governing the Control and Practice of
Naturopathic Physicians

Approved by the Lieutenant-Governor in
Council, 26th day of January
1938

Secretary's Office:
603 W. Hastings St., Vancouver, B.C.

and comprised such early practitioners as naturopathic doctors Lee Holder, James Perrin, Frank Dorchester, (Mr. and Mrs.) Moore, W. Castes, Arno Kruger, Everly Rogers, Marshall and Arthur Dennis. It was at this meeting that the decision was made to form an association which was called the Association of Naturopathic Physicians of British Columbia (ANPBC).

Initially the difficulties that the association faced were "stool pigeons" from the conventional medical associations that claimed that naturopathic physicians were practicing medicine without a license. In one such incident, one member, refusing to pay the fine, served a month in prison. These activities serviced the purpose of alerting the members of the need to stick together and to have a common voice.

In 1921 the first approach to the provincial legislature for legal recognition was made. The association presented petitions bearing 36,000 signatures and in a short time spent around $25,000 - which was a lot of money in the 1920s. The bill was defeated on second reading by one vote. In 1923 the B.C. Medical Association put a bill through the house to legalize naturopathic physicians under a committee of their naming, with only one appointee from the naturopathic group. So in 1923, naturopathic doctors and chiropractors in B.C. became regulated under the Medical Act.

The profession battled on through the years until 1936 when the Naturopathic Physicians Act became law in B.C. It was clear that the legislative intent was to enhance the social status of naturopathy as

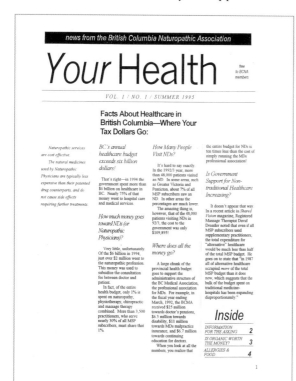

news from the British Columbia Naturopathic Association

Your Health

free to BCNA members

VOL. 1 / NO. 1 / SUMMER 1995

Facts About Healthcare in British Columbia—Where Your Tax Dollars Go:

Naturopathic services are cost effective.

The natural medicines used by Naturopathic Physicians are typically less expensive than their patented drug counterparts, and do not cause side effects requiring further treatments.

BC's annual healthcare budget exceeds six billion dollars!

That's right—in 1994 the government spent more than $6 billion on healthcare in BC. Nearly 75% of that money went to hospital care and medical services.

How much money goes toward NDs (or Naturopathic Physicians)?

Very little, unfortunately. Of the $6 billion in 1994, just over $2 million went to the naturopathic profession. This money was used to subsidize the consultation fee between doctor and patient.

In fact, of the entire health budget, only 1% is spent on naturopathy, physiotherapy, chiropractic and massage therapy combined. More than 3,500 practitioners, who serve nearly 30% of all MSP subscribers, must share that 1%

How Many People Visit NDs?

It's hard to say exactly. In the 1992/3 year, more than 48,000 patients visited an ND. In some areas, such as Greater Victoria and Penticton, about 7% of all MSP subscribers saw an ND. In other areas the percentages are much lower.

The amazing thing is, however, that of the 48,000 patients visiting NDs in 92/3, the cost to the government was only $109,895!

Where does all the money go?

A large chunk of the provincial health budget goes to support the administrative structure of the BC Medical Association, the professional association for MDs. For example, in the fiscal year ending March, 1992, the BCMA received $25 million towards doctor's pensions, $6.3 million towards disability, $11 million towards MDs malpractice insurance, and $6.7 million towards continuing education for doctors.

When you look at all the numbers, you realize that

the entire budget for NDs is ten times less than the cost of simply running the MDs professional association!

Is Government Support for Non-traditional Healthcare Increasing?

It doesn't appear that way. In a recent article in *Shared Vision* magazine, Registered Massage Therapist David Dressler noted that even if all MSP subscribers used supplementary practitioners, the total expenditure for "alternative" healthcare would be much less than half of the total MSP budget. He goes on to state that "in 1987 all of alternative healthcare occupied *more* of the total MSP budget than it does now, which suggests that the bulk of the budget spent on traditional medicine-hospitals has been expanding disproportionately."

Inside

1

a medical profession distinct from allopathy, homeopathy and osteopathy. In the Act, "Naturopathy" was defined broadly as "the art to healing by natural methods." The passing of this act, which was piloted through largely by the untiring efforts and skill of Dr. Arthur Paskins ND marks the end of the individual practitioner's struggle for professional existence. From that time, it became the responsibility of the association and its executives to continue to press for wider recognition by raising the professional standards of the professions, by lobbying for better legislation, and by establishing legal precedents through the courts.

Two of the early influential naturopathic doctors were Ron Holtum and Arthur Hilton. Dr. Holtum ND was exceptionally brilliant and had served on the B.C. board as chairman of education before becoming president. He was responsible for a tremendous amount of progress in B.C. Dr. Albert Russell ND who came into the profession later on, had considerable external contacts. He'd been vice-president of the Vancouver Junior Board of Trade, and had established many political contacts. Another key member was Dr. Douglas Kirkbride ND. He was a pharmacist, and his skills proved very helpful in getting the preparations straightened out. These three doctors worked on rebuilding the Act, making it more coherent, pushed to have it revised, and got a lot of amendments accepted. Dr. Kirkbride worked on the Act mainly in the areas of ethics while at the same time working toward bringing a feeling of fellowship amongst members. Another active member was Dr. Joseph

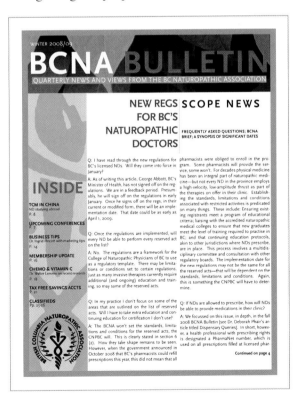

Boucher ND who contributed an enormous amount of time to the profession. Following the war, Dr. Boucher was instrumental in encouraging Dr. Robert (Bob) Fleming ND to enter the profession.

Dr. Boucher's sister was Ann Fleming, Dr. Fleming's wife. Although Ann was never a member, she dedicated herself to the profession and her administrative skills were invaluable.

The initial naturopathic doctors in B.C. were a close knit group. Annual meetings were like a family reunion and there was a real sense of unity and team work. The provincial and regulatory work was spearheaded by a few, but the profession was supported by the majority of its members. The initial struggles and challenges were instrumental in holding the professions together.

Educational Standards

High educational standards have been part of the B.C. Act since its inception in 1936. The initial legislation stated "a recognized school or college of naturopathic medicine shall be deemed to be an institution which teaches a residence course of not less then four calendar years of eight months in each year and not less than four thousand school hours in the four years." The initial colleges that were approved included: the National College in Chicago and the Western States College in Portland. The initial act also stated that all members must past board exams prior to be entitled to registration and to practice as a naturopathic physician within the province.

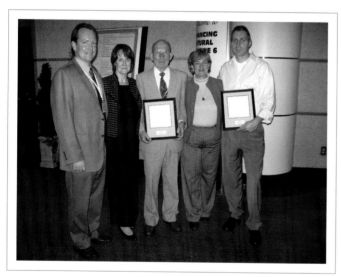

Dr. Christoph Kind ND, Shawn O'Reilly, Dr. Gerry Farnsworth ND, Dr. Iva Lloyd ND, and Glenn Cassie. At the BCNA 2006 convention Glenn Cassie, Executive Director of the BCNA was recipient of the 2006 Award of Appreciation for his years of hard work and dedication to the profession; Dr. Gerry Farnsworth ND was awarded the Verna Hunt award for his continual contribution to the CAND and the profession.

Amendments to the British Columbia Naturopathic Act

The original Act of 1936 contained a separate section covering physiotherapists and masseurs, who were regulated by the board of naturopathic physicians. This proved unsatisfactory to all groups and in 1947 the practitioners of physiotherapy and massage were placed under their own separate acts.

One of the provisions of the original Act was the inclusion of a board of supervision whose purpose was approving the schools. This board was comprised of three members: the provincial secretary, the dean of the Faculty of Arts of the University of B.C., and the registrar of the University. The original board proved very valuable and there was close co-operation between these three members and the board of naturopathic physicians.

In 1938 the regulations were changed to cover a more comprehensive examination schedule which included clinical and laboratory diagnosis, bacteriology, medical jurisprudence, dietetics and biochemistry, obstetrics and gynecology, endocrinology and remedial psychology. The schedule of the practice of naturopathic medicine was specified as including electrotherapy, light therapy (helio and photo), hydrotherapy, physiotherapy (mechanotherapy), orthopedics, phototherapy, anatomical manipulation, manipulative surgery and homeopathic materia medica.

Naturopaths Permitted to Treat Compensation Cases

Naturopathic physicians, for the first time in the 50-year history of their profession, will be allowed to treat injured workmen under the B.C. Workmen's Compensation Board Act.

Dr. Albert L. Russell, president of the B.C. Naturopathic Physicians' Association, said Thursday the WCB has granted the association parity with the medical doctor on all injured worker cases.

He said the new ruling will widen treatment available to WCB patients without conflicting in the field of medical physicians.

"The broadening of the act gives the workman advantage of all treatment fields, helping save man-hours, reduce cost of care and relieve pain," he said.

Dr. Russell, with Dr. R. M. Grant and Dr. R. A. Holtum, both of Victoria, has formed a committee that spent more than a year in negotiations with Adam Bell, WCB chairman.

All three were in Vancouver Thursday to address a special meeting of the NPA on the new WCB ruling.

They said there are 45 to 50 trained naturopathic physicians in B.C. The profession, 50 years old, was first recognized in B.C. in 1936.

Permission received from the Vancouver Sun December 1986

In 1948 the regulations were further amended to include increased educational requirements for entrance into a naturopathic college. During this time it also became mandatory for all members of the B.C. Association to take post-graduate studies each year, or to attend an educational symposium conducted by the B.C. board of governors, and submit proof of such attendances to qualify for membership in the association for the ensuing year. Also, stipulations respecting control of advertising by members of the profession were added to the regulations.

In 1958 the Act was amended to improve scope of practice and to enhance legal protection for the members. At that time, a legislative mandate for a schedule of preparations was established and in 1979 the *Naturopathic Materia Medica*, which outlined the range of products, herbs and supplements used by naturopathic physicians was updated. This document became a component of many government submissions. In 1984, the ANPBC prepared and presented a brief to the Caucus of the Government of B.C. The aim of this brief was to further educate the government on naturopathic medicine and to highlight the benefits that would be achieved it there was greater cooperation between the various health care disciplines.

In the mid 1990s, the B.C. government began work on revising its health care system. Two initiatives were started. The first being the Canada Health Protection Act (CHPA) and the other being the Health Professions Council (HPC). The goal of the CHPA was to consolidate out-dated and disparate acts representing health issues including tobacco regulations, wearing of hockey helmets, food and water regulations and, of special interest to naturopathic community, regulations with regards to natural health products.

The Health Professions Council (HPC) was devised to look at a number of different groups and determine if they required their own separate Acts and if so, what changes and revision were needed. The brief that the ANPBC submitted in 1995 included answers to over fifty questions. The main focus of the ANPBC was to address the issues of scope of practice with an emphasis on laboratory privileges, prescription rights, access to natural health products, referrals to specialists and enhancing the role of NDs within the provincial health care system. They could not visit or treat their patients in hospitals or other institutional settings – even if a patient specifically requested their care. They also did not have access to the diagnostics that they needed and had to send laboratory samples to Alberta or Washington State. These issues were addressed in all documentation to the government, members and to the public.

In 1995 the naturopathic profession was involved in consultations with the government concerning moving to the Health Professions Act, which was an umbrella Act that would regulate many different health professions under one Act. The members of the ANPBC and the BCNA were not in favor of such a move. Naturopathic physicians had been regulated under their own act for almost sixty years and in a letter written to the government it stated, "The BCNA is skeptical that there are tangible benefits for inclusion in the Act. We feel that inclusion under an umbrella Act is a slight on our individuality, uniqueness and historical right to self-regulation."

The work which began under the Health Profession's Council review process has continued for over 14 years, and is still ongoing. It has involved the dedicated efforts of many individuals including naturopathic physicians Eugene Pontius, Braven Rayne, David Wang, Christoph Kind, Brian Martin, Garrett Swetlikoff, Lorne Swetlikoff and others. Glenn Cassie, the Executive Director of the BCNA has been involved for over ten years. The BCNA and the ANPBC have hired public relations consultants, government affairs consultants, lobbyists, and have maintained a letter writing campaign for over ten years. There have been numerous meetings with government officials, letters, written submissions and attendance at government functions. The physicians in B.C. realized that no matter how dragged out the process and how much it monopolizes the focus of the ANPBC (now CNPBC) and the BCNA, they can never give up; both groups continue to ensure that they have a strong presence both publically and with the government.

In April of 2009 the B.C. Ministry of Health approved a new set of regulations which now recognizes naturopathic doctors as primary health-care providers. The new regulations bestow on naturopathic doctors, sweeping changes to their authority with respect to compounding, prescription authority, dispensing, ordering of laboratory and diagnostic services, and other priviledges.

Laboratory Access

Naturopathic physicians in B.C. had enjoyed access to provincial laboratory services since the early 1920s. Yet, in April of 1995 they started to receive letters from the provincial laboratories indicating that their access had been cancelled as a result of a ruling by the College of Physicians and Surgeons of British Columbia (CPSBC). The president of the BCNA, Dr. Eugene Pontius ND wrote to the health minister on many occasions requesting the reversal of the this restrictive and discriminatory practice. Eventually the issue was deferred to the HPC. Over the next several years, there were various writ-

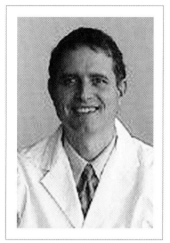

Dr. Lorne Swetlikoff ND

"The vision of once and for all aligning the ND's training and education with accurate and up to date regulations (that don't discriminate against our training) is at our doorstep here in British Columbia."

LORNE SWETLIKOFF ND, CHAIR CNPBC, JANUARY 2009

ten submissions, expert testimony, meetings, and phone calls with no resolution. Following the publication of the final HPC reports, the committee was disbanded and the issue was once again a government issue. In response to a request made by the deputy health minister a third party evaluation was completed and in 2004 a document titled, *The Naturopathic Scope of Practice Gap Analysis* was presented to the health ministry. This document addressed all facets of scope of practice, specifically re-affirming the integral nature of laboratory testing (and access) in respect to naturopathic medicine. As a result of the regulatory changes that occured in April of 2009 the door for laboratory access for naturopathic physicians in B.C. has been opened.

Medical Services Plan

Up until the 1950s, Canadians paid for all health care services out-of-pocket; consequently much health care was done at home. After the Great Depression there was increased demand for publicly funded health care. Saskatchewan was the first province to adopt a medical services program (MSP) (also known as medicare) in 1946, followed by British Columbia in 1965. A national medicare program was instituted across Canada in 1968. This meant that the provincial programs currently in place would now receive assistance from the federal government. As medicare was implemented, the

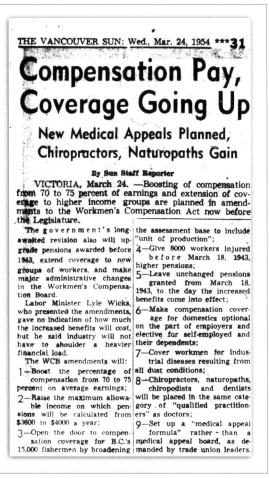

Permission received from the Vancouver Sun March 24, 1954

expectation became that all medical services in Canada would be covered.

For years the provincial and national associations, especially in the West, spent most of their energy and focus on having naturopathic services included under medicare. The results were mixed. Some provinces such as British Columbia had limited success, others not at all. At no time did any provincial government allow for full inclusion of naturopathic services under medicare and over time, the profession realized that inclusion would be detrimental as the compensation and restrictions were out-of-synch with the time-intensive, patient-focused premise of naturopathic medicine. By 1990, only B.C. maintained any MSP coverage. However, the patient visit fees were increased incrementally while government subsidies decreased. Most NDs opted-out of the plan entirely. By 2002, MSP subsidies were modified to include only certain individuals, such as those that were on premium assistance, refugees, and individuals with eligible First Nations status registered with Health Canada.

CHAMPION:
DR. GERALD ROSS FARNSWORTH (GERRY), DC ND
Written by Dr. Ronald Grant ND and Dr. Kelly Farnsworth ND

GERALD ROSS FARNSWORTH WAS BORN in Moosejaw, Saskatchewan on January 24th, 1928. He is the youngest member of a family of one sister and two brothers. At an early age he gave promise of his ingenious, competent, enterprising and proficient manner which would become the trademark of his life. As a young man the "great outdoors" presented a tremendous attraction to which he responded by becoming an ardent and well-rounded sportsman – fishing, hunting and horseback riding over range and hill.

Gerry graduated from the Canadian Memorial Chiropractic College and pursued post graduate training at National College in Chicago and subsequently at the Page Foundation of Antropometric Medicine in Florida. He moved to Kamloops, B.C. in 1950 and began practice as a naturopathic physician and coupled an enquiring mind with abundant physical and mental energy. He obtained his pilot's license shortly thereafter enabling him to explore the wide open spaces and providing him with transportation to attend many professional functions.

Dr. Farnsworth soon became an active and enthusiastic member of the ANPBC serving on the board twenty-seven consecutive years commencing in 1952. He was also a founding member of the National College of Naturopathic Medicine (NCNM) serving on its Board from 1956 to 1979, principally as Chairman. While this statement is easy to read, his involvement in the early days with NCNM meant a 40 hour return drive each month on the roads of that time, to and from Kamloops, B.C. to Portland, Oregon. And he was seldom, if ever, late for his meetings. This often meant driving all night. He also served on the

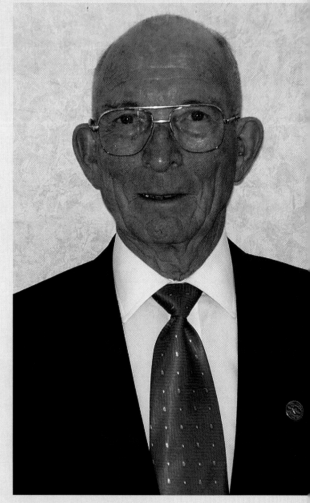

Board of the John Bastyr College of Naturopathic Medicine for five years and is Trustee Emeritus of that College. He is a Charter and Lifetime member of the Canadian Association of Naturopathic Doctors serving in almost all executive positions. Dr. Gerry Farnsworth has also been honoured by his profession by being given Lifetime memberships in both the British Columbia Naturopathic Association and the College of Naturopathic Physicians of B.C.

The Canadian Naturopathic Foundation (CNF) owes its continued existence to Dr. Farnsworth's unrelenting commitment. The Society nearly failed due to lack of funding in recent years. Its continued existence and current revitalization owes its success to the almost single-handed fund-raising efforts of Dr. Farnsworth. He has nurtured the growth of the CNF and overseen its transition under the CAND umbrella.

One of his on-going passions has been the North West Naturopathic Physicians Convention (NWNPC) of which he is a founding member. The NWNPC just recently saw its 53rd consecutive Convention take place in Seattle W.A. Dr. Farnsworth has sat on its Board, directing naturopathic education and camaraderie, continuously since 1957.

Dr. Gerry Farnsworth has been blessed with family and support. He fathered five children and had a loving relation with his wife, Penny, who recently passed away. His brother, Dr. Early Farnsworth DC, ND was his partner in practice and one of Gerry's closest friends. His son, Dr. Todd Farnsworth ND followed his father into the profession. As a tribute to his father, Dr. Todd Farnsworth now chairs the North West Naturopathic Physicians Convention.

In recent years, Dr. Gerry Farnsworth authored a history of the Naturopathic Physicians Convention and he has completed a comprehensive history of the naturopathic profession BC from the 1950s to the present.

According to his colleagues and his many friends both in Canada and the United States, Dr. Farnsworth has given of himself far beyond the call of duty. He has and still is, after almost sixty years, tirelessly and selflessly serving his profession ignoring the time and dollars which his work demanded. To sum up, Dr. Gerry Farnsworth has been and continues to be dedicated and committed to his profession – a true champion of naturopathic medicine.

CHAMPION:
DR. ALLEN N. TYLER, MD, DC, PhD, ND
Written by: Dr. Ted Sleigh ND

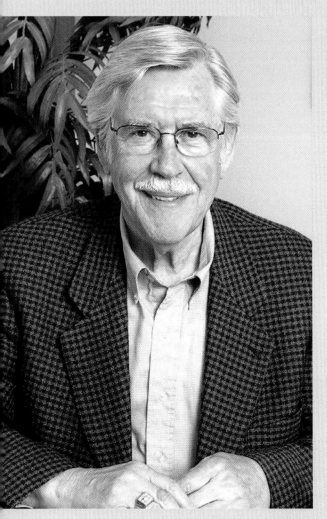

THE HISTORY OF NATUROPATHIC MEDICINE in British Columbia would be incomplete without including the contributions of Dr. Allen Tyler ND. He has been a tremendous influence in the field of naturopathic medicine in administrative, political, educational, research and commercial capacities.

But first, a little bit about his background. Dr. Tyler received his MD degree from Universidad Libre Americana in Mexico City in 1943. Then, while serving in World War II as a paratrooper he was impressed how effectively a chiropractor treated the soldiers' backs. This inspired him, after the war, to attend Canadian Memorial Chiropractic College in Toronto from 1945-1949; he graduated with his chiropractic degree (DC) in 1949. During 1946-1949 he was also studying naturopathic medicine at Philadelphia College of Naturopathic Medicine from which he graduated in 1949 with his naturopathic degree (ND). Dr. Tyler practiced as a chiropractor in Ontario from 1945-1965, then moved to British Columbia in 1965 where he continued to practice in Victoria, B.C..

Later he was accepted into medical school at the University of Washington in Seattle and he moved to the United States, where from 1971 through 1974 he completed his master of science degree in physical medicine and rehabilitation. He worked as a hospital resident at the University Hospital and ultimately became Chief Resident. In 1976 he moved back to British Columbia where he began his practice of naturopathic medicine in Langley. He worked in this community until his retirement in 2002.

Upon his return to B.C. in 1976 he became politically involved and active in the administration and regulation of the provincial naturopathic association. Almost immediately he was elected President of the Board of the ANPBC, (now known as the CNPBC) and subsequently continued to serve the profession in various capacities including the ANPBC for a number of years.

Dr. Tyler has been generous with sharing his skills and talents; these included helping new ND graduates get established by providing opportunities to work in his busy private practice. Over the years, one at a time, he helped many become successful naturopathic doctors including myself as well as Drs. Brian Vallee, Timothy Taneda-Brown, and his own son, Scott Tyler, also a naturopathic physician in Langley. I recall from working with him for six years that Allen Tyler was an excellent clinician, brilliant diagnostician, astute businessman and extremely knowledgeable in many types of therapies. Patients and colleagues alike admired and respected these qualities.

Dr. Tyler also shared his knowledge and professional experience with students at the Canadian College of Naturopathic Medicine by commuting from British Columbia to Ontario to teach in the school's early years. Always thirsty for knowledge, Dr. Tyler continued his own personal quest in education and research. He earned a PhD in 1983 from West London University, England. His research and interest centered on the neurological evaluation of patients with various diseases.

Dr. Tyler was pleased to lecture periodically at the naturopathic college in Toronto and flew out there for a few days at a time. On one of these occasions he was told that the then dean of the college—Dr. Sandy Wood ND —one of the leading professionals in naturopathic medicine, was hospitalized at the Toronto General Hospital in a comatose condition. As he had had a lot of training in this field, he felt that he should go in and see him. Dr. Wood was held in isolation, when Dr. Tyler walked in, touched his forehead and spoke his name much to his surprise, Dr. Wood opened his eyes and smiled. After a few days Dr. Wood was released from the hospital and he laughingly stated that he knew he was not in heaven because Tyler was standing there looking down at him.

In the commercial arena Dr. Tyler has also been a pioneer and an innovator. He was the first Canadian distributor of Nutridyn and Seroyal nutritional products, then he co-founded Thorne Research, and subsequently founded his own nutritional supplement company, A.N. Tyler Distributing in 2000.

Throughout his career Dr. Tyler has been a faithful, constant supporter of the naturopathic profession. He has invested extensive amounts of time, sharing his talents with his colleagues, and has been a generous financial contributor to the profession. For these reasons the profession is indebted to Dr. Allen Tyler for his dedication, contribution, influence and commitment to the advancement of naturopathic medicine in both British Columbia and Canada.

Alberta

Alberta has always been a hub for naturopathic activity in Canada and for many initiatives it has been on lead. It was instrumental in supporting and growing the profession and it has encountered and overcome many obstacles. Alberta is the home of the first naturopathic convention in Canada, it spear-headed the initiative to create a national organization and it is also the only province that had to regain its naturopathic regulation.

Regulation and Amendments

Alberta was the home of many naturopathic doctors in the early 1900s, but from 1935 to 1942 there were only a handful still practicing. These doctors, many of them men who had served in the war and were prepared to fight for what they wanted, spent much of their time ensuring that naturopathic medicine became a recognized profession. In 1945 The Naturopathic Association of Alberta under the 'Societies Act'. In 1948 legislation for naturopathic medicine was acquired under the "Drugless Practitioners Act". The original register lists naturopathic doctors Fred E Parson, Ross Skaken, Ruth E. Budd, Lambert Kenneth Grube, John Edward Davies, Abram John Penner, Gordan Biswanger and Colin Skaken as members. The initial Act covered naturopaths, masseurs and physiotherapists. Similar to other provinces, this did not serve any profession well and in 1950 the act was replaced with the "Naturopathy Act" and only included naturopathic doctors. At the same time the association was renamed and incorporated as the Alberta Association of Naturopathic Practitioners (AANP). The association had the dual responsibility of a provincial association and a regulatory board.

Supplied by Queen's Printer Edmonton — Price 25c

GOVERNMENT OF THE PROVINCE OF ALBERTA

THE NATUROPATHY ACT

with amendments up to and including 1955

OFFICE CONSOLIDATION

DEPARTMENT OF PROVINCIAL SECRETARY

Membership in the profession fluctuated through the 1950s and 1960s with as little as 16 members to as many as 36. Part of the fluctuation was because many of the older practitioners had dual licenses as both a naturopathic and chiropractic practitioner. When the chiropractic colleges dropped their naturopathic programs the number of licensed naturopathic doctors in Alberta decreased substantially. During these years the Alberta government left naturopathic doctors virtually alone to practice within their "Scope of Practice" as taught in the schools of naturopathic medicine at that time.

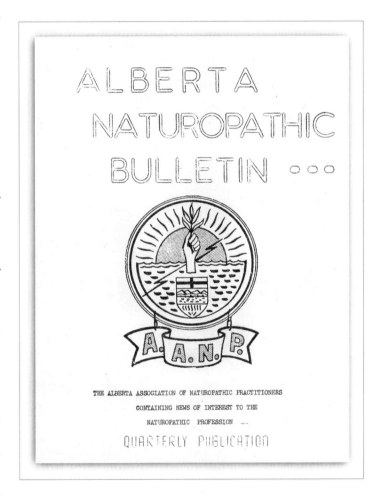

In 1949 Dr. Ross Skaken ND, chair of the Alberta association, spear-headed the initiative to form a national organization. Over the next six years much of the efforts and resources in Alberta were spent on ensuring that this happened, for the first thirty some years the office of the Canadian Naturopathic Association (CNA) was located in Alberta and many of the Alberta practitioners were instrumental in ensuring that both their provincial association and the national association survived.

It wasn't until the early seventies that naturopathic medicine started to gain attention and resurgence especially from the younger people in Alberta. The Naturopathy Act was revised and updated in 1980. Soon after, the Legislative Assembly of Alberta passed the Health Occupations Act which was intended to provide a means of regulating a variety of health occupations and it provided for the establishment of the Alberta Health Occupations Board. One of the major functions of the Board was to conduct investigations to determine which health occupations should be regulated. Naturopathic medicine in Alberta was one of the professions that was slated to be deregulated. To assist with this threat, the association sought the help of Majorie Zingle, who was the current Executive Director of the Canadian Naturopathic Association.

During this time, there were about ten naturopathic doctors in the province, but only two were members of the provincial association - Dr. Ross Skaken ND, and Dr. Jutte Roy-Poulsen ND. As tension, fear and panic manifested, the association members and Majorie worked hard to keep the Association alive and to increase the membership of the Association. Finally, after much time passed, the government stated they did not know where to place naturopaths in this new act. Adding to the challenges at that time was the unfortunate death of a child, who was under the care of a naturopathic doctor in Alberta.

In 1984, the Alberta association received notice from the government that their act was to be rescinded. The government put an advertisement in the paper requesting that the public and patients write to the government indicating why they chose naturopathic health care, and asked for their viewpoint. It was stated that the Naturopathy Act was being repealed because it did not adhere to the standards for professional legislation and it contained a very broad definition of the scope of practice of naturopaths that had proved to be almost unmanageable to enforce and investigate. In 1986, Alberta became the first province to have its regulation repealed.

Members of the AANP including naturopathic doctors: Ross Skaken, Sinnoi Skaken, Robert Pearman, Pat Wales, Karen Jensen, Raj Rahkra, Michael Nowazek worked throughout the late 1980s and 90's to reestablish relationships with the government and to insist that naturopathic medicine be regulated in the province. Dr. Dan Labriola ND from the Washington Association of Naturopathic Physicians also participated in some of the meetings. At the time, the Alberta government was establishing the Health Professions Act (HPA) and there was talk that naturopathic doctors would be included. Finally in 1999, after many government meetings, the AANP were notified that they would be regulated under the new: "Health Professions Act". Regulation would not come into force until regulations were written and approved, a process that was delayed due to a change in Health Ministers. The regulations were finally approved in 2009.

As part of the work with the government, specifically with the Alberta Health and Wellness department, the development of a competency document - a system of assessing, sustaining and overseeing the ongoing competencies of the profession to ensure excellence of expertise, aptitudes and ethics.- was undertaken. The writing of this document involved 16 Alberta naturopathic doctors representing all aspects of the profession meeting without textbooks or written material at hand, and outlining step-by-step what the practice of naturopathic medicine entails and how naturopathic doctors are educated and trained to practice competently. While the project was anticipated to take about six months, Alberta's NDs accomplished the task ahead of schedule, indicating the coherence and co-operation within the profession. The result was the 122 page *Continuing Competence Profile* that is probably the most comprehensive look at the naturopathic skill set that has ever been compiled in North America. Dr. Mike Nowazek ND, who was the chair of the AANP at the time, was instrumental in this effort. The intention is that this profile will serve as a template for all other provinces in the future. The process also produced a state-of-the-art computerized program and website to assess and track continuing competence activities of naturopathic doctors in Alberta.

The Alberta Association of Naturopathic Doctors also produced a 300 page document *Monographs of Products Prescribed by Doctors of Naturopathic Medicine* that provides comprehensive information on Schedule I and II substances for naturopathic doctors.

"Unless we give freely – our time, our efforts, our pleasures for the sake of helping someone with a view of no reward we shall never partake of the glory and graces that the medical professional possesses."

LAWRENCE F. SCHNELL, ND

CHAMPIONS:
FOUR GENERATIONS OF SKAKEN'S
As told by Dr. Sinnoi Skaken ND

THE FOUR GENERATIONS OF SKAKEN doctors started with Colin Skaken's mother who had a special gift of healing and ultimately became a doctor and teacher in spite of many hardships. That gift was passed to her son, Colin Skaken (birth name: Dimitri M. Skakun) and then to his son Ross Skaken and daughter Luci Skaken. Ross' son Sinnoi continued the family tradition.

This is Dr. Sinnoi Skaken's story. After being a prisoner of war in the World War II in Germany, and serving with the International Red Cross in Switzerland after the war, my father, Ross Skaken, returned to Alberta in 1948 to join his father, Colin Skaken ND and other members who were working on the legislative steps needed to ensure that naturopathic medicine was regulated in the province of Alberta.

My father, Ross had received his degrees from Southern California College of Naturopathic Physicians and Surgeons in Los Angeles, California in 1947. He then returned to Alberta and quickly became active in the profession. In 1949 he was one of the organizing members for the CNA and was one of the select few who helped to keep it alive when the number of Canadian naturopathic physicians reached an all-time low.

In the 1960's, naturopathic medicine was witnessing a "changing of the guard" as practitioners from the pre-antibiotic days retired and many schools and associations fell into low membership. During this period, many members, like my father and grandfather continued to be active in provincial, national and international naturopathic associations, often in executive positions. My dad served on executive positions with the following organizations: Alberta Naturopathic Association, Alberta Association of Naturopathic Practitioners, Canadian Naturopathic Association and International Society of Naturopathic Physicians. As a younger man, I remember my grandfather, Colin, coming to Calgary for association meetings. I did not see my grandfather very much, so I took every advantage to go with my mother to pick up my father and grandfather from council meetings.

At a young age of 13, I started working at my father's clinic after school as a shipping and receiving clerk as my father had patients from all over Eastern and Western Canada. After seeing my dad help and heal so many people, young and old, I knew this was the kind of medicine I wanted to practice. Education of new physicians was a primary focus of my dad and he provided financial support and was a devoted instructor at three of the naturopathic colleges in North America. Fortunately for the profession my dad had a deep appreciation for the historical importance of the profession in Canada and maintained a basement full of files and reference material.

In 1984, I started at National College of Naturopathic Medicine. During my 2nd year, I received a disturbing phone call from my father. He had told me that the new government intended to put all the Health Care Acts under one "Umbrella Act" to better be able to police the Heath Care Professions. This new act was initially called the "Health Occupations Act" and later named the "Health Professions Act". I remembering asking what this meant for the Alberta Association. Dad did not know, and like others he was waiting to see what happened over the next few months as this new act was explored in more depth. Seeing as this would have a major impact on myself and many other graduates, I went to every council and board meeting I could. I remember many discussions with members like Roger McHan ND, Carl Peterson ND, my father and Marjorie Zingle as to the new regulations and how to proceed with them. Upon graduation, my dad said, "Now I pass the torch to you." I was up to the job as I wanted naturopathic medicine to succeed in Alberta.

Through the 80's and early 90's, board members and Government Health Ministers changed, it was always a "new playing field". In the mid 1990's naturopathic doctors Pat Wales, Karen Jensen, Robert Pearman and Raj Rahkra continued to put in countless hours preparing and attending meetings with bureaucrats. I remember many times taking a day off from my busy practice to board the Air Bus for Edmonton to meet with bureaucrats over association politics and to negotiate new regulations.

In conclusion, it was a pleasure to follow in the footsteps of my father Ross, Grandfather Colin, and many other senior members who committed themselves and work endlessly to ensure that the profession was regulated in Alberta.

CHAMPION:
DR. MICHAEL NOWAZEK ND
Written by Dr. Mona Zarei ND

BORN AND RAISED IN BRANDON, Manitoba, Michael Nowazek originally set out to follow in his father's footsteps and study dentistry. As a reservist of the Canadian Forces Maritime Command (the Canadian Navy) he was able to study part time and earn a Bachelor of Science with a chemistry major and a mathematics minor. The late 80s marked the end of the Cold War and downsizing of the fleet which enabled Michael's discharge from service.

Like many doctors, Michael was introduced to naturopathic medicine when conventional medicine was unable to provide viable solutions to personal health issues. As an avid athlete, he suffered a serious knee injury during martial arts training. Medical doctors and surgeons outlined a poor prognosis – surgery was required and he would never again walk properly. Michael accepted his mother's suggestion and consulted a naturopathic doctor. Despite being the ultimate skeptic, he followed the treatments which included acupuncture, diet and nutrition. Within a short span he was able to walk again and before long regained the ability to pursue his martial arts training. Encouraged by his experience, he began to investigate naturopathic medicine and was soon inspired by the work of Dr. Linus Pauling on vitamin C therapy. With a newly inspired focus, he pursued an education at the Canadian College of Naturopathic Medicine in Toronto and graduated in 1997.

That same year Dr. Nowazek relocated to Edmonton, Alberta to begin his naturopathic career. Three years after establishing a full-time practice, he became the president of the Alberta Association of Naturopathic Practitioners (AANP). Undaunted by the massive learning curve, Dr. Nowazek sacrificed many aspects of his private practice and family life,

to attend biweekly government meetings, confer with lawyers and consult fellow naturopathic doctors.

Dr. Michael Nowazek spent years dedicated to building relationships with other health
professions and enriching the awareness and appreciation of naturopathic medicine in
Alberta. During this time he maintained a full time private practice.

The perception of naturopathic medicine in Alberta has undergone a staggering evolution. A profession that was once erroneously regarded as no more than "hippies handing out
herbs" has gained a new level of awareness and understanding in the community — health care
professionals now understand that naturopathic doctors are highly trained physicians with
unique points of view; the government envisions naturopathic medicine as worthwhile part
of the health care solution; and the public has come to notice that naturopathic medicine is
a real and valuable health care alternative.

Saskatchewan

Saskatchewan first received regulation under the Drugless Practitioner's Act in 1948. This act regulated the practice of naturopaths, physiotherapists and masseurs. In 1952 the naturopathic doctors wanted to break away from the physiotherapists and masseurs and requested a separate act which they received - *The Naturopathic Act*. At this time the Saskatchewan Association of Naturopathic Physicians (SANP) was formed as both the member association and the regulatory body. The initial members of the association included Lambert K. Grube, Bernard R. Hansen, and Vernon B. Norman. It is of interest that in 1955 the Act was amended to change the definition of Naturopathy and to create the Naturopathy Appraisal Board.

In the initial regulations it was stated that Saskatchewan would only license naturopathic physicians who had taken basic science examinations set by the medical faculty of the University of Saskatchewan. These examinations included anatomy, physiology, chemistry, pathology, histology, sanitation and hygiene, general diagnosis and the principles and practices of naturopathy.

Bill (William) McGill, a Doctor of Osteopathy who was

Naturopaths ask for participation

Saskatchewan naturopathic physicians have asked that their services be included in the proposed government medical care plan.

In a submission presented Thursday to the Thompson committee on medical care in Regina, the Saskatchewan Association of Naturopathic Physicians said the public has an inherent right to choose any qualified practitioner or physician at any time it wishes to do so.

Patients of naturopathic physicians will be contributing to the provincial health scheme, the submission said. Therefore, where a choice of a naturopathic physician is made, it should be respected by the government and its agencies and maximum assistance accorded both patient and physician to see full and adequate treatment is given.

The presence of the naturopathic physician in the community assures an additional facility. The more facilities for treatment the people of the province can obtain, the greater will be the force promoting the health and well-being of its citizens.

The naturopathic physician does not limit himself to any one treatment, but employs in his services the use of botanical medicines, vitamins, minerals, hormones and a variety of other medications which are beneficial to mankind, but have a low, if not complete absence of toxicity, the submission said. He also utilizes physiotherapy and pays special attention to body mechanics such as manipulation of all the articulations of the human body including the spine in treating human ills.

Many conditions treated by the naturopathic physician are also attended to by other professions which will be under the medical scheme and many of his patients are now covered by private sickness and accident insurance companies, it said. If the government scheme does not cover his services it will mean such a drastic cut in his income that he will not be able to stay in practice, as patients will no longer buy private insurance from which the naturopathic physicians can collect their fees.

Present naturopathic services are rendered in connection with the Workmen's Compensation Board, sickness and accident insurance claimants, life insurance company examinations and sports organizations, the submission said. Barring the naturopathic physician from the proposed medical scheme would mean the citizens of the province would not have the opportunity to obtain the full health coverage they desire.

In 1954 the legislature enacted the Naturopathic Act which accorded to naturopathic physicians the right to practice in the province, it said. Since then, an increasing number of citizens have learned of the techniques and objectives of the profession and many have benefitted from the skills and services of members of the association.

Permission received from Regina Lender Post. January 26th, 1961.

living in Saskatchewan, was extremely interested and passionate about naturopathic medicine. He was known to have a "colorful" character by a few of the naturopathic doctors that had met him. In many ways he encouraged and guided the new practitioners that came to the province. He is credited for keeping the naturopathic profession alive in Saskatchewan in the 1980s when there were few practitioners in the province. He is also one of the few, if not the only, person to serve as chair of a provincial association who was not a naturopathic doctor.

Dr Peter Gleisburg ND had obtained his training in naturopathic medicine in Germany in 1977 and moved to Saskatchewan around 1983. He set up practice in the town of Battleford. For years he was unaware of other naturopathic doctors in the province or the fact that he had to be a member of the association, a fact which he rectified in 1988.

Dr Norman Wallace ND was the first member of the SANP to write the Naturopathic Physicians Licensing Examinations (NPLEX) and the first SANP member of the Canadian Naturopathic Association (CNA). He was active in fostering the connection of the SANP with other provincial and national associations.

Naturopathic physicians in Saskatchewan have enjoyed continuous regulation for over sixty years and as of 2008 steps are being taken to update the act and to create a separate regulatory body and member association.

Manitoba

Due to the efforts of naturopathic doctors J.B. and Sam Gladstone, Manitoba received its *Naturopathic Act* in 1946. This act defined the practice of Naturopathy as "a drugless system of therapy that treats human injuries, ailments, or diseases, by natural methods, including any one or more of the physical, mechanical or material, forces or agencies of nature, and employs as auxiliaries for such purposes the use of electro-therapy, hydrotherapy, body manipulations, or dietetics."

The Manitoba Naturopathic Association (MNA) was also established in 1946 and it has acted as both the provincial association and the regulatory board. The Act stipulated that the board was to be comprised of five members three professional and two public. The initial responsibility for administering the Act rested with Dr. Fred Ripley ND (President), Frauk M. Gibbs (Secretary), Dr. J. B. Gladstone ND, Henry Hall (Registrar) and Dr. A. Yaremovitch ND.

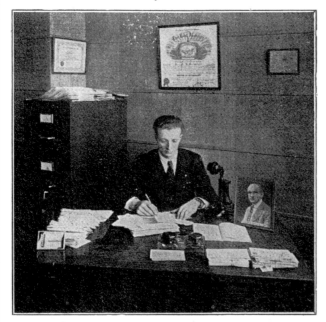

LETTERS

In Praise of the "Handy Home Doctor"

Photo (taken in 1936) of editor J. B. Gladstone at work on the third edition of the "HANDY HOME DOCTOR." The 1957 edition, judging from readers' letters, is the best edition in the past 22 years.

LETTERS ... LETTERS ... AND STILL MORE LETTERS FROM EVERY PROVINCE IN CANADA poured into our office in large numbers during February and March, while advertisements for the "Handy Home Doctor" issue of our Digest were appearing in every leading daily newspaper and weeklies across the country. That special advertising campaign ended on March 30th.

Of course, we still get a lot of mail each day.

Every mail brings many letters containing orders for food supplements and multi-herbal formulas . . . letters asking for answers to

For many years in the 1970s and 1980s the profession in Manitoba was supported by only a few members – naturopathic doctors George Kroeker, Royce Baker, Bert Grube, Frank Amsden and Joseph Bzowy. In 1986 Dr. Chris Turner ND arrived and quickly became active in the association and in the initial formation and implementation of NPLEX in Canada. Later that year, Dr. Grube ND passed away suddenly leaving only two practicing members. On several occasions, Dr. Turner ND and Dr. Kroeker ND were notified unofficially that naturopathic medicine may become slated to be deregulated due to the low number of practitioners. These practitioners continuously worked to ensure that the regulation remained intact.

In the early 1990s a law was passed in Manitoba that stated that all existing acts had to be written in French as well as English. The Manitoba Act was translated but the new French translation did not appear in the Gazette and hence it did

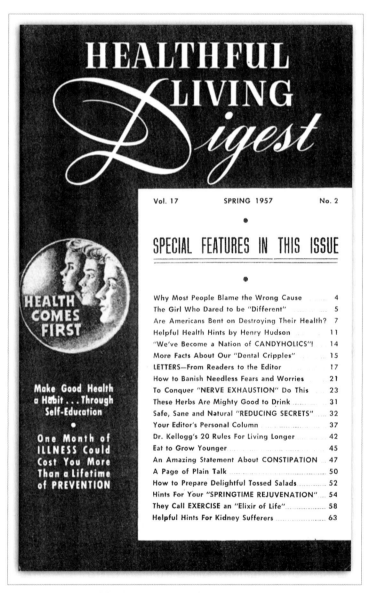

Healthful Living Digest from 1935 to ~1960.

not make it into law. After consultation with a lawyer and other advisors it was decided, due to the few number of members, not to publish the translation as doing so meant that the Act would be opened and hence it might be at risk. In 2008 this situation again came to the attention of the association, it has once again been translated and is slated to appear in the Gazette in 2009.

After a period of many years, new members gradually started to move to Manitoba. In 2008 there were nineteen members in the Manitoba Naturopathic Association. Although the number of practitioners in Manitoba has been small, the members have been active in the development of the profession.

CHAMPION:
DR. CHRISTOPHER TURNER ND
Written by Dr. Iva Lloyd ND

CHRISTOPHER (CHRIS) TURNER WAS BORN in Winnipeg and other than attending private school and College in British Columbia, he spent most of his life in his home town.

He was interested in chiropractic medicine as a result of an illness that his dad had and spent a couple of years at the Chiropractic college in Toronto, but returned home and ran an apiculture (beekeeping) and orchard business for a number of years.

In 1983, still interested in healing and health care, he enrolled at National College of Naturopathic Medicine in Portland, Oregon. After graduation in 1986 he returned to Winnipeg at the request of his ailing grandmother. At the time, his grandmother was terminally ill and had decided to forgo conventional medical treatment. She was sent home, yet home-care was not offered in those days. For a number of months Chris cared for his grandmother and when her health was still critical, but stable, he decided, at her request, to start his practice. Two days after he made an offer on a building she passed away — having achieved her wish of seeing her grandson established in practice.

When Dr. Turner returned to Manitoba there were only three practicing naturopathic doctors — Bert Grube, George Kroeker and Frank Amsden - all over the age of seventy-five. He was informed that he was the first "new blood" in over thirty years. In the 1980s naturopathic medicine was not well known in Manitoba and one of the concerns was that the regulation required at least five board members. He recognized that if Manitoba was to retain its regulation he would have to take the lead in legislative and provincial issues.

Dr. Turner set up a private practice and started offering lectures for the College of Physicians and Surgeons and for the community at large. Over time he developed a relationship with the medical community and with the government. He also flew to different schools and associations to teach. He had strong opinions and an equally strong dedication to the profession. He served on the Manitoba board for over 15 years and also served on the CNA and NPLEX board. The year that he graduated was the first year of NPLEX exams and Chris, after experiencing the difficulty in flying to the different jurisdictions to write all the exams, was instrumental in centralizing and implementing the NPLEX exam process in Canada and in the creation of NABNE. Over the years he has financially supported the CNA, American Association of Naturopathic Practitioners and the MNA and is a founders member of all three. One of his primary initiatives while on the MNA board was to recruit new practitioners to the province, which he did.

In 1995 Dr. Turner married Darlene Schmidtke and has two step daughters and four grandchildren. Despite his busy professional life, he finds time for wood-working and has built a timber-frame cabin which he intends to live in part-time when he retires. He also skis and stays involved in various community groups.

Dr. Turner believes strongly in the eclectic nature of naturopathic medicine. In his practice he uses all naturopathic therapies and continues to expand his skills all the time. He embraces the holistic nature of naturopathic medicine and believes in the value of a practitioner integrating physical treatments, psychological therapies and treatments that address functional concerns. Dr. Turner practices according to the principles of naturopathic medicine and he uses diet, detoxification and tonification as the fundamental basis of his treatments. He has never advertised and to this day still does not have a sign on the outside of his office. His practice has grown by word-of-mouth and he is well-known for his work with patients that have cancer and AIDS. He also provides naturopathic services, primarily volunteer, to the First Nations community.

Dr. Christopher Turner has dedicated years to the profession and has financially supported its growth. But more importantly, he has maintained the focus and intention of the founders of naturopathic medicine and has assisted it in acquiring the professionalism, stability and recognition that it sought.

Ontario

Ontario practitioners were the first naturopathic doctors regulated in Canada, they were responsible for the development of the first naturopathic school in Canada, and they spear-headed one of the largest letter writing campaign in naturopathic history. Between the 1950s and the 1980s, the practice of naturopathic medicine in Ontario was fraught with identity crises and continual battles with the government with regards to regulatory status.

The early start of naturopathic medicine in Ontario was closely tied to that of chiropractic. Most of the early naturopathic physicians graduated from the Canadian Memorial Chiropractic College (CMCC) which was located in Toronto. After graduation from CMCC, practitioners could take additional courses and then write Drugless Therapy (DT) exams – naturopathic doctors in Ontario were initially referred to as DTs. In 1953 there were 309 Ontario naturopathic doctors and about 85% of these held dual licensure as chiropractors and drugless therapists. In the 1960's, as the chiropractic profession stressed the need for chiropractors to follow the 'straight' model of practice, the number of naturopathic doctors dropped dramatically. In 1977 when CMCC ended the naturopathic component of its program the door was opened for the Ontario Naturopathic Association (ONA) to start a school in Ontario dedicated to naturopathic medicine.

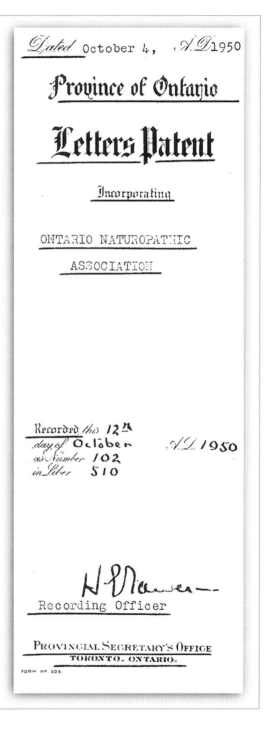

Although regulation of naturopathic doctors in Ontario started in 1925, it wasn't until 1950 that the Ontario Naturopathic Association (ONA) and a separate regulatory board were formed. Six of the eight founding members of the ONA also held a chiropractic license and while the ONA was overtly a naturopathic association, the implicit intent of the association was to provide a vehicle to protect the rights of chiropractors to employ drugless therapies. In 1954 Dr. John LaPlante ND a former president of the ONA warned: 'We must not let up for one minute and we must be on our guard at all times. Remember that majority who attend our meetings are CHIROS at heart and are liable to see things "chiropractically" and think of things in such a way as chiropractic being the drugless profession. I cannot make this too plain.'

In 1974 the ONA was very active in ensuring that acupuncture remained as a treatment method that naturopathic doctors could access. They also requested the National College of Naturopathic Medicine (NCNM) add acupuncture to their curriculum. In 1978 the ONA established the Ontario College of Naturopathic Medicine (OCNM) and continued to play an active role in the College's administration until around 1986.

In 1997 the ONA changed its name to the Ontario Association of Naturopathic Doctors (OAND) to better reflect the mandate of the association. The OAND is currently the largest provincial naturopathic association in Canada. It remains pro-active in provincial regulatory concerns, offers continuing education for its members, promotes the naturopathic profession in Ontario and provides a number of member benefits.

Ontario Regulatory Battles

When the Drugless Practitioner's Act first came into effect in 1925 it was an umbrella legislation to govern all drugless practitioners including: chiropractors, chiropodists, drugless therapists, masseurs, and osteopaths. At that time the terms 'drugless therapist' and naturopath were synonymous and according to the 1944 regulation was defined as any person "who practices or advertises or holds himself out in any way as practicing the treatment by diagnostic methods, direction, advice, written or otherwise, of any ailment, disease, defect or disability of the human body by methods taught in colleges of drugless therapy or naturopathy and approved by the Board."

In 1944 the Act was amended to designate major and minor classifications. Chiropractors, drugless therapists, and osteopaths were designated as major classifications and masseurs and physiotherapists (added at that time) were designated as minor classifications. The minor classifications could only undertake treatment under the prescription of a medical doctor or a member of one of the major classifications.

In 1952, an Act authorizing separate boards for each classification was passed which now allowed each group to be administered by their own board of directors. The Board of Directors of Drugless Therapy – Naturopathy (BDDT-N) was then established to regulate the activities of naturopathic doctors and drugless therapists. The first meeting of the BDDT-N was held on January 28th, 1953. At that time the board consisted of naturopathic doctors Leonard Bailey (Chairman), Eric Sjoman (Vice-Chairman), Victor Tomlin (Secretary-Treasurer), Henri Avonde (public member) and Robert B. Farquharson (public member). The other groups also established their own regulatory boards yet until 1986 they all remained under the Drugless Practitioners Act.

Between 1953 and 2007 there were four major commissions affecting health professionals in Ontario: the Royal Commission on Health Services (RCHS) appointed in 1961; the Committee on the Healing Arts (CHA) appointed in 1966; and the Health Professions Legislative Review (HPLR) appointed in 1983 and the Health Professions Regulatory Advisory Comittee (HPRAC) in 1990. Although naturopathic doctors had been regulated continuously since 1925, it was not until 2007 (83 years after first being regulated) that naturopathic doctors in Ontario finally received the commitment that they would be included under the same regulatory act as all other health professionals in Ontario, the Regulated Health Practitioners Act (RHPA).

Royal Commission on Health Services (RCHS)

The RCHS was introduced in 1961, just shortly after the ONA and the BDDT-N had been established and hence the profession was vulnerable and due to inexperience and limited resources. Adding to the challenges was that many members had split loyalties with the chiropractic profession, the number of naturopathic doctors was dwindling and many were not members of the ONA. Another challenge was that the legislation of the Drugless Practitioners Act (DPA) was based on what was taught in the schools and the only naturopathic school in North America was located on the west coast in the United States. The profession had heart, but lacked political clout and experience on how to deal with government and regulatory issues.

Both the ONA and the BDDT-N presented separate briefs (documents) to the RCHS committee, but neither was well argued. The ONAs five page brief simply made several very general and sometimes contradictory comments. During the first hearing before the committee in June of 1967, representatives from both the ONA and the BDDT-N appeared. The naturopathic doctors were no match for the legal minds of either members of the committee or the committee's legal counsel (who later became the legal counsel for the College of Physicians and Surgeons of Ontario (CPSO). The hearings began poorly as the naturopaths were accused of deliberately flaunting the laws by introducing each other as doctors. During the hearing, Dr. Harold Drescher ND the ONA president at the time, was questioned about the use of radionics machines in a naturopathic practice. At the time it was quite common for naturopathic doctors to use these machines in their practices. Yet, conventional medicine felt that they were unscientific and the RCHS committee chose to make this point the focus of their discussion with the ONA. At the time, the government's knowledge of naturopathic medicine was particularly lacking and the beliefs and understanding of Committee members regarding health and disease were certainly more congruent with those of conventional medicine than with those of naturopathic. The extensive liaison between the Ontario Department of Health and the CPSO continued during the period under discussion, with the CPSO often being asked to clarify issues regarding drugless practitioners. It was clear that the ONA and the BDDT-N had a lot of work to do to establish themselves as the experts in the field of naturopathic medicine.

Although the experience had been a difficult one for the ONA and the BDDT-N, during the final recommendations it was noted: "It is surely going much too far to refer to the naturopaths' concept of treatment "by the use of nature's agencies, therapeutics, processes and products" as "meaningless jargon" . . . If a doctrine attempts to stress the benefits of nutrition and vitamins but fails to use the right medical jargon, does this make it unscientific? . . . In our opinion, the evidence presented by the medical profession in Ontario is not sufficient to warrant their recommendation that the practice of naturopathy should be banned . . ."The result of the RCHS was that the naturopathic regulation under the DPA be maintained.

Committee on the Healing Arts

In 1967 the Ontario Government set up the Ontario Committee on Healing Arts (CHA) to investigate the various health care professions. The Ontario Medical Association (OMA) urged that the naturopathic act be rescinded; the chiropractic profession supported the decision of the OMA. The ONA and the BDDT-N prepared a response to the Committee, but the relationship between the naturopathic profession and the Ontario government was still not strong.

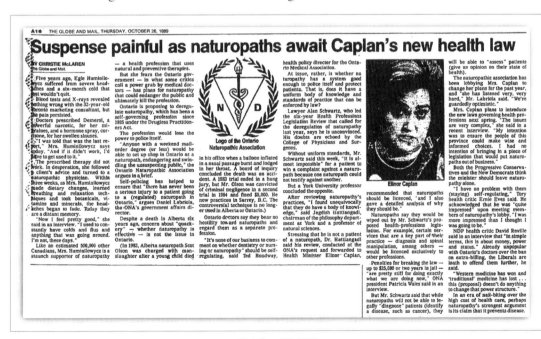

October 26, 1989
with permission from the *Globe and Mail*

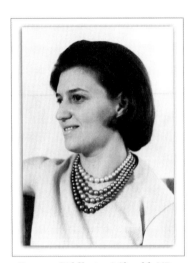

Frances (Eddleston) Shrubb ND A passionate bright light in the naturopathic profession. Dr. Eddleston always had time for students, patients or fellow NDs. Full of energy and ideas Frances was tireless in her support of her profession.

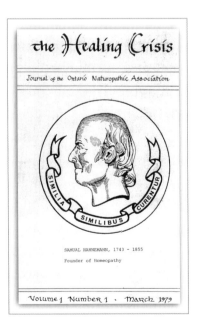

the Healing Crisis

Journal of the Ontario Naturopathic Association

SAMUAL HAHNEMANN, 1743 - 1855
Founder of Homeopathy

Volume 1 Number 1 · March 1979

In a letter from the CHA to the British Columbia naturopathic association, the statement was made that "in 1969 there were 79 practitioners of naturopathy in Ontario and of these 70 were registered also with the board of chiropractic and practiced both as chiropractors and naturopaths. Thus, although naturopathy is not included as a benefit, nearly 90% of its practitioners can submit claims to the Plan under the terms of the limited chiropractic benefit. Our inquiries have led us to the conclusion that the merits of naturopaths are limited… we have not found any distinctive feature of the practice of naturopathy which has a particular merit on its own…" In June of 1972 it was recommended that the Health Disciplines Act, which was the outcome of the Ontario Committee on Healing Arts, would allow those already licensed to continue, but no new practitioners would be licensed. At this point a joint submission was prepared by the ONA, BDDT-N and the CNA.

Dr. Lawrence Schnell ND who was president of the CNA, spear-headed an 85 page treatise on naturopathic medicine and initiated a campaign that concentrated on sending letters and information to the provincial premier, to the Minister of Health, to ministry officials, and to members of parliament. There was also a public relations booklet that was directed to the patients of naturopathic doctors in Ontario in order to inform them of the legislation and to solicit their assistance. The response from members and their patients was impressive. Dr. Norah Stewart ND secretary of the ONA, received responses from the British Naturopathic & Osteopathic Associations, as well as The New Zealand Association of Naturopaths and Osteopaths. One comment from the letters was that "All the countries seem to be having a fight with the governments to stay alive." In response to the deregulation concerns, two members of the ONA, Dr. Gord Smith ND and Dr. Asa Herscoff ND, established the "Friends of Naturopathy". This group included a number of public members and it created newsletters and ran fundraising programs to support the regulatory efforts in Ontario. In 1980, "Friends of Naturopathy" became a non-profit arm of the ONA and the newsletter was renamed *The Healing Crisis.*

When the Health Disciplines Act became law in 1974, the section about removing naturopathic doctors had been deleted. The principle reason appeared to have been the political action campaign spearheaded by Dr. Schnell ND and the public support that was received.

Health Professions Legislative Review (HPLR)

In 1982, just prior to the next government review, an Ontario naturopathic doctor was charged with practicing medicine without a license. Instead of the complaint being forwarded to the regulatory board to investigate, the CPSO intervened directly. thus circumventing the authority of the BDDT-N and raising the question as to whether or not they were able to adequately regulate their own members. Instead of the case being resolved and a fine paid, the Regulatory board interpreted the actions of the CPSO as harassment of the profession and hired a lawyer for consultation. Months later, when the ONA became aware of all details, they took over the strategy and funding of the case. The case received a lot of publicity and it impacted the legislative actions in Ontario. The case was eventually settled out of court, yet the fall-out for the practitioner involved and the profession lasted for a long t ime.

During the years 1983 to 1985, naturopathic doctors Verna Hunt, John Cosgrove, George Roth and Kim McKenzie worked with an organizational consultant to improve the effectiveness of the ONA and to ensure stronger political relationships. Up to that time much of the ONA activities were handled on a volunteer basis with individuals such as Dr. Norah Stewart ND who held the association together as secretary for over 35 years.

When the Ontario Government created the Health Professions Legislative Review (HPLR) in 1983, its purpose was to review all legislation pertaining to healthcare, paying special attention to the "legal and procedural issues associated with the self-regulation of health professionals" and to make recommendations to the Ministry of Health about updating health care legislation. Ontario practitioners were concerned that once again there was a threat of being deregulated especially as a result of the ongoing public court case and the strained relationship between the regulatory board and the government.

In the spring of 1986, the Minister of Health released a list of 25 occupations recommended by the HPLR review committee for regulation under new legislation. While such occupations as chiropractic, midwifery, and massage therapy were included, naturopathy was excluded. What was interesting was that there were seven professions that were being regulated for the first time; naturopathy was the only profession that was currently regulated where the recommendation was to deregulate. The Minister stated that naturopathy was omitted because: ". . . . naturopathy is based on a philosophy of natural healing that makes it extremely difficult to define standards of practice. As a result the continued regulation of this profession would not enhance protection to the public." It was also stated that "procedures which require advanced training and skill to prevent harm to patients will be regulated." The naturopathic profession found that statement contradictory to the recommendation of deregulation as the training of naturopathic doctors consisted of over 4500 hours of classroom instruction and supervised clinical practice. The naturopathic curriculum was surely evidence of the advanced training and skill required of naturopathic doctors.

Due to the threat of deregulation, the government with the co-operation of the ONA replaced the board members of the BDDT-N. In 1989 the ONA and the new BDDT-N board mounted a public campaign to prevent deregulation. Mr. Schad, the father of a naturopathic doctor, was instrumental in the funding and hiring of Dr. Dan Labriola, a naturopathic doctor from the state of Washington, who had had considerable experience in regulatory matters. Dr. Pat Wales ND, the ONA President at the time and Dr. Dan Labriola ND worked continuously for years to rebuild relationships with the Minster of Health and other government officials, ensuring that the naturopathic profession in Ontario did not lose its regulation. Their letter writing campaign resulted in over 80,000 letters and signatures, one of the largest responses that the government had ever seen. Drs. Wales and Labriola were also successful in meeting with many levels of government. Naturopathic Drs. Pam Snider and Edie Pett were actively involved in initiating a

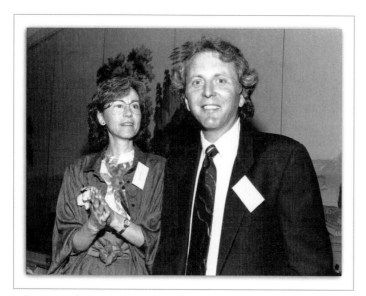

Dr. Pat Wales ND and Dr. Dan Labriola ND. Dr. Labriola was an engineer, pilot and legal advisor to the aviation industry before becoming a naturopathic physician in Washington State, USA. He was a key person in assuring continued regulation of naturopathic medicine in Washington State in that state's sunset review process. His dedication to naturopathic medicine plus his extensive political experience played a crucial role in retaining regulation in Ontario.

grass roots movement with patients. The Citizen's Alliance for Naturopathy was also formed in 1986 under the efforts of Gail Fisher-Taylor, a patient of one of the practitioners, which was instrumental in creating tremendous public awareness.

In January 1989 when the HPLR Committee released its final report titled, *Striking a New Balance: A Blueprint for the Regulation of Ontario's Health Professionals* the Committee recommended that naturopathic medicine be deregulated. In June of 1990, following over seven years of research and consultation, the Government of Ontario introduced the Regulatory Health Professions Act (RHPA) into the legislature. Naturopathic medicine was not included in the RHPA, but remained under the Drugless Practitioners Act. The efforts of Dr. Wales and Dr. Labriola had paid off and once again the regulation of the profession had been saved.

Naturopathic doctors were not included in the new Regulated Health Practitioners Act (RHPA) as they had desired. The decision was to continue to regulate the naturopathic profession under the Drugless Practitioners Act until the RHPA was opened the next time and a professions specific act could be created.

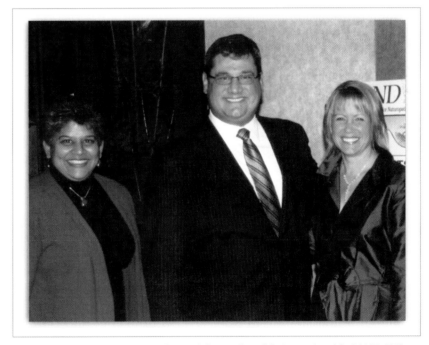

The Honourable David Caplan, Minister of Health (centre), with OAND CEO, Alison Dantas (left) and OAND Chair, Shelley Burns ND (right) at the OAND Convention 2008

Health Professions Regulatory Advisory Committee (HPRAC)

In response to the recommendations made by the HPLR Committee, the Health Professions Regulatory Advisory Council (HPRAC) was formed in 1992. Shortly after this, the ONA's government affairs chair, Dr. Pat Wales ND and Dr. James Spring ND chair of the BDDT-N met with the chair and staff of the HPRAC in preparation for a joint presentation to the new Committee. Throughout 1993 the ONA and BDDT-N were focused on ensuring that their submission to the Ministry of Health requesting inclusion for Ontario naturopathic doctors under the RHPA was received favourably.

Over the next fifteen years there were three separate submissions made to HPRAC. Throughout the years, the relationship between the ONA/OAND and the BDDT-N with the government improved. In all three submissions HPRAC recommended that the naturopathic profession be included under the RHPA with a broad scope of practice. One of the challenges was that the Ontario government went through a number of elections during this period and the governmental power repeatedly changed hands which may have contributed to the recommendations not being acted upon. The second challenge was that the recommendations of HPRAC were privileged information to the Minister of Health and were not made public until years later.

It was only after the third submission which was made in 2006 that any action was taken by the Ministry. At the time the government was committed to legislative reform of health-care and the OAND and BDDT-N worked closely with them to ensure the legislation moved forward. Also in 2006, Dr. Angela Moore ND chair of the BDDT-N invited the OAND, CAND and CCNM to form an Ontario coalition. The coalition sponsored a survey of Ontarians to determine the interest in naturopathic medicine and they worked co-operatively to ensure that the profession had a common voice. The OAND also hired Alison Dantas as their Chief Executive Officer to assist with their regulatory efforts.

In June of 2007, Bill 171 was tabled and approved. Under this bill a transitional council will be appointed and the intention is that by 2010 the naturopathic profession will have its own act under the RHPA, at which time the DPA will no be repealed. There is still much work to be done with respect to scope of practice, prescribing rights for naturopathic doctors and access to substances. In January of 2009 HPRAC completed a review of the prescribing authority for health professionals and has recommended that Naturopathic doctors in Ontario be awarded prescribing authority.

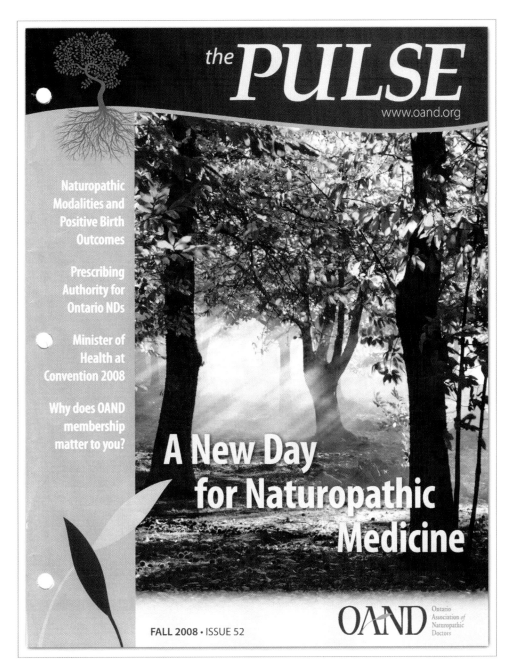

the **PULSE**

www.oand.org

Naturopathic
Modalities and
Positive Birth
Outcomes

Prescribing
Authority for
Ontario NDs

Minister of
Health at
Convention 2008

Why does OAND
membership
matter to you?

A New Day
for Naturopathic
Medicine

FALL 2008 · ISSUE 52

OAND Ontario
Association *of*
Naturopathic
Doctors

OAND Pulse 2002...

CHAMPION:
DR. ROBERT BOWDEN FARQUHARSON DC, ND

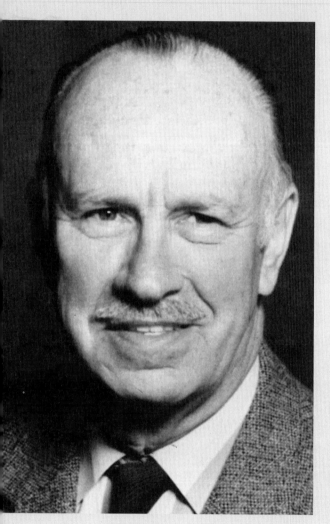

"GOD, FAMILY, PATIENTS AND THE PROFESSION." Those were Bob Farquharson's priorities and he lived by them every day. He was born in Toronto on November 8, 1919 and received his early education there. He developed an interest in chiropractic and naturopathic medicine early in life due to the influence of his father and two cousins who practiced these professions.

His education at the National College of Chiropractic and Drugless Physicians in Chicago, Illinois, was interrupted by World War II, during which time he served overseas in the Royal Canadian Medical Corps. While overseas, he married Margaret.

On his return from the war he completed his training in Chicago and graduated in 1947. Returning to Canada, he bought a chiropractic practice in the town of Orillia, north of Toronto. He and Margaret had five children. The reason for his success in practice was that he worked hard, he set high standards of integrity for himself and he became involved with his profession and his community.

Dr. Farquharson's practice was primarily chiropractic when it was established, but evolved with time into the practice of naturopathic medicine. In the mid 1950's he decided to make a statement regarding his support of naturopathic medicine. Dr. Farquharson removed the chiropractic sign on the lawn of his home where he practiced and replaced it with a naturopathic medicine sign. This was a major risk as naturopathic medicine was virtually unknown at this time. However, his practice continued to thrive and his wife Margaret joined the practice to help with the increased patient load.

Dr. Farquharson practiced the naturopathic therapies – homeopathic medicine, clinical nutrition and chiropractic manipulation. He was also skilled in the use of an instrument developed by Albert Abrams which often guided him in his assessment and treatment of patients.

Dr. Farquharson supported the profession in many ways. He served as secretary/treasurer of the Board of Drugless Therapy – Naturopathy for over ten years. In 1978 he was one of the six founders of the Ontario College of Naturopathic Medicine (changed to Canadian College of Naturopathic Medicine in 1992). He realized that the profession needed a professional college to survive and for naturopathic medicine to continue to be regulated in Ontario. Using personal funds, he was one of the college founders who guaranteed a line of credit at the bank for the fledgling school. He served on the Board of Directors of the college as Chair from 1981 –1983.

Dr. Robert Farquharson started to slow down in 1985 at age 66, and was looking forward to retiring. At that time, his son Jim decided to change careers and enrolled at OCNM. Jim graduated in 1990. Due to his son's involvement in the profession he developed a renewed interest in the college and served as Chair for a second time from 1987 to 1990.

His dream of a family practice materialized in 1990 when he joined Jim in practice in Ayr, Ontario. They practiced together until he passed away on October 22nd, 1991.

CHAMPION:
DR. PATRICIA J. WALES, BSc ND
Written by Dr. Verna Hunt ND

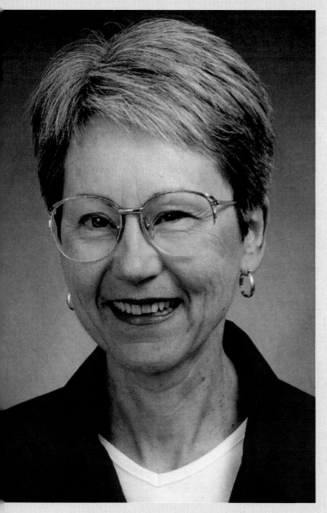

PAT WALES WAS BORN IN CALGARY in 1944, the oldest of three children. When she was young her family lived in house with 5 other families, each one had their own apartment and they all shared a garden and a root cellar. It was a very close-knit community where helping and taking care of each other was the norm. It really ingrained in her the importance of working together and appreciating the little things in life. It wasn't until Pat became an adult that she realized that her family had lived below the poverty line, what she remembers is that she grew up in a very safe place and that her parents encouraged her ambitions to go to University.

Pat was able to attend the University of Calgary due to scholarships and by working part-time. In 1965 she graduated with a Bachelor of Sciences Honors in Chemistry and was offered two jobs. One of the jobs involved doing laboratory research for the Food and Drug Directorate in Ottawa. After four years she realized that lab work was too isolating for her and while she figured out what she wanted to do next she and her sister spent 4 years in New Zealand and Australia.

Pat returned to Canada with the desire to work in the field of natural healing. She attended the Canadian Memorial Chiropractic College (CMCC) as both she and her dad had been helped by chiropractors in the past. Pat herself had fallen on the ice during her first year at University. Eventually she went to see a chiropractor and it helped. While at CMCC she took a number of courses in nutrition, Applied Kinesiology (AK) and Touch for Health. The triad of muscle-organ-meridan, which was taught in AK, was a concept that resonated with Pat and that provided a frame-work for how she approached the integration of all aspects of the body. After graduating from CMCC in 1977 Dr. Pat Wales started her practice in Thunder Bay, Ontario with Dr. Dan Gleeson, DC. She was interested in the energetic, spiritual and nutritional side of health care and her practice grew quickly.

Dr. Wales wanted to ensure that she would be able to retain a broad scope of practice and when John Cosgrove informed her that a naturopathic program was opening in Toronto, she traveled to

Toronto 40 times over 3 years to take the accelerated OCNM program and graduated in 1981.

In 1985 the Ontario naturopathic profession was in the midst of tremendous change and there were concerns about its lack of infrastructure and ability to deal with the threat of deregulation. Dr. Wales had built a reputation of being tactful, organized and inclusive-minded and hence she was approached by NDs Verna Hunt, Kim McKenzie and George Roth to run for president of the ONA. Dr. Wales moved to Toronto and, for the next ten years, became the person leading the cause to ensure continued regulation of naturopathic medicine in Ontario, which then affected decisions made in other jurisdictions around the world. Dr. Dan Labriola ND, was a key mentor as he worked with Pat and others, teaching them political strategies that successfully retained regulation.

Dr. Wales organized the MPP meetings, fund raising, letter campaign (with major help from NDs Pam Snider and Edie Pett), media training, the first press conference and media interviews, to name some of her accomplishments. Protecting the regulation of naturopathic medicine in Ontario was a full-time job and Dr. Wales chose to put her practice on hold for two years during a critical period of time for the ONA. Along with Dr. Dan Labriola ND and Dr. Jim Spring ND she wrote, edited and produced the joint ONA/BDDT-N briefs to HPRAC, providing the historical roots and modern scope of naturopathic medicine to the Committee and government. Under her guidance the ONA successfully ensured the ongoing regulation of naturopathic medicine in Ontario.

From 1989 to 1994, Dr. Wales worked part-time at a manufacturing site, Husky Injections Molding Systems Ltd. Husky was establishing a wellness centre for its employees and was one of the first companies to offer naturopathic services as part of an in-house corporate health program. In 1996 she returned to her roots in Calgary where she still practices today. She quickly became involved in the regulation efforts in Alberta.

Dr. Pat Wales has been an ongoing board member for the CNA (now CAND) since 1996 serving in many positions including Chair of Government Affairs. She has assisted in developing good relationships between the provinces and the national organization.

Dr. Wales generously donated time, energy, intelligent insight, money and humour that was key in assuring the longevity of naturopathic medicine as a profession in Canada and as a body of knowledge in the world today. She continues to mentor new graduates and teach on many topics including laboratory diagnosis, breast health and muscle response testing.

Quebec

The titles 'naturopathic doctor', 'naturopathic physician', 'ND', 'naturopath', etc are not reserved titles in Quebec. As such, anyone can use these titles, creating much confusion in this province. In this text regarding Quebec's history, the use of the terms 'naturopathic medicine', 'naturopathic doctor' and 'ND' will be consistent with the use of those titles in regulated jurisdictions (i.e., naturopathic medical education that is recognized by NABNE). The use of the terms 'naturopathy', 'naturopath' and 'nd' refer to the practice of natural therapies where the training is not consistent with the requirements of regulated jurisdictions.

The practice of naturopathic medicine in Quebec began in the 1920s and 1930s. Up until the late 1960s there were very close ties between the Quebec naturopathic practitioners and the rest of the naturopathic profession in Canada. Quebec practitioners were members of the CNA and were active in the development of the profession. As the profession worked on increasing its educational standards across Canada, there became two 'camps' in Quebec. One 'camp' did not embrace the increased educational standards, the other 'camp' followed the direction of the other provinces and adopted and adhered to the increased educational standards. The latter 'camp' is known as the Quebec Association of Naturopathic Medicine (QANM).

Quebec Provincial Association

Quebec is an unregulated province and unlike any other province, there is more than one provincial group that claims to represent the interests of naturopaths and naturopathic doctors. For years there have been ongoing struggles between the different groups in Quebec. The issues revolve around the differences in educational standards, the qualifications of the persons practicing without any legitimate degree, ongoing court cases and differences in terminology. Many of the different groups have been involved in public meetings and demonstrations, which have served the purpose of increasing the knowledge on natural health care but also added to the confusion about the different groups.

During the early years, many of the practitioners in Quebec were involved in battles with the College of Physicians, and were threatened with fines proposed from $200 up to $5000 and possible six month jail penalties. One of the early naturopathic practitioners (J. Thuna) who had practiced for 50 years received a fine every November. This was simply considered to be an "Illegitimate tax".

In 1968 Quebec naturopaths submitted and defended two briefs (documents) before the Claude Castonquay's Royal Commission of Inquiry into Health Care and Social Welfare - one about the recognition of the naturopathic physician in Quebec, and the other titled, the Philosophy of Natural Health. When the brief was first released naturopathic doctors intended to apply for registration, yet the College of

Physicians was seeking complete exclusion of all forms of medical services other than their own.

In 1970 three Quebec naturopaths, Raymond Barbeau, Hervé Boisvert and Lucien Vallieres, approached the CNA stating that they represented a new order of naturopaths in Quebec. They claimed to be completely organized, unified and ready to receive regulation. The CNA accepted the organization on this basis only to find later that it was not so. The CNA then withdrew its official recognition. Therefore, throughout the 1970s and 1980s the CNA did not recognize any group in Quebec, as the internal struggles had not changed. During this period of time only individual bona fide applications could be accepted but no Quebec association was affiliated with the national association.

In June of 1995, the naturopathic doctors in Quebec who were in line with the educational standards set by the rest of Canada formed the Quebec Professional Association of Naturopathic Physicians (QPANP)/ Association professionnelle des médecins naturopathes du Québec (APMNQ). At the first meeting the following naturopathic doctors were present: André Saine (President), Lise Maltais (Secretary), Michèle Lafond, Autumn-Louise Drouin and Tutti Gould. This group decided that it would only accept members who were graduates of a CNME accredited school. On August 28th 1995, the QPANP was registered by the Quebec government. Over the next few years the QPANP attempted to work with other groups in order to strengthen the overall position and education of complementary and alternative therapies in Quebec. The affiliation with the other groups did not happen as it was felt that the QPANP posed a threat to the other professionals.

The QPANP was accepted as a constituent member of the Canadian Naturopathic Association at the October 15, 1997 CNA meeting. In 1998 the QPANP changed its name to Quebec Association of Naturopathic Medicine QANM)/ Association de médecine naturopathique du Québec (AMNQ). From 1999 to 2002 the association was not very active and a few of the members decided to leave Quebec to practice in regulated jurisdictions. Activity began again in 2002 when new graduates of CCNM established practices in Quebec. In 2002 and 2003, members of QANM visited a number of members of the National

Assembly in an effort to educate politicians about naturopathic medicine and the need for government regulation. In October 2002, the QANM requested that naturopathic medicine be regulated in Quebec and in December the director of communications for the Office wrote back stating that a 1992 report on naturopathy/naturopathic medicine showed that it did not pose a threat to the public and that the file would not be reopened. Since that time QANM members such as naturopathic doctors Andre Saine, Stephanie Ogura and Anne Hélène Genné continue to meet with members of the government to educate them on naturopathic medicine and to work on achieving the regulation of naturopathic medicine in Quebec. In 2008, the QANM estimates that Quebec has 5-10 schools of naturopathy, 8-10 associations of naturopaths and naturotherapists and there are about 2,000 individuals who call themselves naturopath, naturopathic doctor, or naturotherapist.

Educational Struggles

One of the main challenges in Quebec has been that there has never been, as of yet, a 4 year French program that adheres to the educational standards set by the naturopathic profession. In the 1950's, Quebec practitioners responded to the need for educational facilities by starting up a number of naturopathic schools. Over time, the schools were successful in that they graduated a number of students, but the educational standards were never at the level set by the profession at large.

In the 1960s the CNA had an educational committee that recognized colleges that met certain standards. In 1967, one of the Quebec associations hoped their college, l'Institut de naturopathie du Québec, would gain recognition from the CNA and from NCNM in Portland, Seattle. Their application was conditionally granted, but it was withdrawn a couple years later as the Institute was not able to adhere to the standards set.

Other colleges were also founded over the years yet there was never any affiliation with the CNA or CNME accredited schools . In the fall of 1995 the QPANP (later renamed QANM) started discussing and planning the establishment of a school for naturopathic medicine in Quebec. They formed an affiliation with the Southwest College of Naturopathic Medicine and discussed with its President Dr. Michael Cronin ND the possibility of opening a Quebec campus of the SCNM that would become an independent school within 5-10 years. This project did not move forward as SCNM had other pressing issues.

In 2003 The QANM met with representatives from the Université du Québec à Trois-Rivières. The goal of this meeting was to establish a CNME accredited school at the university (chiropractic and midwifery programs were taught at this university). CCNM was to facilitate the implementation of the program at the university. The university concluded that such a program could not be taught in Quebec until naturopathic medicine was regulated in the province.

In 2007, the QANM, CCNM and the CNME were approached by the École d'enseignement supérieur en naturopathie du Québec (EESNQ). The EESNQ graduates naturopaths in Quebec and was interested in raising the education such that it met CNME standards. As of 2008 the feasibility of this initiative is still being discussed.

CHAMPION:
DR. ANDRÉ SAINE, ND, DHANP
As told by Joseph Kellerstein, DC, ND, FCAH, CCH

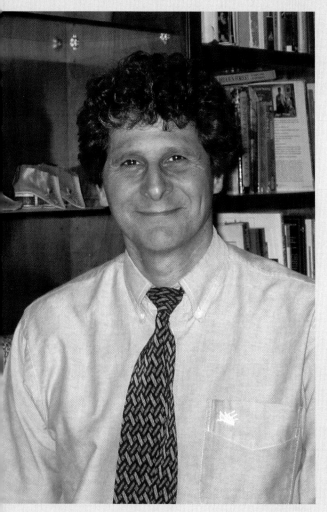

ANDRÉ SAINE WAS BORN IN MONTREAL, Quebec, one of eight children. His father was a holistic medical doctor who raised his family without any vaccinations, white bread, or junk food, and instead had their table and root cellar full of fruits and vegetables year round. He even bought a fruit farm on the Niagara Peninsula so that his children could benefit from the sun and fresh air while learning to work on the farm.

After graduating from college with a degree in health sciences, André chose to live in a pristine part of Quebec close to the ocean and far into the woods of the Gaspé Peninsula. He was three miles from a small fishing village of about 100 people. The village had been isolated without a road and electricity until about 10-15 years before his arrival and it was like stepping back into the 19th century. There, he built himself a log cabin and lived without electricity, a calendar or a clock. He ate from his garden, and fished the lakes, rivers and ocean. He hunted deer and small game all year round. He built a sauna and discovered the amazing benefits of sitting by the fireplace after having taken a sauna and having rolled in the snow and jumped in the river still covered with ice. He learned much from the wisdom of the elders and witnessed some amazing spiritual healing among the local folks. One day while André was visiting with his brother, he dislocated his shoulder cutting wood. This was almost a daily occurrence as a result of previous sports injuries. His brother suggested that he consult a chiropractor. At the chiropractor's office, he picked up a brochure which mentioned two self-evident truths: one, that the body can heal itself; two, that there are causes to disease and they must be dealt with. After two chiropractic treatments, and six months without dislocating his shoulder he decided to go and explore this profession.

In September 1976, he left his cabin and his idealistic way of living to attend courses at the Canadian Memorial Chiropractic College (CMCC) In Toronto. In his first week of classes, he met Dr. Joseph Bonyun DC ND (Hom.). Curious about the ND and Hom designations, André was invited to observe Dr. Bonyun in his clinic. While at the clinic he picked up a brochure from the National College of Naturopathic Medicine (NCNM) in Portland and said to himself: "This profession fits me like a glove". While observing Dr. Bonyun, André was introduced to the healing power of homeopathy when a skeptical dermatologist was prescribed one pellet of Zincum metallicum 10 M for his eczema. André learned that this patient had an aggravation of his eczema that was then followed by a complete disappearance of his lesions. He was intrigued by the fact that such a tiny single influence could trigger such a reaction for the body to heal itself. He knew then that he had to study homeopathy.

André pursued his education at NCNM in 1980. On the first day of class Dr. John Bastyr, NCNM's President emeritus, had been invited as a guest lecturer. André was able to convince Dr. Bastyr to take him as a preceptor. During one of his visits, André was introduced to hydrotherapy and Dr. Bastyr recommended André visit Dr. Harold Dick ND in Spokane, WA. André went and learned the values of hydrotherapy and gathered all the information he could from the only four doctors who had learned from O.G. Carroll, namely, Drs. Harold Dick, Leo Scott, John Bastyr and Bill Carroll (O. G. Carroll's son). André went on to teach hydrotherapy at the four existing naturopathic colleges and co-published with Dr. Wade Boyle ND *Lectures in Naturopathic Hydrotherapy*. While studying at CMCC and NCNM, André continued to preceptor in his father's clinic where he learned how to manage "incurable" cases. As a third and fourth year student at NCNM, he was asked to teach manipulation, and received the Hahnemann scholarship for his paper on the placebo effect and its implication for homeopathy. He also traveled to various libraries to research the old homeopathic literature. After graduation from NCNM, Dr André Saine taught manipulation, hydrotherapy, introduction to research and naturopathic philosophy.

In December 1986, Dr. Saine left NCNM and Oregon with the goals to research spiritual healing and continue visiting old naturopathic doctors throughout North America. Instead, he began his family and relocated on his father's fruit farm in Ontario. This location was very convenient as it was close to many of the best homeopathic libraries in the world and permitted him to continue his research of the homeopathic literature. Once in Ontario he was asked to begin a three-year postgraduate course in homeopathy. And thus he co-founded the Canadian Academy of Homeopathy which has offered training in genuine homeopathy for the last 22 years. A year later the National Center for Homeopathy asked him to join the teaching staff for its summer school. He taught philosophy of homeopathy and chronic prescribing for the next 18 years until they offered it for the last time in 2004.

Since the early 1980's, Dr. Saine has been giving regular seminars and taught courses in the Americas and in Europe. His busy academic and clinic schedule has been keeping him away from further researching spiritual healing, one of his older interests, and even further from his cabin on the Gaspé Peninsula.

In 1995, Dr. Saine relocated permanently in Montreal. His practice focuses in the use of classical homeopathy in difficult cases. Dr. André Saine continues to research, teach, write and since 1995 has been the president of the Quebec Association of Naturopathic Medicine. In addition to his tremendous contribution to the profession, the literature and his patients he is the father of five children and married to Dr. Lisa Samet ND.

Nova Scotia

As told by Dr. Lois Hare ND

Naturopathic medicine was birthed in September 1987 with the return of Dr. Lois Hare ND a recent graduate of OCNM. Dr. Hare was joined by naturopathic doctors Manon Bolliger in 1992, Cheryl Lycette in 1993 and Margot Kleiker in 1994. Together, these four NDs gathered and officially formed the Nova Scotia Naturopathic Association in December 1994.

The primary purpose of the Association was to educate the public about Naturopathic Medicine and also to be a support for the practitioners who were pioneering this new form of medicine in Nova Scotia. The Association met monthly sharing the joys and frustrations of practicing in an unregulated profession. This newly minted organization created a network of support for practitioners, allowing its members a place to share challenging cases and generate solutions.

The association grew by nine members in the 1990's. Ten new naturopathic doctors joined the profession in 2000 - 2001, and by 2008 there was a total of 29 practicing naturopathic doctors in Nova Scotia. In 2006 the association adopted a new image and name, the Nova Scotia Association of Naturopathic Doctors (NSAND) and created a new logo and website www.nsand.ca.

NSAND made history on July 2, 2008 with the proclamation of the Naturopathic Doctors Act. The bill was passed unanimously by all three political parties making Nova Scotia the first Atlantic province and the sixth province overall to legislate the practice of naturopathic medicine. The unopposed support in the legislature and the speed with which the bill passed, speaks to the strong desire for Naturopathic Doctors to be recognized in Nova Scotia. Acclamation of the Bill was welcomed by the Nova Scotia Association of Naturopathic Doctors (NSAND), the professional association of naturopathic doctors.

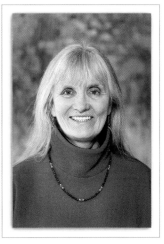

Dr. Lois Hare ND

"Prior to the government's support and the introduction of the Bill, naturopathic medicine was a 'Buyer Beware' market in Nova Scotia. Nova Scotians had no way of knowing who was or was not a properly trained and educated ND. The new law will now protect against unqualified individuals practicing in the area of naturopathic medicine."

NSAND CO-PRESIDENT JYL BISHOP VEALE ND, 2008

Eastern Provinces

As of 2008, there are naturopathic doctors in every province in Canada and each province has a provincial association that is part of the CAND. In 2001 the New Brunswick Association of Naturopathic Doctors (NBAND) was established, in 2004 the Prince Edward Island Association of Naturopathic Doctors (PEIAND) and in 2006 the Newfoundland and Labrador Association of Naturopathic Doctors. Although there are only about 20 naturopathic doctors in these provinces, they are working to achieve regulation.

Yukon

As told by Dr. Michael Mason-Wood ND

Long before the introduction of naturopathic medicine in the Yukon, traditional healers were alive and well. First Nation traditional medicine was passed on from generation to generation in the form of stories that the healers would tell eager pupils. The tradition of being a medicine healer was usually bestowed to women, who were known as gate keepers. The gate keepers would keep the medicine connected to the land from where it came and when needed they would know the location of plants and go in search of obtaining the medicine even in the winter. A pupil wishing to learn about traditional medicine would normally undergo an intensive apprenticeship with an medicine elder. In today's society, with the advent of computers and TV, many young people are not interested in learning in this fashion.

Naturopathic medicine as we know it today officially started in the Yukon in 2001 when CCNM graduates, naturopathic doctors Janice Millington and Joanne Leung, arrived and soon after started the Yukon Naturopathic Association (YNA). In 2002 Dr. Lianne Erikson ND arrived and Dr. Michael Mason-Wood ND in 2003. Both Dr. Mason-Wood and Dr. Erikson have since relocated to other areas. In the summer of 2006, Dr. Gordon Smith ND relocated to the Yukon to be closer to his children who live in Whitehorse. With him he brings his 31 years of experience in clinical practice and in government and regulatory work. Although the YNA is a young association with few members, it is actively involved in pursuing regulation.

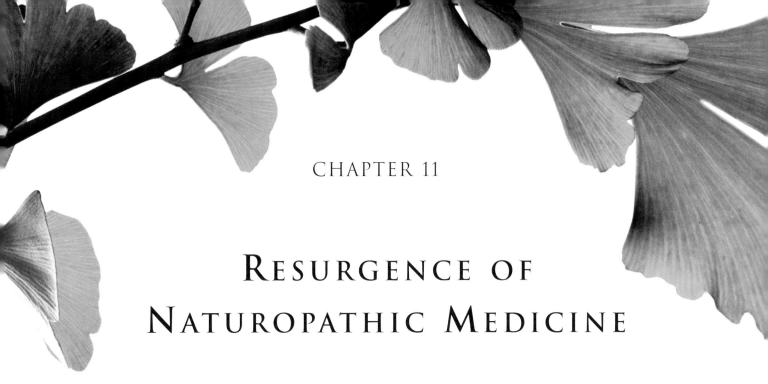

CHAPTER 11

RESURGENCE OF
NATUROPATHIC MEDICINE

RISING RATES OF CHRONIC and degenerative diseases, dissolution with the promise of a 'magic bullet'; growing concern with the drug-based conventional medicinal system; the internet explosion; the renewed awareness that health and disease were interrelated with a person's lifestyle and environment; a focus on preventive medicine; and growing concern about the health and future of the environment all contributed to the resurgence of naturopathic medicine.

The Fraser Institute completed a study entitled *Complementary and Alternative Medicine in Canada: Trends in Use and Public Attitudes, 1997 – 2006*. According to this study the dollars spent on alternative practitioners increased from 2.8 billion dollars in 1997 to 5.6 billion dollars in 2006. It also reported that for some conditions, such as anxiety and allergies, Canadians were actually seeking alternative practitioners more often that conventional and that 17% of people visited an alternative provider first and 32% visited both an alternative and conventional practitioner for the same health concern. This study also reported that 81% of people use naturopathic medicine for wellness. This is one of many studies that has illustrated the rise in awareness and interest that Canadians have in complementary and alternative medicine, including naturopathic medicine.

Chronic and Degenerative Diseases on the Rise

"Too often in politics, what we cherish most we inadvertently destroy by believing that protecting something means freezing it in time, when in fact protecting it may require dramatic change. Protecting children, for instance, means encouraging them to grow and adapt to the world in which they have to live. If we are going to save Canada's health care system we will have to change it, and the sooner we embark on the road to change, the smoother the journey will be."

JANICE McKINNON (MINISTER OF FINANCE, PROVINCE OF SASKATCHEWAN 1993-1997)

Prior to the introduction of sanitation and the use of antibiotics and surgery, acute illnesses were the primary cause of death. Over time, the death-rate from acute illness dramatically decreased, yet the incidence of chronic, debilitating and degenerative diseases continues to grow at an alarming rate.

There are many proposed reasons including unhealthy stressful lifestyles; the destruction and alteration of the food and water supply; the increase in environmental toxins, heavy metals and chemicals in food, personal care products, cooking utensils, toys, etc.; and the increasing use of pharmaceutical medicine. Decisions affecting farming, environment, manufacturing, industry, even school cafeterias have been made based on economics – not health. Is it any wonder that health - whether personal, social or environmental – is in such a dire state? If you do not make your decisions based on health; you can not expect health as the outcome.

In today's society, too often the same approach is used to treat disease as what caused it – quick, fast, expedient, short-termed, single focused. The common practice of medicine is to treat the body as individual parts instead of an interconnected whole; to treat every symptom with a new drug without looking for the underlying pattern or cause of illness; to suppress acute healing responses; and to 'kill the bug' versus to support the healing ability of the body.

Promise of a 'Magic Bullet' Proved Invalid

Antibiotics and hormones were initially believed to be 'magic bullets' that would eradicate and cure diseases. Creating a drug to kill a bug makes sense when a profession holds the belief that microorganisms are the cause of disease. It promotes the idea that disease can be prevented by taking a pill. These "magic bullets" have saved lives, but the problem is that this belief is far from the whole story.

The promise of a "magic bullet" was one of the primary factors that contributed, and still contributes, to the lack of personal responsibility that many people take with respect to their own health. The abuse and over prescribing of antibiotics have contributed to new strains of microbes and to drug-resistant viruses and bacteria.

Hormone replacement therapy, although sometimes effective in relieving menopausal symptoms, has its own risks and adverse effects. What is being recognized is that many drugs are over prescribed and used in place of lifestyle changes.

The current 'magic bullet' of conventional medicine is the use of vaccinations as a form of preventive medicine. True prevention comes from living a lifestyle that promotes health and involves making healthy choices throughout one's life; not by taking a drug.

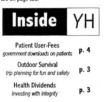
Concern with Conventional Medicine

Concern with the conventional medical system has been growing over time. Canadians are questioning the drug-approach to disease management, the shortage of medical doctors and the increased wait times. Ongoing research also refutes the value of some medical treatments and surgeries and highlights the adverse effects and associated risks, thus increasing the caution that many feel.

The use of drugs to treat disease has been part of medicine for centuries. It is a natural habit for medical practitioners and patients to connect the onset of symptoms with the need to take something. A common belief is that drugs cure disease with minimal or no lifestyle or behavioural changes. This fallacy continues to be questioned. Yet this habit of 'taking a pill' when sick is a difficult one to break. The naturopathic perspective is that health starts by asking "what do you change?", not "what do you take?" The focus is not necessarily on the management of symptoms or diseases but on regaining self-responsibility over your health and on addressing the underlying causes.

The growing concern has been attributed to a perceived lessening of interest on the part of physicians to see their patients as people. There is less time during medical visits for a patient to talk, to discuss not only what their chief concerns are, but the impact on their life and there is little time for a patient to gain insight into the factors contributing to their current state of health. There is much discussion in medical journals about this. The challenge appears to be the restrictions of medicare and insurance, not necessarily practitioner desire. At the same time, there is growing research showing that the patient-practitioner encounter has an impact on the therapeutic outcome. There is a greater chance of healing when the relationship is strong and there is an element of trust. Part of the reason many people seek naturopathic medicine is because they are not bound by many of the same restrictions, the visits are longer, and there is the time for the practitioner to assess not only what is happening but why.

In the 2004 report written by Glover, he states

"If we look at the system from the citizen's perspective, two critical issues stand out: (1) Canada does not have a health-centered system, but an illness-centered system; (2) the Canada Health Act is not a health act, but an insurance or financial act and it is not based on principles of health, but on insurance principles. As a result, citizens are care providers and not served as well as they should be. It is time to design a system around health."

Focus on Preventive Medicine

Focusing on prevention has always been one of the key principles of naturopathic medicine. For years, naturopathic doctors have discussed the merits of prevention in all their discussions and communications with the government and in any information that they disseminated. The conventional medical profession started to make strides along preventive lines since the 1970s.

Many diseases, especially chronic, are due to the wear-and-tear of having to cope with a constant lifestyle of excesses and deficiencies which eventually cause the body to 'break down'; for example, a history of eating poorly, not drinking sufficient water, being too sedentary, having poor posture, ineffective breathing, not having enough sleep and relaxation, not spending sufficient time outside or holding onto unhealthy thoughts and emotions.

Prevention from a naturopathic perspective involves hygiene, sanitation, living a healthy lifestyle, and ensuring a 'clean' and non-toxic environment and food supply. Each person is an individual and part of preventing disease is to understand each person's unique constitution and what is right for them. Prevention is a process that starts at birth and continues throughout life, not one that is employed at the first sign of trouble. The maintaining of health and prevention of disease is achieved by living a healthy lifestyle, by ensuring the health of the environment, by decreasing the exposure to chemicals and toxins and by using natural products to support the healing power of the body.

Concern About the Environment

Global warming and the exhaustion of natural resources is on the minds of politicians, environmentalists, consumers and even young school children. Due to the growing prevalence of toxins in food, soil, water and air, there is reason to be distressed not only about the health of the environment but its impact on the health of people.

The human body is constantly being bombarded with 'foreign' and toxic chemicals and substances that enter it through the air we breathe, the water we drink, the food we eat and what we put on our skin. Normally the body 'takes-in' substances, keeps what it needs and excretes the rest. Yet, the body is unfamiliar with many of these toxic chemicals and is unable to naturally excrete them. Toxins and foreign

"We have created a medical-industrial complex that is pretty darn good at diagnosing disease, and sometimes curing disease – but not nearly so good at preventing disease. And sometimes it is only too good at creating disease."

RONALD DAVID, MD
(1927 – 1989)

"An ounce of prevention is worth a pound of cure."

AUTHOR UNKNOWN

chemicals often result in modifications of body functions, such as the hormone disrupting impact of plastics (phenols). Heavy metals disrupt the normal functioning of many systems and impact the body's ability to absorb nutrients. Toxins are increasingly associated with different diseases and health concerns. Other factors impacting health are the abuse and over-use of computers, television, cell-phones and other electromagnetic frequency (EMF) producing devices.

There is, and needs to be, an increased focus on improving the health of the environment, on decreasing environmental toxins and chemicals, and on improving the quality of natural resources. Addressing the impact of environmental factors needs to become an integral part of living a healthy lifestyle and part of the assessment of all health concerns. The desire to work with doctors that are aware of the interrelationship between a person's health and the health of the environment increases as individuals are becoming more aware and health conscious.

Internet Explosion

The internet has changed the information available to both patients and doctors. There are many advantages to the internet, but there are also challenges and cautions that are often overlooked. Many people search the internet for information on their symptoms and disease. Yet, the information retrieved can be misleading, erroneous and taken out of context. Instead of identifying the factors that are contributing to the symptoms, individuals are too often jumping to the worse case scenario – replacing reason and logic with fear and uncertainty. This results in people requesting, sometimes demanding, expensive medical testing that is not indicated. This impacts the access for people who truly are in need. There is a logic, a flow chart per se, to medical diagnosis which walks a doctor through the most common or logical explanation to the more rare. The value of doctors (and patients) following this flow chart is to easily and quickly diagnose a majority of symptoms and diseases, reduce costs, decrease fear and increase trust in the healing process.

Health and disease are logical; they happen for a reason. The naturopathic 'flow-chart' starts at lifestyle, external, social and environmental factors. Naturopathic doctors utilize and refer patients for needed laboratory tests, ultrasounds and MRIs, yet not in place of listening to the whole story and its timeline and addressing the most obvious causes first.

"Although many health professionals agree that the internet is a boon for consumers because they have easier access to much more information than before, professionals are also concerned that the poor quality of a lot of information on the Web will undermine informed decision-making."

OFFICE OF DISEASE PREVENTION AND HEALTH PROMOTION (2000) HEALTHY PEOPLE 2010, 2ND EDITION.

Naturopathic Medicine: *Its Time has Come*

There were different economic and external factors that initiated the resurgence of naturopathic medicine. What also contributed was that the naturopathic profession continued to build a solid infrastructure and foundation during the years that it was not as popular. The profession has accredited naturopathic colleges; it has achieved provincial legislation in six provinces and has maintained an active national and provincial associations.

The early pioneers of naturopathic medicine always believed that healthcare would return to its roots. They knew that healthcare that was outsourced to the pharmaceutical companies would be short lived and eventually people would embrace the old values of healthy living and return to nature and more natural forms of treatment.

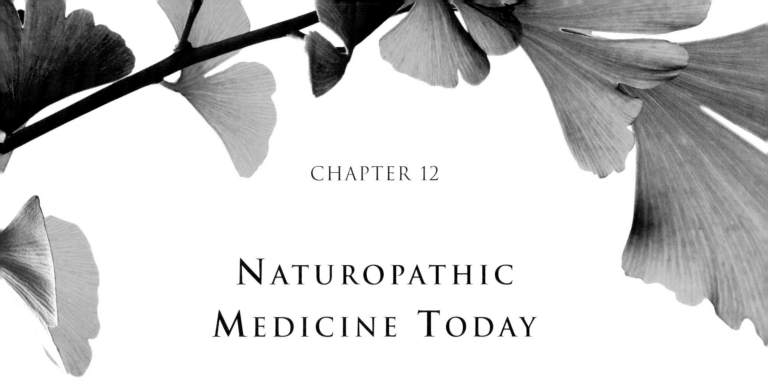

CHAPTER 12

NATUROPATHIC
MEDICINE TODAY

NATUROPATHIC MEDICINE IS ON THE FOREFRONT of the paradigm shift occurring in healthcare. Scientific tools now exist to prove and appreciate many aspects of naturopathic medicine. Naturopathic doctors are the experts of natural medicine and, as the naturopathic profession develops and expands, there are increasing numbers of practitioners that are involved in education, government, research, private industry and in health care initiatives around the world.

Naturopathic Clinics

Naturopathic practices were first established as 'old fashion' clinics, with practitioners typically having their own clinic and working one-on-one with patients. In the last ten years, the practice of naturopathic medicine has embraced the concept of integrated clinics. It is common to find multiple naturopathic doctors working with other health care practitioners, including medical doctors, chiropractors, osteopaths, registered massage therapists and others in the same clinic.

The focus of the naturopathic visit remains a strong patient-practitioner relationship. The initial visit with a naturopathic doctor is often one to two hours in length with subsequent visits being twenty to forty minutes. The length of visit allows the practitioner time to listen to the patient's story and to understand the role that a patient's life and lifestyle play with respect to the causal factors of disease and the process of healing.

Naturopathic medicine remains an eclectic practice. Some practitioners focus extensively on lifestyle changes; others more on mind-body medicine; some use energetic therapies such as acupuncture; others use functional medicine such as nutraceuticals, botanicals and homeopathics; some focus on structural therapies such as naturopathic manipulation, and remedial exercises; and still other practitioners focus on intravenous therapies and other forms of treatment. Most naturopathic doctors offer a combination of therapies. What unites the practice of naturopathic medicine is the philosophy and principles in which these therapies are applied.

Naturopathic doctors are general primary care practitioners. Recently, some NDs are choosing to focus on specific areas of healthcare, such as cancer, environmental medicine, women's health, pediatrics, etc. Other doctors are establishing associations or creating journals, magazines and books.

There are also many ways that cooperation between naturopathic and medical doctors is increasing. For example, hospitals are starting to include alternative therapies in their clinics and, as they do, it is common for naturopathic doctors to fill these positions. Referrals are now permitted resulting in NDs and MDs working together more frequently. There is an increasing number of medical doctors who are supporting their patient's desire to approach health concerns from a naturopathic perspective. Addressing the root cause of diseases and making lifestyle changes are being encouraged prior to prescribing drugs or other medical interventions.

Naturopathic adjunctive cancer-care clinic

By Heather Gibson

The Robert Schad Naturopathic Clinic (RSNC) at the Canadian College of Naturopathic Medicine is offering a cancer-focused clinic, created to provide a range of adjunctive complementary and alternative (CAM) therapies to cancer patients.

With more than 10 years of experience in helping individuals living with cancer, Associate Professor Peter Papadogianis, B.Sc., M.Sc., ND, is leading fourth-year interns in this new adjunctive cancer care clinic."We have developed this cancer-care program to help ensure people accessing complementary cancer care receive the best possible, evidence-driven care and approach for their particular cancer type," says Papadogianis.

The clinic provides treatment that is complementary to, not a replacement for, conventional therapies. Treatment goals include minimizing the side effects of those therapies, increasing patients' overall well-being, and the inhibition of the spread of cancer. Natural medicine can be supportive of conventional cancer care, or if used improperly can inhibit the effectiveness of other treatment. This shift serves to provide expert advice on reasonable naturopathic medical interventions, based on the most current research evidence.

"The RSNC clinical team values the collaborative approach when treating patients and will actively communicate and work with oncologists and other relevant health-care practitioners," says Papadogianis. "In that respect, everyone benefits - from the patient, who receives the best in collaborative care, to the interns, supervisors and other health-care practitioners, who garner a greater appreciation of appropriate complementary cancer therapies."

"We'll also consider utilizing CAM diagnostics that may not have reached the level of mainstream medicine, but have ample supportive indications for their use," explains Papadogianis. Thermal imaging is an example of one such diagnostic.

A patient's first visit takes approximately 90 minutes and includes a full history intake, a physical, and lab work.

Subsequent visits are one hour long. Naturopathic therapies include nutritional and lifestyle counselling, intravenous nutrition, botanicals, and traditional Chinese medicine including acupuncture. "We anticipate that NDs and other health-care practitioners in the field will welcome a referral centre for therapies such as intravenous cancer protocols, and we anticipate that people living with cancer will welcome a facility that provides evidence-based care, standardized intakes and cancer-specific therapies in an academic environment," says Papadogianis.

The Canadian College of Naturopathic Medicine (CCNM) is Canada's premier institute for education and research in naturopathic medicine. CCNM offers a rigorous four-year, full-time doctor of naturopathic medicine program.

Naturopathic doctors (NDs) are primary healthcare practitioners. Interns at CCNM's Robert Schad Naturopathic Clinic improve their patients' health by identifying and treating the underlying causes of illness, integrating acupuncture/Asian medicine, botanical medicine, nutrition, homeopathic medicine, hydrotherapy/massage and lifestyle counselling.

Heather Gibson is a Communications Officer with the Canadian College of Naturopathic Medicine.

The Adjunctive Cancer-Care Clinic at the Robert Schad Naturopathic Clinic is just one of the specialty shifts offered at CCNM's teaching clinic.

Publications

The ability to capture the wisdom and knowledge of any profession is an essential component of its survival. There were many naturopathic books written between 1900 and the 1930s, but only a few between the 1940s and the 1980s. In 1985 Dr. Joe Pizzorno wrote a naturopathic textbook, the *Textbook of Natural Medicine,* that was instrumental in rejuvenating the writing of naturopathic doctors. This textbook was one of the first to articulate the latest research that was available on natural medicine. Since that time there have been many new books, both textbooks and consumer-based books, that articulate and share the principles and therapies of naturopathic medicine. For a listing of the books written by naturopathic doctors visit the CAND website at www.cand.ca

CCNM Press was founded at the Canadian College of Naturopathic Medicine in Toronto in fall 2003 and first released books in spring 2004. CCNM Press is dedicated to publishing college texts, clinical reference materials, scholarly monographs, consumer trade books and corporate wellness guides in the field of naturopathic medicine to further the advancement of the profession of naturopathic medicine and to teach the principles of healthy living and preventive medicine, better enabling naturopathic doctors to assist patients in the healing process.

CCNM Press publications are based on current medical and health research, fully referenced and peer reviewed. They are authored by foremost scientific authorities and professors of naturopathic medicine. The production qualities of each publication are set at the highest standards for clear presentation of the information and ease of reader access. For all editorial, marketing and financial inquiries, please contact ccnmpress@ccnm.edu.

In 2002, Dr. Jared Zeff, a naturopathic doctor that practises in the United States, decided it was time to write a history and philosophy textbook on naturopathic medicine. He contacted Dr. Pam Snider ND who was in the process of doing the same thing and had already been in touch with a publisher. The vision quickly grew into *The Foundations of Naturopathic Medicine Project.* The textbook will be over 700 pages and involves over 200 writers, mostly naturopathic

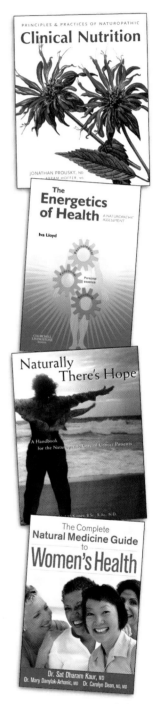

Above are a few of the recent books written by Naturopathic Doctors in Canada.

doctors, and editors from six different countries. The textbook is planned to be published in 2010 and it will provide an in-depth, research-based, look at naturopathic medicine. For more information on this project visit the website www.foundationsproject.com.

Public Awareness

Public awareness has always been a focus of the naturopathic profession. Historically, the limited resources were either focused on regulatory concerns or simply ensuring survival. The focus on public awareness initiatives increases as the profession becomes larger and more financially secure. These ini-

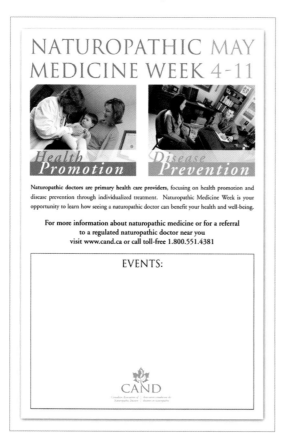

In 2001 Dr. Ingrid Pincott ND a CAND board member, initiated and organized the first Naturopathic Medicine Week. This event is now an annual public awareness campaign that occurs in the first week of May each year.

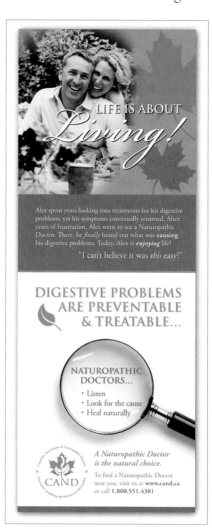

Appeared in Macleans magazine in November 2008

tiatives are carried out by the provincial associations, the CAND, naturopathic Colleges and individual NDs. The initiatives currently underway include television shows, radio talk shows, a national commercial, print advertising, public lecturers and information brochures and documents.

Some of the future public awareness initiatives planned include expanding the offering of public and educational seminars and the production of health documentaries. To find out about the current public awareness initiatives, visit the CAND website at www.cand.ca and the websites of the individual naturopathic colleges and provincial associations.

Global Involvement

Many naturopathic doctors in Canada have a strong sense of international responsibility and have been instrumental in spreading naturopathic medicine to other countries, both in the form of naturopathic educational institutes and as health-care clinics. Organizations such as Natural Doctors International www.ndimed.org ND Global Network www.ndglobalnetwork.com, the International Naturopathic Students' Association and Homeopaths Without Borders www.homeopathswithoutborders-na.org coordinate efforts in different countries in order to offer naturopathic services.

There are also many naturopathic practitioners who personally operate and support clinics in South Africa, Vietnam, Thailand, Saudi Arabia, South Korea and other places. For example, Dr. Laura Louie ND is involved with Thai AIDS workers and works in rural hospitals incorporating acupuncture and other complementary therapies into standard allopathic regimes. She also teaches local practitioners and nurses how to administer the therapies she employs. In 2006, her project expanded to Africa. Dr. Heather Eade ND opened a 200 bed hospital in Saudi Arabia. Dr. Alexander Yuan ND graduated from OCNM and is currently the director of the Optimum Health Centre, the Hong Kong Colon Hydrotherapy Centre and the Green Concepts Health Shop in Hong Kong.

Dr. Hong Keun David Oh, MD ND, PhD graduated from OCNM in 1991 and in 1997 he established The Korean Association of Naturopathic

Medicine in which over 100 medical doctors are now members. Apart from monthly academic meetings, the association runs various seminars and workshops where naturopathic modalities like homeopathy, hydrotherapy, chiropractic and qi (chi) energy medicine are introduced.

Dr. Alfono Wong ND, after receiving his naturopathic training at OCNM in 1988, moved to China and established the Asian College of Naturopathy (ACN) in 1999. The college offers a 4,000 hour program on naturopathic medicine and, within the first ten years has graduated over 1000 students. Many of the professors at ACN are graduates from Canadian and US naturopathic colleges. The College is also involved in joint-research with a number of State universities in Asia, such as Chinese University of Hong Kong, Polytechnic University, Malaysia HUKM Medical University, Italy Ferrara University and has journal publications in "International Journal of Molecular Medicine". Dr. Wong ND has also been involved in pursuing the regulation of naturopathy in Hong Kong, Malaysia and China. His vision is for everyone who is continuously suffering from their discomfort under the care of Conventional Medicine, to be relieved and cured by Naturopathic Medicine.

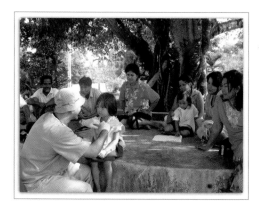

Dr. Gurdev Parmar ND of Fort Langley, established The HELP Foundation in 2005; soon after the disastrous 2004 tsunami ravaged South East Asian coastal countries. Drs. Karen and Gurdev Parmar ND were in India with their two boys at the time of the tsunami and vowed, while there, to do something.

The HELP Foundation's mission is to provide integrated healthcare services, both medical and dental, to people living in poverty, both locally and in developing countries. HELP Foundation designs, develops, and maintains integrated medical teams capable of delivering quality medical care and medical relief and plans to continue its support as long as there is a need.

Over the past 2 years, the HELP Foundation has been working diligently at the Pak Koh Health Center and is proud to report that, after three years, they have successfully transitioned the clinic to the Phangna Provincial Public Health Office (PPPHO). The clinic is now being managed and staffed by Thai employees year-round in what is now a well-updated clinic. Sites are now set on providing free healthcare to residents of a new homeless shelter being built in Langley, BC. HELP Foundation also gives many thanks to all the Thailand Health Officials, nurses, and doctors that made their work there so enjoyable and memorable.

PART 3

NATUROPATHIC
MEDICAL EDUCATION

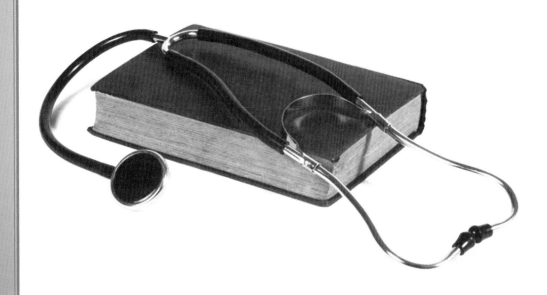

CHAPTER 13

ESTABLISHING NATUROPATHIC
MEDICAL EDUCATION

IN RESEARCHING AND STUDYING the formation of the naturopathic medical institutions, one can not help but sense the dedication, sweat and tears that so many have poured into this profession. Early in its formation, there was a deep understanding and appreciation for the need to ensure that the educational standards were strong and held true to the principles of naturopathic medicine and that they met the requirements of accrediting boards and government agencies. The balancing of all of this for any profession, let alone a young profession is not an easy task. It was accomplished by a small group of practitioners consistently putting their profession ahead of their personal lives and sacrificing much in order to ensure that the profession remained alive and strong. These goals were finally achieved in the 1980s and since then the educational standards have remained strong.

Early Years

The development of the naturopathic medical institutions started very much like that of conventional medical colleges - a few charismatic practitioners starting schools, initially apprentice-ship based and privately funded. Dr. Benedict Lust established the first naturopathic educational institution, the American School of Naturopathy in New York City in 1900 which offered several branches of nature cure in a two-year general course. Dr. Forster founded a similar institution in Idaho a few years later.

Within twenty years there were about 20 schools in existence. The naturopathic education in the early part of this century was unique and powerfully vitalistic, yet it suffered because it had not reached maturity in the context of professional unification or in uniform accreditation standards. Some of the naturopathic colleges offered four-year programs; others offered shorter programs that did not live up to the standards that were being set by the governing bodies of the profession.

The years between 1920 and 1960 were difficult for the profession. Many of the naturopathic schools had either closed or their naturopathic program had been merged within a chiropractic school. Difficulties within the profession itself and its relationship with the chiropractic profession made matters worse. The number of practising physicians was in rapid decline as the retiring doctors were not being replaced by equal numbers of graduating physicians.

By the early 1950s the situation was dire. Most of the chiropractic colleges that had been offering a naturopathic curriculum cancelled that part of their program. National College of Drugless Physicians in Chicago, which graduated over 85% of the naturopathic doctors practicing in western Canada, closed its naturopathic program and only offered chiropractic in 1952. By 1953 Western States Chiropractic College (WSCC) in Portland, Oregon was the only institution offering an approved ND program.

DR. BENEDICT LUST
Founder and President of American School of Naturopathy and American School of Chiropractic

A Dignified Profession — Doctor of Naturopathy

You are ambitious—you are intelligent; do not allow the lack of an extensive and long college education stand in your way of entering a wonderful, handsome paying profession. Study the new marvelous science of Naturopathy at our School of Biological Healing. Covers the entire field of Natural Methods, as Diet, Chiropractic, Osteopathy, Hydrotherapy, Massage and Physical Culture. Study under enthusiastic, earnest professors with the best of modern equipment. Day and night classes. Busy, practical clinics. Students can pursue studies on self-supporting plan.

Founded 1896 by Dr. Benedict Lust. Incorporated 1905 under the Laws of the State of New York.

Our Graduates are recognized by all Naturopathic State Boards of America, Canada, and foreign countries.

START TODAY ON A HELPFUL AND PAYING CAREER
SEND 25c FOR FULL EDUCATIONAL LITERATURE

American School of Naturopathy and American School of Chiropractic
DR. BENEDICT LUST, President and Dean
Dept. L., 7 West 76th Street   New York, N. Y.

This ad appeared in "The Naturopath" magazine in the early 1900s

Dr. Budden, president of WSCC was a staunch supporter of naturopathic medicine and refused to discontinue the program. He was knowledgeable in accreditation and knew that as long as his college met the standards, approval could not be withdrawn. The naturopathic program as WSCC was short-lived and in 1955 the program was cancelled following the passing of Dr. Budden. Once this happened, the naturopathic profession had no means of replenishing its ranks especially in the western provinces. Of tremendous consideration was that the licensing law in British Columbia would only remain active if there was an approved college in operation. Despite all of the ongoing obstacles, if the profession were to have a chance at survival, it was imperative that a new college dedicated to naturopathic medicine come into existence.

In 1956 National College of Naturopathic Medicine, a school dedicated to naturopathic medicine opened its doors. It was not until 1978 that a naturopathic college opened in Canada.

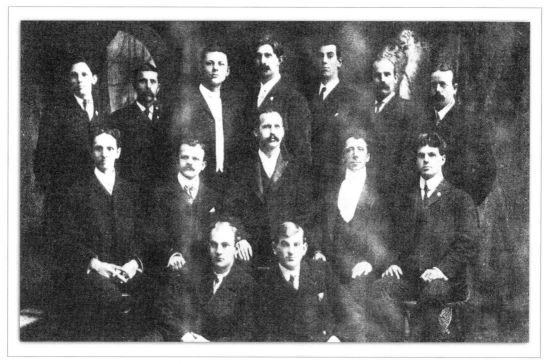

1902 Graduating Class of American School of Naturopathy

The School that Saved the Profession

Adopted from a write-up provided by Dr. Sandesh Singh Khalsa ND

Starting in early 1950s, officers of the naturopathic associations of British Columbia, Oregon and Washington began meeting to discuss what would happen when the program at Western States College was cancelled and to consider the founding of a new school. They were committed to seeing naturopathic medicine survive and on May 28th, 1956 the charter for the new school, National College of Naturopathic Medicine (NCNM), was privately incorporated. Naturopathic doctors Charles Stone, Martin Bleything, Frank Spaulding, Joseph Boucher, Elizabeth B. Murray, Gerald Farnsworth, Carl Kennedy Sr., Dorothy Johnstone and Henry Merritt successfully took the first step to establish a naturopathic college dedicated to naturopathic medicine. A major reason for choosing Oregon over Washington or British Columbia as the home for the new school was the strong licensing law and broad scope of practice in that state.

The initial board of trustees had members from each of the founding associations. This was intended to allow input from physicians throughout the Northwest and ensure the college was responsive to the needs of the profession rather than to one individual or a small group.

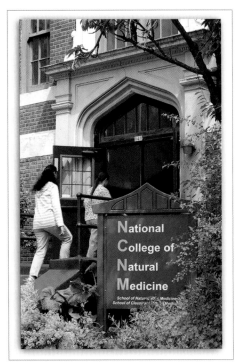

National College of Natural Medicine

The college was started on a shoestring and prior to opening there had been no advertising or formal recruiting process for students. To help provide resources for the fledgling institution, donations were solicited from naturopathic physicians throughout the country. During the first year of operation, there were five students - one was a first year student and other four were post-graduate chiropractors seeking the ND degree. There was no money to pay faculty, administration or staff. For the first number of years the small number of staff would often pay College bills from their own pocket and await payment until tuition money or donations came in. Faculty and administration did not receive a salary for many years to come.

During the early years NCNM was academically successful but there was incompetence due to inexperience. A weakness in the program was the lack of medical and laboratory equipment; a strength was the close student contact and apprentice-like training that the student's received.

The number of naturopathic physicians who were available and/or willing to teach was few. Doctors from British Columbia and Washington travelled from their homes on weekends to teach classes and participate in Board meetings. Travel by car in the late 1950s was much slower than today. There were no interstate highways in place and air service was unreliable or unavailable, even if you could afford it. As an example; it was sixteen hours by car from Kamloops, BC, the home of Drs. Gerald and Earl Farnsworth ND to Portland, Oregon – a trip which they made monthly, sometimes weekly, for years. In addition NDs Joseph Boucher, Robert Fleming, Fred Loffler, Al Russell and Ron Holden traveled to Portland from British Columbia on a frequent basis. From Seattle came NDs Walter Adams, John Bastyr, George Rombough, O.G. Carroll, Robert Carroll and others. Dr. Arno Koegler ND from Ontario, was also a significant financial contributor and occasionally travelled to teach at the college. The heart of any school is its faculty. They impart knowledge to the students, but more importantly they set an example for attitude and behaviour. NCNM has been fortunate to have had so many exemplary faculty over the years.

The struggles of NCNM were significant in the late 1950s. The financial picture was bleak, students numbered only a few per class and the facilities were marginal. In 1958 the decision was made to move the main program to Seattle, closer to more of the teaching physicians. The 1960s to the 1970s were almost a lost generation for the profession due to the low number of graduates each year. However, those who did go through the program developed a strong sense of comradeship and commitment to the profession and were active in ensuring the survival and growth of the profession for years after. By the early 1970s the classes began to grow in size. The college was still struggling financially, but it was able to stay afloat due to the continual efforts of its founders, faculty and administration. If there is a common view expressed by those who attended NCNM in the early years, it was that they were fortunate to have had the opportunity to learn from a group of highly skilled and dedicated naturopathic physicians. In the late 1960s and into the next decade, doctoral and post-doctoral teachers from the University of Washington were added to the faculty. They taught biochemistry, neuroanatomy and physiology and were the first paid faculty at the college. During this time, there was a lot of focus on the basic science component of the curriculum since passing the basic science exams was linked to licensure in many states and provinces. At that time, there was one group of basic science exams for all types of physicians seeking licensure, including medical doctors, chiropractors, osteopaths and naturopathic physicians.

As it is today, the course of study was demanding. The graduates felt that they received a good education overall and were sufficiently prepared for practice. It was also common for new graduates of that era to spend a year or two in an established doctor's office observing and assisting in order to develop additional confidence and experience before licensure and setting up their own practice.

In 1973 NCNM entered into an agreement with the College of Emporia in Kansas to transfer the first two years of the naturopathic program, the basic sciences. Later that year, due to financial difficulties at the College of Emporia, the students were transferred, yet again, to Kansas Newman College (KNC). The environment at Kansas College was very different than NCNM. It was a very conservative and a much larger campus where most of the students and faculty knew little, if anything, about naturopathic medicine. The feeling and learning experience was quite different than that offered at NCNM. During the day, students took basic science classes taught by professors of Kansas College and two to three evenings a week attended additional classes taught by naturopathic physicians in topics such as naturopathic philosophy and history, pathobiology, introduction to pathology, and clinical and physical diagnosis.

The tuition for Kansas College was $2,090 per year, compared to the $1,500 that students had paid in Seattle. One major advantage to the unity with Kansas was that NCNM students now had access to Federally Insured Student Loans. Professors at Kansas College contributed greatly in strengthening the basic science component of the naturopathic education. Yet, the gains realized in the basic science education came with a price. There was no naturopathic clinic associated with the campus and there was only one naturopathic physician with whom the students could interact most of the time. However, there were guest lectures from visiting NDs, such as NDs John Bastyr, Joseph Boucher, Gerald Farnsworth, Robert Fleming, George Rombough, Bill Mitchell and Joe Pizzorno.

With every change and growth the increased need for clinic space, classrooms, equipment, staff, supervisors and faculty required more funding and resources. There were many fundraising initiatives proposed, such as requesting that every physician in Canada and the licensed states donate $20 a month for two years to upgrade and update the physical structure and appearance of the College. Even though most of the fundraising initiatives were not very successful, it was due to the continual support of naturopathic doctors and their families that NCNM was able to stay afloat.

By the late 1970s, it was becoming increasingly obvious that it was important for naturopathic doctors to have their full training in a naturopathic environment. Therefore, in 1976 NCNM's Seattle campus closed and the operation was moved back to Portland. The basic sciences portion was united with the Portland curriculum in 1979. When the students from Seattle arrived at the new building in Portland, the rooms were undeveloped and the clinic had not yet been established. This small group of students took classes during the day and worked on interior construction of the classrooms and clinic at night and on weekends. In 1978 when Ontario College of Naturopathic Medicine (OCNM) in Toronto and the John Bastyr College (Bastyr) in Seattle opened, NCNM provided the curriculum details and supported the development of both schools.

The late 1970s was a challenging time for NCNM. Differences in educational philosophy and management style were emerging and there were differing opinions about how the constant change should be handled. The internal struggles almost resulted in its closure. In the end, the College emerged intact and ready to move onto the next phase of its development.

By 1980 NCNM was beginning to meet the standards of stability and accountability needed for an institution of higher education. The future of naturopathic medicine appeared much brighter than it had twenty-five years earlier. The vision and dedication over many years created NCNM and allowed it to succeed in spite of tremendous obstacles. The naturopathic profession owes a wave of gratitude to a small group of men and women who put their hearts into supporting NCNM and, at great personal sacrifice, contributed the time, money and knowledge required.

All of us who practice naturopathic medicine and have benefitted from its services, owe these doctors a tremendous debt of gratitude. Although there continue to be individuals that are dedicated to the growth and development of the profession, the level of commitment, generosity and sacrifice that the founders and elders exhibited will never be matched.

Academic Accreditation

Adopted from information provided by Joseph Pizzorno ND, Co-Founder CNME and founding president, Bastyr University.

Accreditation is recognition granted to educational institutions and professional programs indicating that a high level of quality and integrity has been achieved. Accreditation also provides the general public, the educational community, governmental agencies, other organizations and potential students' confidence in a specific program and institution.

Since the 1920s many of the provincial and state regulations required that a naturopathic doctor graduate from a school that both provided a four-year naturopathic medical program and was approved by the states and provinces licensing naturopathic medicine in order to achieve licensure. This caused some difficulties within the profession, as not all of the states and provinces agreed on which schools should be approved and what the academic standards were. Hence, graduates were restricted from practicing in various jurisdictions.

Due to the decline in the naturopathic profession and the dominance of the political environment by the medical profession, the late 1970s were a challenging time for naturopathic medical education. Only National College of Naturopathic Medicine (NCNM) was recognized by the states and provinces as an acceptable naturopathic medical institution and yet there were new colleges being started. There was tremendous need to ensure that the profession had consistent accreditation standards recognized not only by the profession, but by the government and the public.

In 1978, the National Association of Naturopathic Physicians called together the presidents of NCNM, John Bastyr College of Naturopathic Medicine (now Bastyr University) and the Ontario College of Naturopathic Medicine (now Canadian College of Naturopathic Medicine), presidents of the non-residential, non-degree granting "naturopathic" programs, select members of the profession and interested influential public members. At this meeting the Council of Naturopathic Medical Education (CNME), the Federation of Naturopathic Boards and the Federation of Naturopathic Colleges were formed. The purpose of this was to provide curriculum standardization, a central accreditation body and ongoing unity of naturopathic medicine across North America. The doctors involved in the foundation of CNME included: NDs Joe Pizzorno, John Bastyr, R. Boyce, Richard Finley, A.H.W. Norton, Cyrus Maxfield, M Loftin, M Shelton and Eric Shrubb and Jeffery S. Bland PhD.

There were three colleges that provided a 4-year residential education leading to a degree or diploma. Other schools offered mail order programs and "naturopathic" education that was not recognized or considered credible by any state or province. The residential colleges wanted high, graduate-level academic standards and to achieve recognition by the U.S. Department of Education while the others wanted few or no standards. Happily, after several years of argument and struggle, academic standards won. Naturopathic Drs. Carlo Calabrese and Joe Pizzorno, with the help of others, wrote the rigorous academic and institutional standards, carried them through the gauntlet of review by state and provincial licensing bodies and colleges, developed a comprehensive application, and appeared before tough governmental committees. All the hard work paid off in 1987 when the CNME was granted recognition by the U.S. Department of Education. This was an historic achievement for the profession and began laying the foundation of credibility that allowed the profession to blossom in the 1990s.

CNME continues to uphold strict curriculum and educational standards that encompass a four-year full-time program that leads to a Naturopathic Doctor (ND) or Naturopathic Medical Doctor (NMD) degree or diploma, depending on the school. It is also the only accrediting agency that is recognized by the Canadian and American national associations of naturopathic medicine and the US Government.

CNME has established itself as a strong accrediting body, but its growth and development has endured its own challenges and lessons. In 2000 CNME's recognition by the US Secretary of Education was withdrawn due to perceptions of how specific CNME policies were being enforced. CNME remained the accrediting agency recognized by the national naturopathic associations and in 2003 its recognition was re-established with the US Secretary of Education. For further information on CNME visit their website at www.cnme.org

Standardized Exams

The requirement for naturopathic standardized licensing exams has occurred in a few provinces since naturopathic medicine was first regulated.

Similar to the accrediting concerns, there were issues around the inconsistency in the standardized exams written by NDs within the different provinces and in 1986 this issue threatened the licensing of Hawaii. They were informed that, in order to maintain licensure, the profession had to establish standardized exams to ensure that practitioners licensed in one state could transfer to another. Naturopathic doctors from Washington, Oregon, Hawaii and Connecticut, in conjunction with representatives from Bastyr and NCNM formed the Naturopathic Physicians Licensing Examinations (NPLEX). Over the next few years they worked with different national testing companies to establish standardized exams for the naturopathic profession. The original nine-member NPLEX Board had representatives from the states Arizona, Connecticut, Hawaii and Washington; the provinces British Columbia and Manitoba; from Bastyr and NCNM; and from the American Association of Naturopathic Physicians. Representatives from CCNM and the Canadian Association of Naturopathic Doctors were added in 1993.

Initially the exams only included the clinical component. In 1990 the decision was made to bring the exam production in-house and to have NPLEX establish standardized exams for both the basic medical sciences and the clinical component which they have done ever since. Dr. Christa Louise, PhD, the executive director of NPLEX and NABNE, has spear-headed this project for the last 19 years. It is thanks to her dedication and high standards that the naturopathic profession has developed standardized exams that are comparable to any other medical profession.

Originally the various jurisdictions determined who was eligible to write the standardized exams. In 1999 it was decided that there was too much inconsistency between the different jurisdictions and the North American Board of Examiners (NABNE) was established to set policies regarding the qualifications and administration of the exams. Since then, only graduates of a CNME approved school are eligible to write the NPLEX exams.

Naturopathic doctors from Western Canada have written NPLEX exams since the early 1990s. OCNM renamed CCNM started using the exams in 1993. Currently, graduates of accredited schools who wish to practice in Canada and in most States, must take and pass NPLEX. The current exams consist of three sections: basic medical science exam (anatomy, physiology, pathology, biochemistry, microbiology and immunology) that is written after 2nd year; clinical science exam (clinical and physical diagnosis, laboratory diagnosis and diagnostic imaging, botanical medicine, pharmacology, nutrition, physical medicine, psychology and lifestyle counselling, homeopathy and emergency medicine), and add-on exams (acupuncture and minor surgery) that are written after 4th year of study. Jurisprudence and the provincial practical examinations are prepared and administered by the separate regulatory boards in Canada and the United States. For more information on NPLEX exams or NABNE visit their website at www.nabne.org

Naturopathic Curriculum

Four-year naturopathic curriculums have been offered since the 1920s. Part of the regulation of naturopathic medicine in different provinces and in the United States included the accreditation and recognition of schools that met specific standards.

Naturopathic Doctors undergo training similar to medical doctors. Following three years of pre-med sciences at a recognized university, a student would then complete four years of full time study that includes more than 4,500 hours of classroom training and 1,500 hours of supervised clinical experience. It is during this four year intensive program that students are trained on the following four areas of study:

Basic Sciences - This area of study includes anatomy, physiology, histology, microbiology, biochemistry, immunology, pharmacology and pathology.

Clinical Disciplines - Diagnostic medicine areas of study include physical and clinical diagnosis, differential and laboratory diagnosis, radiology, naturopathic assessment and orthopaedics.

Naturopathic Disciplines - Each discipline is a distinct area of practice and includes diagnostic principles and practices, as well as therapeutic skills and techniques. They include: clinical nutrition, botanical medicine, traditional Chinese medicine and acupuncture, homeopathic medicine,

Western States College and the National College in Chicago, Illinois, were approved under the BC Naturopathic Physicians Act of 1936 as accredited educational institutions for NDs. Both colleges taught residence courses for at least four years of eight months per year for a total of at least 4,000 hours as required by the Act. Western States graduated naturopathic doctors through 1959.

Curriculum in Naturopathy

Prescribed Work

FIRST YEAR

Fall Quarter

Course No.	Course Name	Term Credits	Class Hours
Anat. 111	Osteology	2	60
Chem. 101	Inorg. Chemistry	2	60
Anat. 151	Histology	2	60
Nat. 101	Introduction to Naturopathy	2	60
Phys. 101	Physiology	4	120

Winter Quarter

Course No.	Course Name	Term Credits	Class Hours
Anat. 112	Osteology	1	30
Anat. 113	Syndesmology	1	30
Chem. 102	Inorganic Chemistry	2	60
Anat. 152	Histology	2	60
Phys. 102	Physiology	4	120
Anat. 211 & 212	Angiology & Lymphatics	2	60

Spring Quarter

Course No.	Course Name	Term Credits	Class Hours
Chem. 120	Organic Chemistry	2	60
Anat. 114	Myology	2	60
Bact. 131	Bacteriology	2	60
Phys. 103	Physiology	4	120
Nat. 103	Splanchnology	2	60
Nat. 117	First Aid	1	20
		35	1110

Page 20

Western States College: Curriculum in Naturopathy, 1952

Western States College First-year Curriculum from 1952

hydrotherapy, naturopathic manipulation and lifestyle counselling.

Clinical Experience - All students must complete 1,500 hours of clinical requirements and demonstrate proficiency in all aspects of Naturopathic Medicine prior to graduation. Naturopathic doctors complete this supervised clinical experience at the student clinics that are part of the school or at satellite clinics that are affiliated with the schools.

Course Listing

Course Code	Course Name	Credit Hours
First Year		
ASM102	Asian Medicine Fundamentals	2.0
ASM103	Asian Medicine Point Location I	2.0
BAS100	Anatomy	13.0
BAS103	Biochemistry	3.0
BAS107	Physiology	12.0
BAS108	Embryology	1.5
BAS112	Histopathology	3.0
BAS115	Immunology	4.0
BOT101	Botanical Medicine I	2.5
CPH101	Public Health	2.0
HOM100	Homeopathic Medicine I	2.0
NMS101	Ethics and Jurisprudence I	1.0
NPH101	Naturopathic History, Philosophy, Principles	2.0
NPH102	The Art and Practice of Naturopathic Medicine	2.0
NUT102	Clinical Nutrition I	3.0
PHM104	Massage/Hydrotherapy	3.0
PSY103	Health Psychology I	2.5
RES100	Principles in Research	3.0
TOTAL YEAR ONE		**63.5**
Second Year		
ASM202	Asian Medicine Diagnosis and Pathology	2.5
ASM203	Asian Medicine Point Location II	1.0
ASM204	Asian Medicine Point Location III	1.0
BAS205	Microbiology	4.0
BAS206	Pathology	6.0
BAS208	Pharmacology	5.0
BOT202	Botanical Medicine II	5.0
CLE200	Clinic I	1.0
CLS201	Differential Diagnosis	8.0
CLS202	Laboratory Diagnosis	5.0
CLS221	Physical and Clinical Diagnosis Theory	3.0
CLS222	Physical and Clinical Diagnosis Practicum	2.5
FNM200	Foundations of Naturopathic Medicine	1.5
HOM202	Homeopathic Medicine II Advanced Fundamentals	3.0
HOM203	Homeopathic Medicine II Clinical Applications	1.0
NUT202	Clinical Nutrition II	5.0
PHM201	Naturopathic Manipulation I	2.0
PSY203	Health Psychology II	1.5
TOTAL YEAR TWO		**58.0**

Academic Calendar 2008/2009   45

**Canadian College of Naturopathic Medicine Curriculum from 2008
(Years 1 & 2 of their 4 year program)**

Conventions and Continuing Medical Education

In the early 1900s naturopathic conventions attracted thousands of practitioners from many systems of medicine. During the 1930s to the 1950s the number of conventions decreased dramatically to the point of extinction. In 1957 the Northwest Naturopathic Physicians Convention, organized by NDs Joseph Boucher, Doug Kirkbride and Gerry Farnsworth, was considered the reawakening of naturopathic conventions for Canada and the United States. The three associations – British Columbia, Washington and Oregon – participated in the organization. Overtime Alberta and Idaho have also become participants. The initial conference was held in Nanaimo, BC and to this day there continues to be yearly conferences that alternate between Washington, Oregon and British Columbia.

The Ontario association has held yearly naturopathic conferences since 1963 and the B.C. association has held seminars and conventions for its members since 1994. The CAND also holds the biannual naturopathic conference Health Fusion.

All the regulated provinces in Canada have mandatory continuing education as part of their licensing requirements. Continuing medical education is offered by the schools, by the associations and by some of the professional health product companies. In the last few years many of the continuing education

The first Northwest Naturopathic Physician's convention in 1957 was considered the reawakening of naturopathic conventions for Canada and the United States.

courses and conferences have been extended to external practitioners, such as medical doctors, chiropractors, and other primary care providers that are interested in the naturopathic approach to health and healing.

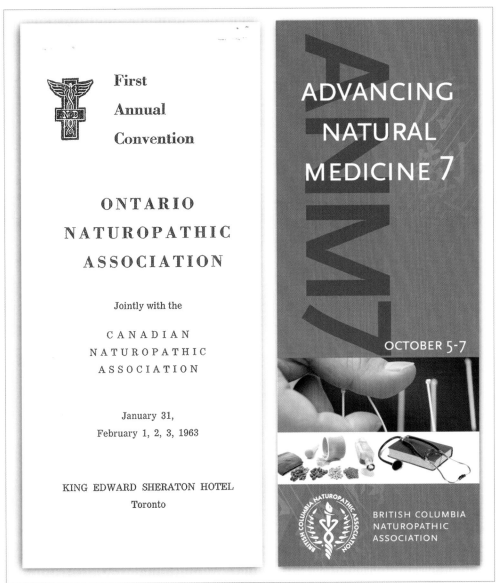

1963 conference   conference 2007

CHAMPION:
DR. JOSEPH AIME BOUCHER,
DC ND (1916-1987)

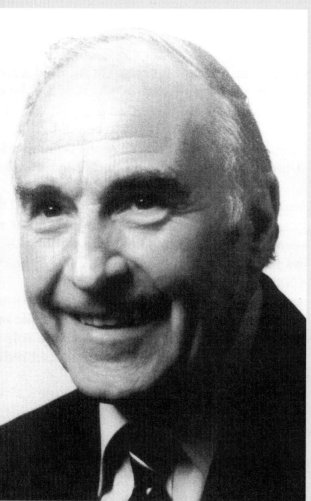

JOSEPH AIME BOUCHER WAS BORN in Edmonton, Alberta on October 17, 1916. He was an eleventh generation Canadian and the second eldest of eight children. At the age of four he moved to British Columbia where he lived for most of his life. He had a varied career: a caddy for golfers, cook, construction worker and a dairy truck driver. He did these odd jobs while attending business college at night. He was also a deck hand on a coastal freighter and after that worked in a large wholesale grocery firm where he met Patricia, his future wife. They married in 1941 and had three children.

When the war broke out in 1939, Joe transferred to the Royal Canadian Navy Coastguard Service with the rank of Petty Officer. He spent the next two and a half years patrolling the west coast of British Columbia. His ship was the first to investigate the only incident of shelling by a Japanese submarine of Canada at Hesqueth on the west coast of Vancouver Island.

Joe subsequently received a medical discharge from the navy due to severe ulcerative colitis. At the age of twenty-nine, he was faced with the threat of surgery and a colostomy. The thought of this was far too frightening for him to accept. He decided to try an alternative approach by visiting a naturopathic physician. This proved to be a good decision since he completely recovered a year later.

Being an individual who did nothing in half measures, Joe decided to enter the field of natural healing and in 1949 he moved with his family to Portland and enrolled at the Western State College of Chiropractic. He also enrolled at

Lewis and Clark College to complete his requirements for a Bachelor of Arts in Psychology.

Despite his gruelling work load, he graduated with honours in all three categories – BA, DC and ND. Dr. Boucher returned to Vancouver with his family and opened a practice. He was immediately selected to the Board of Directors of the Association of Naturopathic Physicians of British Columbia (ANPBC) and held continuous office in the different associations for the next thirty-two years: including Board member, Secretary, President, Chairman of the Examining Committee, Executive Secretary and a term as President of the Canadian Naturopathic Association.

Dr. Boucher was completely dedicated to the cause and support of naturopathic medicine. He was a pioneer of naturopathic medicine in both Oregon and British Columbia and he was one of the founders of National College of Naturopathic Medicine in 1956. He, along with the other co-founders, travelled every month (quite often even weekly) to teach, attend Board meetings, act as a carpenter and painter and oversee the school's operations. This was done at his own expense. During all of this time, Dr. Boucher conducted a busy practice promoting the teachings of earlier naturopathic pioneers. Dr. Boucher often spoke of NDs Claunch, Kleiner, Tilden, Shelton and many other pioneers. He was always a bold promoter of naturopathic principles, even during the darkest years, and became a sought after public speaker.

Despite his busy professional life, he was an avid outdoor sportsman, becoming a formidable contender for anyone challenging him at tennis, badminton, racquetball, cross-country skiing and especially at his favourite pastime, hiking. His two most loved hiking areas were the rugged West Coast Trail on Vancouver Island and the Black Tusk in Garabaldi Park. He also became a skilled cine photographer, producing two feature length films recording his love of hiking.

Dr. Joe Boucher was a paragon of health, fitness, positive mental attitude and love of service. His practice was truly holistic, blending psychology with natural medicines and exercise. He was a true Hippocratic Physician who taught correct living.

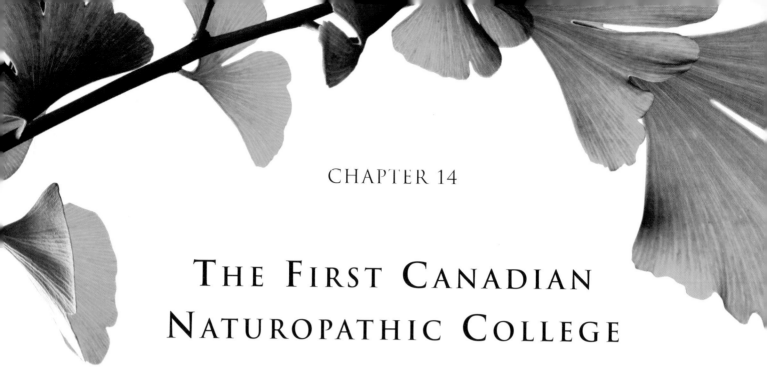

CHAPTER 14

THE FIRST CANADIAN NATUROPATHIC COLLEGE

IN THIRTY SHORT YEARS the Ontario College of Naturopathic Medicine (OCNM), renamed in 1992 to the Canadian College of Naturopathic Medicine (CCNM), developed from just an idea into the largest naturopathic program in North America.

OCNM developed as an educational institution within a challenging economic, political and legislative environment in Ontario – the profession was under threat of deregulation. The number of practitioners was dwindling and since the underlying principles of the naturopathic curriculum were not in line with conventional medicine, all funding had to be acquired personally or through donation. In fact, in the late 1970s, the Ontario government felt that the naturopathic profession was likely to disappear due to the small number of practitioners and a lack of educational institution. Members of the Ontario Naturopathic Association (ONA), in conjunction with support from others, did what needed to be done to ensure that naturopathic medicine survived in Ontario.

Creating and managing a school are two parts of a "professional formation" balancing act. There are accreditation standards that are set by the profession that have to be met; government standards for educational institutions; funding considerations; staff and student expectations and the ongoing challenge of ensuring that it all works together as a seamless process. The formation of OCNM, like most new enterprises, has enjoyed significant growth and recognition, but it has also endured recurrent financial hardships and internal challenges. The institution learned not only how to overcome operational difficulties but also how to manoeuvre though the tricky waters of political conflict as the complexities of administering both full- and part-time programs emerged. Today the College is a solid and strong institution of naturopathic medical education, thanks to the efforts of a number of dedicated people.

Prior to having a naturopathic college in Ontario many of the naturopathic practitioners and drugless therapists were graduates of the Canadian Memorial Chiropractic College (CMCC) which opened in Toronto Ontario in 1945. In CMCC's founding charter it included the right to teach naturopathy. Graduates of CMCC could take additional courses and then write an exam which would give the practitioners a dual license of DC-DT. DT stood for "drugless therapist" which was the term under which naturopaths in Ontario were originally regulated. The operation of a dual chiropractic-naturopathic program was offered in Canada for over twenty years after similar programs in the United States had ended. Dr. Earl Homewood, a chiropractor and a naturopath, was the administrator of CMCC from 1952 to 1961 and then the president of the college from 1968 to 1969. He gave the following reasons for including naturopathy in the college's charter document: (a) Ontario statute provided for Drugless Therapist (DT); (b) The majority of Ontario chiropractors (DCs) held a dual registration (DC-DT); and (c) To forestall the competition from a separate naturopathic college. In 1958 and again in 1963 the ONA, with the support of the other provincial associations, requested that CMCC institute a chair of Naturopathy. Due to ongoing political challenges and internal issues, CMCC was unable to accommodate the request. In 1977 CMCC dropped the ND component of their curriculum. This gave way for the start of the Ontario College of Naturopathic Medicine.

Where it Began

(Adapted from the stories written by Dr. Eric Shrubb, DC ND, co-founder of OCNM, and Dr. James L.Wilson DC ND, Ph.D. class of '81)

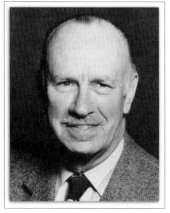

Dr. Robert Farquharson ND

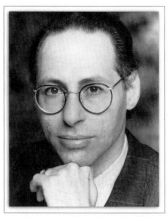

Dr. Gregory (Asa) Hershoff ND

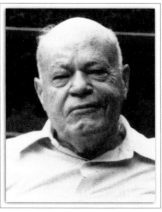

Dr. John LaPlante ND

Before the Canadian College of Naturopathic Medicine (CCNM) came to be, there was the Ontario College of Naturopathic Medicine (OCNM). This was preceded by a small group of doctors who met every couple of weeks to discuss various health issues, the politics involved, and to hope and dream of one day having a naturopathic college in Canada. This group started meeting in the mid 1970s and was affectionately known as "the Bridge Club" because there were usually about as many people at the meetings as it takes to play a couple hands of bridge. They were the true pioneers of the College who dreamed the dream and held the vision that eventually manifested itself into OCNM. The Bridge Club was started by naturopathic doctors John LaPlante and Bob Farquharson and grew to a group of about twelve practitioners including Drs. Eric and Frances (Eddleston) Shrubb, Norah Stewart, Gregory Asa Hershoff, Muriel Grant, Leo Roy, Bill Morris, and occasionally Wilmot Browett. All were members of the ONA and were outstanding naturopathic practitioners and mavericks in their own way.

The Bridge Club knew there was an immediate need for a naturopathic school to augment the number of ND registrants in Ontario and to provide access to the naturopathic therapies for an increasing contingent of chiropractors and drugless practitioners who were losing scope due to changes in provincial legislation. The OCNM was founded at a general meeting of the ONA at the Chelsea Inn in June of 1978.

Robert B. Farquharson, G. Asa Hershoff, John G. LaPlante, William Morris, Eric Shrubb and Gordon F. Smith officially started the OCNM as a division of the ONA. Other members, such as naturopathic doctors Frances (Eddleston) Shrubb, Muriel Grant, John Cosgrove, Ken Dunk, Alexander (Sandy) Wood, Susan Rohn and James Wilson were also very involved in a lot of the background work and in financially supporting the efforts of the college. Dr. Eric Shrubb was the first Chairman of the Board of Governers and Dr. Arno Koegler ND was appointed to the role of honorary President. Dr. Koegler's involvement was widely regarded as a strong endorsement for the school since he had been a key elder and leader of the profession in Canada since 1926.

The plans for the college involved meetings and phone calls with representatives from the National College of Naturopathic Medicine (NCNM) and with Dr. Joe Boucher, president of the Canadian Naturopathic Association (CNA) to ensure the curriculum standards were in line with those that were already established by the profession. Dr. Ronald Hoye ND, then president of NANP also made frequent visits to Toronto and provided tremendous support and motivation.

The first phase of the plan included a postgraduate program which trained doctors from other health professions to become naturopathic doctors. Before OCNM could begin, official sanction from the Board of Directors of Drugless Therapy – Naturopathy (BDDT-N) to award the special designation of Doctor of Naturopathy (ND) to their future graduates had to be obtained. This done, the more daunting hurdle: finding instructors both qualified and able to teach was undertaken. It may be hard to imagine now, but back then "natural"/"alternative"/"complementary" medicine had not even breached the horizon of public consciousness. There was only one naturopathic college in all of North America and very few towns or cities had physicians knowledgeable in natural healing methods. Finally, enough teachers were found to begin the postgraduate program. Ironically, in order for NCNM to survive in the 1950s and 1960s, many of the Canadian naturopathic doctors travelled to Portland, Oregon to teach. In support of OCNM when it first opened, many of the NDs from NCNM travelled to Ontario.

There were 56 students enrolled in the initial accelerated postgraduate program – 32 who graduated in June of 1981. Most were chiropractors, dentists and medical doctors with full time practices. There were also a number of foreign medical practitioners. The classes were conducted in blocks of three eight-hour days and one weekend a month over three-and-a-half years. The first Registrar of the OCNM was Thomas Foster, BIS, MA. He also served as the administrator and lectured on the history, principles, and philosophy of naturopathic medicine. Dr. Gord Smith ND was appointed as the first Academic Dean of OCNM, as well as, its first Clinic Director. There were many efforts to establish a physical college prior to the onset of the first class but that did not materialize and, instead, the class sessions alternated between the

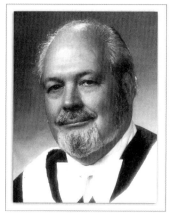

Dr. Bill Morris ND

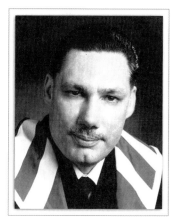

Dr. Eric Shrubb ND

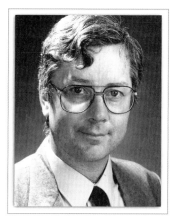

Dr. Gordon Smith ND

Chelsea Hotel in downtown Toronto and the Inn on the Park in Northeast Toronto.

In 1979 Dr. Eric Shrubb ND met with the Council for Naturopathic Medical Education (CNME) and reported that, in order for OCNM to be accredited and recognized as a naturopathic college, at the very least, five key accreditation standards were required to get started:

An official publication generated by the naturopathic college and the profession.

A physical structure in which the college would reside.

A list of faculty members.

A library, preferably located in the college building.

A graduate of an accredited naturopathic college to sign documents on behalf of the College to legitimize its authenticity.

Of these, the most challenging was the physical structure, a building to house OCNM. Real estate in Toronto was prohibitively expensive. Although the College was operating profitably, there were not nearly enough funds to make a down-payment on a building, or even to rent a facility. The second challenge was finding a licensed graduate of a recognized naturopathic college who

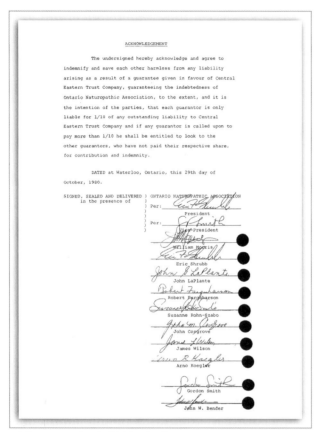

These are the individuals that guaranteed the OCNM mortgage on the Benton Street property in Kitchener.

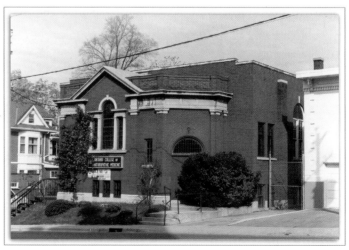

1st home for OCNM - 32 Benton Street, Kitchener

would sign the required documents. This challenge was addressed by a wonderful coincidence. Dr. Gordon Smith had just graduated from NCNM and was moving to Ontario. His arrival acted as the final impetus needed to move toward the establishment of an accredited naturopathic college.

In order to afford a building a fund raising drive was held. Dr. Shrubb committed $5,000 on behalf of the board members. The first fundraising event netted $19,000 towards the building fund and that amount grew to over $40,000 within a month, primarily thanks to the generosity of the students.

After many months of searching, an affordable and suitable building was found on Benton Street in Kitchener. The building had been a church and it was protected by the Canadian Historical Society because of its unique architectural features. This building was the birth site of the longest reigning Canadian Prime Minister, William Lyon Mackenzie King. It seemed like an auspicious place to establish the College. The financing of the building was difficult as the bank did not want

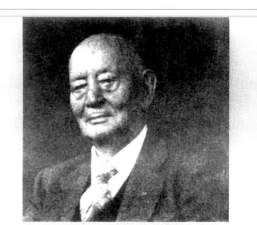

A MESSAGE FROM THE PRESIDENT

After over 50 years of dreaming, wishing and planning we finally have our own College of Naturopathic Medicine in Canada. Previous to this we had to go to the United States to get our training; this is one reason why we have a small number of Naturopathic Physicians in Canada at the present time. Now, anyone wishing to come into the profession will not have to first leave the country to do it.

People are becoming more interested in the natural way of treatment, but above all they are interested in preventive and wholistic medicine. As one who has practiced for over 60 years I have seen many wonderful cures without side effects. While conventional medicine with all its modern drugs has been more interested in relieving symptoms, Naturopathy has been treating the whole person and the cause of the ailments and above all teaching the patients how to keep well by proper eating and by changing their life style for better health. I consider Naturopathy the most rewarding and satisfying occupation and if I had my life to live over again I would select the same profession.

Even though Naturopathic principles are as old as history, they are as new as tomorrow because nature and truth never change. Any system that cured people years ago will help people today, and we can now scientifically validate and explain the clinical success of these approaches. Many people look for an alternative in the healing arts and this is it. In Europe we find many physicians taking up Naturopathy because they are disappointed in some of the new drugs with all their side effects. We are not trying to replace the surgeons (or conventional medical doctors); they have their place, but in many cases Naturopathy can do a better job.

Arno R. Koegler, N.D.
President

Arno Kroegler

to fund an unknown group with an unproven financial track record. In the end, the mortgage was personally guaranteed by ten naturopathic practitioners and students. These people pledged their professional and personal possessions as collateral. They put up their office equipment, personal valuables and even their houses to make certain the College would have a start. Their love for naturopathic medicine and their belief in its importance and future was very strong. The Kitchener property was purchased for $185,000 and in the spring of 1981 it became the first home for OCNM.

Turbulent Years

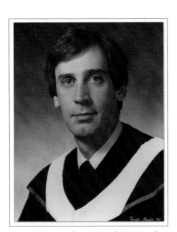

Dr. Alexander (Sandy) Wood ND a passionate visionary who has made many personal sacrifices and has supported the profession through many difficult times.

The years between 1982 and 1992 were a turbulent time for OCNM. In 1982, the college began to formulate its curriculum to be more consistent with the American schools. Dr. Joe Pizzorno ND, who was then president of Bastyr University, aided in this process by providing curriculum materials. Although this was a step in the right direction, there was much debate within the profession as to the content of the curriculum.

Adding to the internal challenges, in 1981 the Minister of Health in Ontario advised that college officials, board officials and members of an association could not be one and the same individuals. This resulted in a shift in naturopathic leadership, as the members that were active often held multiple positions at the same time. The Ontario government passed the *"Degree Granting Act"* in 1983, making it necessary to have authorization from the Ontario Legislature in order to grant degrees. The aim was to encourage new institutions, such as OCNM, to affiliate with currently established colleges or universities. For years board members of the OCNM held discussions with the University of Waterloo with the intention of them providing the basic sciences portion of the naturopathic program. These discussions looked promising, yet did not pan out.

Over the next decade OCNM struggled against the political temperament of the day, not only in terms of regulation of health care professionals under the Drugless Practitioner's Act, but also in terms of the higher education priorities of the time. In 2003, after 25 years in operation, CCNM applied for degree-granting status from the Ministry of Training, Colleges and Universities and, at the time of writing this book, they are confident that the degree-granting status will be achieved in the next few years, as it has been for all the naturopathic Colleges in the United States.

Early in the formation of the College, the decision was made to incorporate OCNM as a non-profit, charitable enterprise with direct links to the profession, but also with an autonomous management group accountable to the executive of the board. Dr. Wood ND spear-headed this initiative and on February 14th, 1984 The Institute of Naturopathic Education and Research (INER) was incorporated. The INER board continues to oversee the management of the College and is comprised of graduates of OCNM/CCNM and public members.

In the early years the growth of the college was difficult as a result of low student enrolment and the high teaching staff turnover. Even though much of the equipment and books for the new College were donated by members or pioneering supporters, the financial state of the college was unstable and those who had guaranteed the College continued to pay the ongoing expenses. In 1983, only two short years after the Kitchener location was purchased, the decision was made to sell the property and move the College to Toronto.

In 1983, an 18-month intensive program was offered and was open to qualified primary health care practitioners. At the same time, the first full-time four-year naturopathic program was also started. Between 1983 and 1989 there were three programs running at OCNM, including the original accelerated program which graduated its last class in 1989. These new programs demanded more resources, classroom space, teachers and infra-structure – all in short supply. In order to ensure that the curriculum demands were met, naturopathic doctors such as Gordon Smith, Alexander (Sandy) Wood, Robert Farquharson, Verna Hunt, John Cosgrove, Dennis O'Hara, John LaPlante, and Robert Gatis, among others, volunteered much of their time to the College for over ten years. The College was also fortunate in that other professors, such as Dr. Plog from Germany, Dr. Jeffery Bland PhD, Dr. Joe Pizzorno ND and Dr. Ronald Hoye ND taught at the College. Dr. Tony Manolis, who held a PhD from England, also volunteered and supported the College at a time when there was little financial compensation. Dr. Manolis was instrumental in setting high curriculum standards for teachers and for students. In 1989 the last group of students graduated from the accelerated program.

When the college moved to Bay Street in downtown Toronto in September 1984, it carried not only the financial burden of the Kitchener mortgage but the new monthly lease payments in Toronto. At this point, the College was in severe financial difficulty and sometimes surviving week-to-week. There were concerns that the bank could confiscate all the professional and personal assets; hurting some and throwing others into financial ruin. If the Toronto expenses were not paid, faculty would stop teaching, the lease on the building might be lost, and the

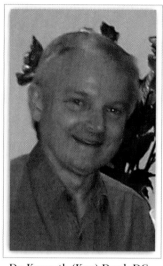

Dr. Kenneth (Ken) Dunk DC, ND a quiet, consistent figure in the naturopathic profession. Dr. Dunk has spent years serving on different Boards and has taught at OCNM/CCNM for about 25 consecutive years.

students, who had paid their tuition in good faith, would be in jeopardy of having neither a faculty nor a location. The college would likely cease to exist. During part of this time period, Dr. Wood ND chair of INER, often personally guaranteed the college's payroll and other expenses.

In 1984 the Kitchener building was finally sold, the debts of the College were covered, and the outstanding expenses were paid. OCNM was still struggling but was out of immediate financial danger. In 1986, OCNM relocated to Berl Avenue in Toronto, Ontario to accommodate the growth in enrolment and need for clinic space.

In the mid 1980s the government of Ontario inquired as to the existence of a naturopathic body of knowledge for the profession. Thanks to the work of Drs John Bender ND and Dr. Martin Kuro ND a 20 inch depth submission, which included over fifteen volumes of information, was assembled and submitted.

Throughout the 1980s, the College struggled with limited resources, internal curriculum-based controversy, disagreements about the management and direction of the College and growing internal and external dissention. Many believed that accreditation with the Council on Naturopathic Medical Education (CNME) would establish the school as a credible institution, adequately preparing NDs to enter the profession; a few others did not.

In 1990 the struggles between the College, the regulatory board and the ONA came to a head. Some of the members of INER included people from the United States who had graduated from non-CNME accredited schools and who did not meet the requirements for licensure as an ND in Ontario. There were concerns that they were abusing their authority without being fiscally responsible to the school. There was another group of

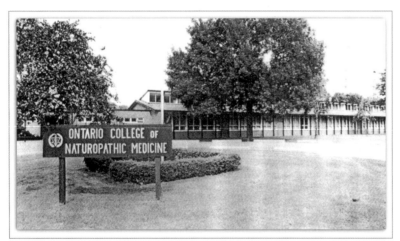

OCNM was located at 60 Berl Avenue, Toronto from 1986 until 1997.

INER members, who had graduated from CNME accredited schools and who had been members of the ONA and INER for a number of years. These members included naturopathic doctors Mark Percival, Richard Tunstall, John Bender, Verna Hunt, Marilyn May and Pamela Snider. They were called "the Requisitionists" as they took on the role of ombudsman for the profession. They were very passionate and very vocal about their concerns with these new members and with the direction that the college was taking with respect to accreditation, regulatory involvement and the growing antagonist relationship between the ONA and the OCNM board. Legal action was taken by the Requisitionists against the College that resulted in the OCNM board being replaced. This situation, and the aftermath that followed, marked one of the darkest moments in the history of the College. The College was near the point of bankruptcy. The respect that the college had built with regards to fiscal responsibility was greatly questioned, and the faith that students and alumni had in the College was almost non-existent. Dr. Don Warren was elected as the new chair of INER and Dr. Kenneth Pownall, DDS, BSc, a former Registrar of the Royal College of Dental Surgeons became the new President in September 1991. Dr. Pownall brought the credibility and network of twenty-five years as a senior officer of a primary health care regulatory body. Mr. Robert Schad, father of Dr. Katherine Willow ND a recent graduate of OCNM, came on board at the same time. He provided guidance, financial support and expertise on business formation and fiscal control. With the new board in place, there was a feeling that the College was back on track.

For the next few years the College focused on rebuilding its credibility with the profession by actively pursuing accreditation from CNME, by supporting the efforts of the Ontario regulatory board and the ONA, and by ensuring that all graduates successfully completed the new licensing exams (NPLEX) that had been put into place. Due to the challenging financial situation of the College, once again, board members such as Drs. Don Warren, Marilyn May, Wayne Scott, and Gerry Farnsworth, and Robert Schad found themselves personally guaranteeing the expenses of the College in order to alleviate student's concern about its solvency. Despite these difficult times, there was an encouraging sense of optimism in the school and in the profession.

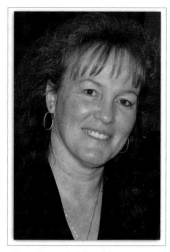

Dr. Pam Snider ND a true visionary and leader for the naturopathic profession. Dr. Snider spear-headed many initiatives and continues to work on strengthening the profession.

A Strong Educational Institution

On September 1st, 1992 the institution's name changed to the Canadian College of Naturopathic Medicine to reflect the national outlook of the College and to indicate the more global perspective that the College was adopting. With increased fundraising efforts, tight fiscal control, clear, strong leadership, and the dedication of a number of NDs and individuals, CCNM was able to meet the challenges that accompanied accreditation and secured the funding to ensure that the College was on solid ground. Once CCNM was financially stable it was able to expand its educational and clinic offerings. In 1996, David Schleich joined CCNM as president. He had experience in College administration and development and was hired with the explicit intention of expanding the funding and enrolment of the College. Within seven years he guided CCNM through tremendous growth and change. CCNM's enrolment increased from approximately 150s students to close to 400 annually.

From 1996 to 1999, CCNM was located at Yonge and Eglinton in Toronto while a suitable permanent location was found. In August 1999, CCNM relocated to 1255 Sheppard Avenue East in Toronto. This new campus included dormitory facilities for students, significantly expanded classrooms, a library

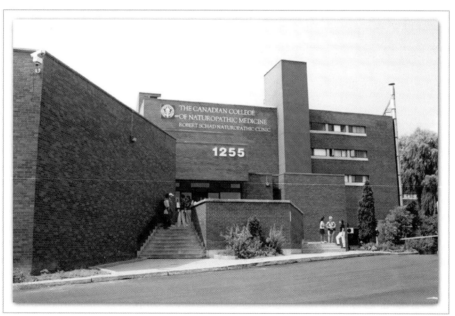

CCNM's current home at 1255 Sheppard Avenue East, Toronto

and student life facilities, a comprehensive on-campus clinic with more than 40 treatment rooms and a laboratory, with a unique courtyard which would eventually house an instructional recreational herbal garden.

In 2000, twenty-one years after the College's first inquiry, CCNM received accreditation from the CNME. CCNM was now one of five accredited naturopathic colleges in North America. It had finally achieved the recognition, financial stability and the status that the original founders had intended.

CCNM's rapid growth had resulted in tremendous changes. In 2004, Bob Bernhardt was hired as president and CEO of CCNM. He was successful in implementing the infrastructure and processes needed to sustain the growth at the College.

CCNM is currently the largest naturopathic college in North America. It continues to expand its educational and clinic offerings and to aid in the advancement of Naturopathic Medicine.

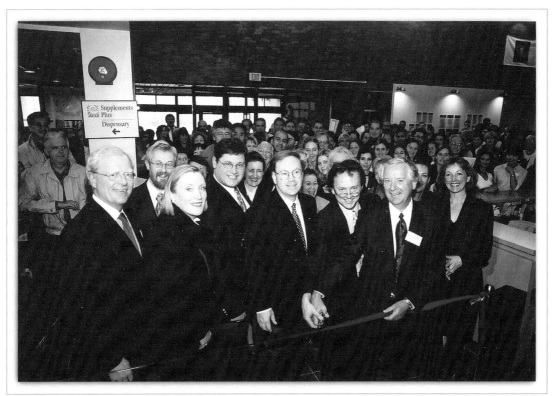

Opening of CCNM location at 1255 Sheppard Avenue East, Toronto

THE CANADIAN COLLEGE OF NATUROPATHIC MEDICINE

naturopathic
C O N N E C T I O N S

Autumn 2000

I N S I D E

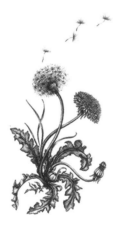

CCNM gains full accreditation

On September 11, CCNM received full accreditation by the Council on Naturopathic Medical Education (CNME) in recognition of the quality and integrity of its educational program. CNME is the accrediting agency for naturopathic colleges in North America.

"The achievement of accreditation is an honour for all CCNM students, staff and faculty," says David Schleich, CCNM President. "Our new status enables us to keep striving to produce leaders in the field of naturopathic medicine.

To achieve accreditation, CCNM underwent a rigorous evaluation process. As a candidate for accreditation, CCNM had to demonstrate to the CNME that its mission and objectives were soundly conceived, clearly stated and in the process of being accomplished. Also, CCNM's educational program had to meet the stringent standards of the council. Finally, CCNM had to show that it was organized, staffed and supported in such a way that it would continue to merit confidence. Now, to maintain its standing as an accredited institution, CCNM will continue to be periodically re-evaluated by the CNME.

Since 1992, when CCNM first achieved candidacy for accreditation status (under its former name, Ontario College of Naturopathic Medicine), CCNM students were eligible to write NPLEX examinations (naturopathic physicians licensing examinations encompassing all North American jurisdictions), as well as provincial licensing examinations. Only students attending and graduating from an accredited program (or program with candidacy status) are permitted to write these licensing exams.

With its newly acquired status, the naturopathic medical education program at CCNM is now part of an

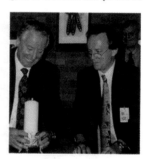

At the accreditation celebration, CCNM Board Chair Jeremy Kendall (L) sets down the Founders candle while David Schleich and Don Warren, ND, look on. Don, who was CCNM President from 1993 to 1996, was instrumental in the early stages of the accreditation process.

elite group of only four accredited programs in North America. CCNM proudly joins the ranks of Bastyr University in Washington, National College of Naturopathic Medicine in Oregon, and Southwest College of Naturopathic Medicine & Health Sciences in Arizona.

CCNM gains full accreditation

Naturopathic Doctor's Oath

I dedicate myself to the service of humanity as a
practitioner of the art and science of naturopathic medicine.

By precept, education and example, I will assist
and encourage others to strengthen their health,
reduce risks for disease, and preserve the health of our planet
for ourselves and future generations.
I will continually endeavour to improve my abilities.
I will conduct my life and practice of naturopathic medicine
with integrity and freedom from prejudice.
I will keep confident what should not be divulged.

I will honour the principles of naturopathic medicine:

First, to do no harm.

To co-operate with the healing powers of nature.

To address the fundamental causes of disease.

To heal the whole person through individualized treatment.

To teach the principles of healthy living and preventive medicine.

With my whole heart, before these witnesses,
as a Doctor of Naturopathic Medicine,
I pledge to remain true to this oath.

Naturopathic Oath

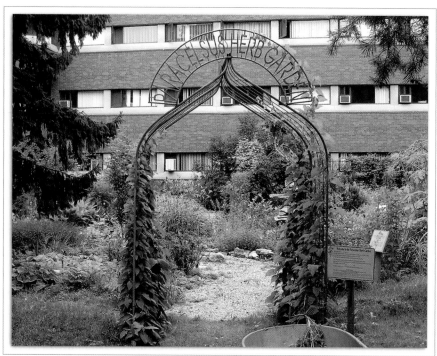

The Paracelsus Herb Garden at CCNM

When the College acquired its new campus at Leslie and Sheppard in 1999 there was, for the first time in CCNM's history, a real potential for a permanent herb garden. The inner courtyard boasted some fine coniferous trees, a nice stand of birch, and two lovely lilac bushes, but not much else. The soil was in miserable shape, nothing more than gravel and weeds-- the previous tenants had obviously had very little interest in gardening.

In the fall of 1999 Christopher Sowton ND, homeopathy instructor at the College and a lifelong lover of botanical gardens, designed and developed the Paracelsus Herb Garden. From the outset the garden was intended to be both an outdoor classroom and a place for meditative relaxation and communion with nature. The Steinke family, parents of Wayne Steinke ND, generously donated the funds to make the vision become a reality. With Chris Sowton ND acting as project director, and with the passion and commitment of several volunteer students and staff, the garden was built. The soil was upgraded with two truckloads of compost, generously donated by the City of Toronto, and the planting began in the spring of 2000.

One of the most dedicated student volunteers was Howie Owens, who designed, dug, and created the meditation pond in 2001. The pond has flourished and become a central and lovely feature of the garden. As a result of all the combined efforts of many individuals the garden now grows over 300 species of plants, and has become one of the best locales in North America to learn about medicinal plants. The garden is home to numerous insects, fish, several varieties of birdlife, and to small animal life as well. The garden is open for visits at all times and should be considered a shared resource for the entire naturopathic community.

Naturopathic Teaching Clinics

Naturopathic teaching clinics have been part of the academic program at OCNM since its inception. CCNM's naturopathic teaching clinic, named the Robert Schad Naturopathic Clinic (RSNC) due to Mr. Schad's contribution to the College and the profession, has 40 treatment rooms for patient visits. Visits to RSNC grows on a yearly basis and in 2008 the clinic experienced more than 26,000 patient visits.

In 2005 RSNC started its first specialty shifts in sports medicine and pain management. It currently has three active speciality shifts, Adjunctive Cancer Care, Sports Medicine and Paediatrics with plans to add more over time.

In 1995 CCNM established a partnership with Lakeshore Area Multiservice Project (LAMP). This represented the first community clinic of CCNM where fourth-year interns are supervised by a practicing naturopathic doctor and work alongside other health-care providers such as medical doctors, nurse practitioners, chiropractors, registered massage therapists and social workers. Community health centres provide services to a specific group, typically service low-income populations that have an array of health problems. These clinics provide access to health care, including alternative health care to which this group would otherwise not have access.

In 1998, CCNM established its second partnership with Sherbourne Health Centre (previously called People With Aids (PWA)). RSNC has partnerships with six satellite clinics: Sherbourne Health Centre, Parkdale Community Health Centre, Anishnawbe Health Toronto, LAMP, Queen West Community Health Centre and 168 Bathurst St. Centre. Every fourth-year student spends a four-month rotation in at least one of the satellite clinics where there are currently around 1,000 naturopathic patient visits per year.

To learn more about CCNM, entrance requirements for school, research activities, continuing education courses, or about the Robert Schad Naturopathic Clinic, visit the website at www.ccnm.edu

CHAMPION:
DR. DONALD G. WARREN ND, DHANP
Written by Dr. Mona Zarei ND

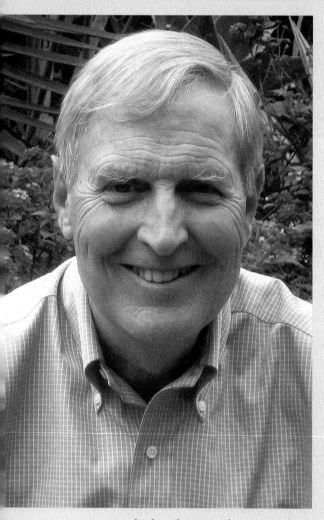

DONALD G. WARREN WAS BORN and raised in Ottawa. Having grown up in a retail clothing family, he pursued business studies at Houghton College in western New York from 1960 to 1964. It was at Houghton that he met his future wife Barbara Wilson - who would become a tremendous inspiration and support in his life. Upon graduation Don returned to Ottawa to begin family life and help run the family business.

As time went on and responsibilities evolved, Don's life became increasingly hectic. He and Barbara became the proud parents of four children. They lived on an organic farm boarding and raising horses. In addition to assisting with the management of a chain of clothing stores, Don was busy directing a church choir and playing trumpet in the Ottawa Civic Symphony. After nearly ten years of being overcommitted in every aspect of his life, Don suffered a major health break. It was a situation for which the conventional medical system could offer no solutions. Not to be discouraged, Don began studying books on natural healing in an effort to find his own answers. It was through these studies and the influence of his wife that Don discovered the field of naturopathy. (A note on Barbara: She was a Massachusetts country girl with a confidence in the body's innate ability to heal itself and a trust of natural and home remedies. Incidentally, unbeknown to her at the time, her parents, Norman and Lena Wilson, had been lay naturopathic practitioners in Texas prior to Barbara's birth and had studied under Benedict Lust.)

Don did his pre-med studies at the University of Ottawa and continued studies in biochemistry and nutrition until it became feasible to move his family to Oregon in order to pursue an education in naturopathic medicine. In 1979 he enrolled at the National College of Naturopathic Medicine (now National College of Natural Medicine) and graduated in 1984. During those intensive five years, Don benefited from the guidance of such visionaries as NDs John Bastyr and Joe Boucher and studied under professors such as NDs Robin Murphy and André Saine.

Following graduation, challenges in the family business required that Dr. Warren return to Ottawa delaying his immediate entry into a naturopathic practice. It was not until a fellow naturopathic doctor referred an individual to him that Dr. Warren started seeing patients out of his business office . . . from which time on he continued to grow his practice in this unique setting.

Motivated by his own profound experiences with health, both as a student and as a doctor, and inspired by the commitment of the forefathers of naturopathic medicine, when a need arose, Dr. Warren became involved in the Canadian naturopathic educational community. Utilizing his business experience, Dr. Warren served as chair of the board of OCNM from 1990-1993, a time when the future of the college was uncertain. He then was asked to serve as the President of CCNM from 1993-1996. It was a position that required setting private practice aside and entailed travelling to Toronto weekly. For three years Dr. Warren would fly out of Ottawa early on Monday morning and return on Thursday evening. The sacrifices proved fruitful as Dr. Warren, along with the new board, revitalized the struggling college and created a secure foundation for its future. Dr. Warren returned to family practice in Ottawa in 1996.

In addition, he served as President of the Council for Naturopathic Medical Education (CNME) from 2001 - 2005. During this time, the CNME gained government recognition as the accrediting agency for naturopathic medical education in the United States. This recognition was an important step for the ongoing licensing and registration efforts in both the U.S. and Canada.

More recently, along with his general family practice, Dr. Warren devotes time as a senior editor to the Naturopathic Foundations Project in the development of a new comprehensive textbook for naturopathic medicine. He is also leading a research project in East Africa, the Rwanda Selenium Supplementation Project for the treatment of HIV/AIDS.

For over thirty years Dr. Donald G. Warren has humbly demonstrated a deep respect for the legacy of naturopathic medicine, a steadfast confidence for a medicine rooted in the wisdom and power of nature, and a conscientious responsibility for this profession.

CHAMPION:
ROBERT D. SCHAD, (HONORARY ND)
Written by KatherineWillow ND (aka Karen Schad)

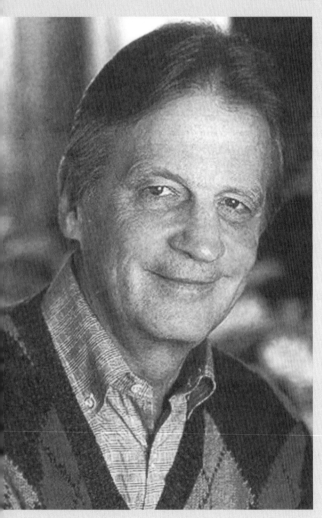

WHEN NATUROPATHIC MEDICINE IN ONTARIO came under threat of de-regulation in the mid 1980's, funds were desperately short. I asked my father, Robert Schad, for support as we have a family tradition of naturopathic medicine in Germany three generations back. He was doubtful about our chances of success and commissioned a lawyer's prognosis on the situation. I remember the two inch bound report containing the conclusion that we couldn't win. Undaunted, we continued our efforts towards what became the biggest letter-writing campaign that Queen's Park had ever witnessed.

Robert did decide to cast his considerable force behind ours – financially and strategically, even to the point of sitting on boards and bringing powerful people in to join the effort to keep regulated naturopathic medicine alive in Ontario. Robert also realized that the college was a crucial factor in growing a strong profession and focussed his energies on pulling that institution out of imminent bankruptcy. His gala fundraiser with David Suzuki raised a whopping two million dollars for the college.

Staff and facilities were made available from his private company at no cost. Robert spent several more years intensively involved with the profession and continues to be a strong supporter of the College where his name graces the clinic and from which he was granted an honourary ND. Robert's strong leadership style wasn't always appreciated, a fact which didn't escape his awareness. "I was probably the most hated man in the profession," he chuckles now. However, the other crucial players in that fight recognized and appreciated his genius.

"Robert Schad was the best friend the naturopathic profession has had in Canada. His contribution to the college has resulted in one of the finest school clinics in North America. He provided tough-minded leadership at a time the college needed it. **DON WARREN ND**

"Robert funded things in a way that made you responsible for the activity and put his expertise into supporting us to do our best." **PAT WALES ND**

"Robert's extensive involvement with the profession has been completely philanthropic. He is savvy about professional formation, how a profession takes shape; he knew what to focus on; which trees to backup and was not afraid to say it. He had the tenacity to *do things properly*. His involvement has resulted in the biggest teaching clinic in North America and the largest jurisdiction of registered naturopaths in the world. Robert D. Schad has singularly done more in North America than anyone else to build and support the profession." **DAVID SCHLEICH PHD**

"Even more important than his critical financial support was that he encouraged LEADERSHIP. He could see far beyond his nose and make decisions not based on immediacy, instead looking 5 – 10 years ahead. Robert was smart and technical and could always get to the heart of the matter." **DAN LABRIOLA ND**

"Robert's fundraising pulled the college from bankruptcy and he hired David Schleich, whose superb management resulted in the college having a net worth of 6 million dollars six years later! Robert really made it all happen." **JEREMY KENDALL ND**

"Robert has an unwavering dedication to naturopathic medicine. He stepped in at a crucial time – without his support we would not be where we are today in any way, shape or form. He contributed with no personal gain, for instance making sure the college had their own building versus buying the building and having the college lease from him. He came down himself or with his team, not just delegating but giving lots of his own time along with Jeremy Kendall, when he was also managing one of the top companies in Canada." **JHON COSGROVE ND**

My father has incredibly high standards and went through understandable periods of frustration with our growing pains as we continually move towards a deeper and more clear integration of our time–honoured fundamental principles and the revelations of science. One of my wishes is that he see the profession stretch into its incredible potential. Even as we are, we witness heart-warming changes in the health and happiness of the many people and families in our practices. Robert D. Schad helped make that possible and we thank him for the essential part he played.

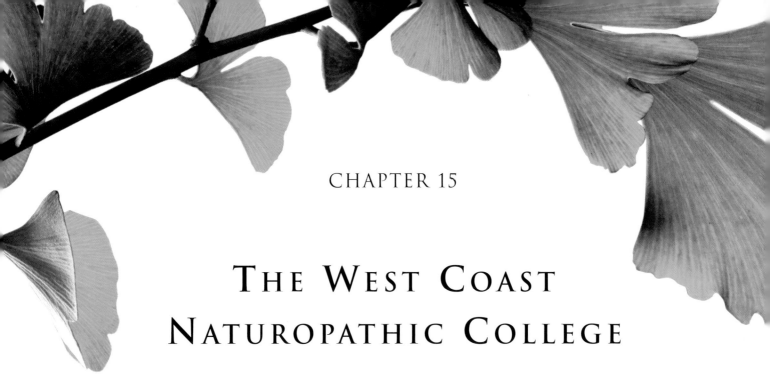

CHAPTER 15

THE WEST COAST
NATUROPATHIC COLLEGE

A Dream Come True
Written by Dr. Pat Wolfe ND

FOR MANY YEARS PRIOR to the 1980's, a number of naturopathic physicians in British Columbia dreamed of the day when they would have their own naturopathic medical school in Western Canada. This was seen as an important way to grow the profession in British Columbia (B.C.), as well as to serve those Western Canadians who did not want to travel to the United States or to Ontario in search of an education in naturopathic medicine.

Although the dream was present, there were few resources in terms of time, energy, money and NDs with the expertise to launch a new school. A few visionaries had drafted a preliminary plan and approached a few established institutions, like the University of British Columbia, but there was no interest from the public sector for such an initiative.

In 1998, the owner of the West Coast College of Massage Therapy (WCCMT), Michael Katigbak, cognizant of the growing interest in Complimentary and Alternative Medicine on the West Coast, mandated his executive director, Cidalia Paiva, PhD bioethics, to establish a program in naturopathic medicine as a subsidiary of WCCMT. Dr. Paiva quickly became a passionate proponent of naturopathic medicine and champion for what was to become the stand alone Boucher Institute of

Naturopathic Medicine. But that was a few years down the line!

One of the first tasks Dr. Paiva accomplished was to create an advisory board of experts to plan and guide the new program, which was christened the West Coast Naturopathic Medical College (WCNMC). In attendance at that first two day planning session, March 4th and 5th, 1999, were the following: Michael Katigbak, Cidalia Paiva, PhD, Neil McKinney ND, Sonya Pederson ND, Julie Pegg ND, Gordon Smith ND (first dean of OCNM,) Eric Yarnell ND, John Yates PhD, Peter Cook and John Magee. This group entered into long and impassioned discussions about the vision and mission of the new program. Key elements that were agreed upon were that the new school was to be founded on a very specific philosophy, embodied by what the ideal naturopathic physician must be: one who has a truly caring nature and a genuine desire to serve, who commits to the ongoing practice of self-reflection and personal growth, who has a passionate belief in the efficacy of naturopathic medicine and a commitment to leading our world toward sustainable health.

This vision of the ideal naturopathic physician underlies specific mission and value statements that were articulated in the very first year of the school's existence and which have been annually revisited and re-validated by the educational community. The founders understood clearly that in order to promote the development of the type of naturopathic physician envisioned, the ND program must be intentionally created on principles of inclusion, integration, integrity, safety, respect, academic freedom, self-responsibility and innovation. It was understood that they were creating a community in which each member felt heard, valued and supported on their journey of self-discovery and academic exploration. It was a conscious decision to steer away from the large, anonymous university model of instruction and to plan instead for small, intimate classes that would allow a mentorship model of instruction and maximum interaction among and between students and faculty.

Over the next several months, more discussions and much work on curriculum development ensued, more members joined (Naturopathic Drs. Dave Scotten and Maylynn Woo joined the board in May), some departed. Dr. Paiva worked hard to garner support for the new program from the local B.C. naturopathic community, but most were skeptical of a program initiated by a for-profit massage school, despite the significant number of well respected NDs comprising the advisory board.

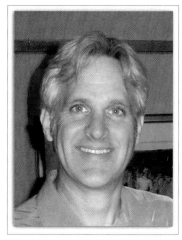

Dr. Dave Scotten ND one of the founding members of BINM and the first Dean of the College.

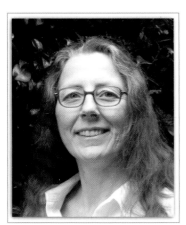

Dr. Isis van Loon ND, Dean of Clinical Studies at BINM

Reception ranged from outright hostility to a non-committal "wait and see" attitude. Nevertheless, the advisory group persevered and supported Dr. Paiva and Dr. Scotten, the new Dean of the naturopathic program, in the huge amount of work that had to be accomplished to prepare to open the doors for the first time. Although it was hoped for a September 1999 opening, it was January 2000 before the WCNMC was ready to welcome its founding class of 15 students.

In April 2000, the West Coast Naturopathic Medical College Society was incorporated, fulfilling the need to be a not-for-profit organization in order to be eligible for Council of Naturopathic Medical Education (CNME) candidacy, as well as seeking to ensure the profession that the school was of the highest integrity. This paved the way for the events that were about to unfold. By May 2000 the parent WCCMT and therefore the subsidiary WCNMC were in financial difficulties. The threat to the survival of the infant ND program and its founding class of pioneering students was substantial. During the summer of 2000, the new Society voted to take full responsibility for the naturopathic program and to offer a transfer agreement to Michael Katigbak to separate from the parent massage school. The turmoil that ensued around this contentious issue placed additional extraordinary stress on the founding students, who were extremely involved in the process. It was largely the commitment, faith and perseverance of these dedicated students that inspired the efforts of the Society board on their behalf.

In December 2000, largely through efforts spearheaded by Dr. Paiva, whose commitment to the students was paramount, a transfer agreement was completed between the WCCMT and the WCNMC Society resulting in a new stand alone naturopathic medical college. To reflect the change in ownership, in May 2001 this new entity was officially renamed the Boucher Institute of Naturopathic Medicine Society (BINMS) in honour of the late Dr. Joseph Boucher, one of the founders of the National College of Naturopathic Medicine and a much respected pioneer in naturopathic medicine in British Columbia.

The Governing Board of BINMS at this time consisted of the following: Bruce Chambers (acting executive director,) Geri Martin, Cameron McIntyre (student rep), Neil McKinney ND, Kevin Nolan, MD ND, Cidalia Paiva, PhD, Ardath Paxton-Mann, David Scotten ND (dean), David Wang ND, and Patricia Wolfe ND. Dr. Scotten was still the only paid employee of the school and was responsible for teaching, hiring other faculty, continuing to develop the curriculum, day-to-day administration, chief handy-man and doer of whatever else needed to be done! In addition, the rest of the dedicated board members met on a biweekly basis for the next year and pitched in to accomplish other administrative duties that needed to be done including, recruitment for the upcoming class (22 students enrolled in September 2001,) securing a new home (3,100 sq feet!) for the school in the Begbie Court Heritage Building in New Westminster, and embarking on the all important task of seeking recognition from our local and North American regulatory and accrediting bodies to gain our graduates access to licensing board exams and entry to practice in regulated jurisdictions.

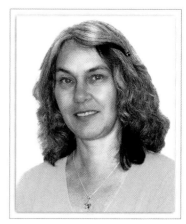

Dr. Pat Wolfe ND, President and Executive Director of BINM

The excitement and enthusiasm for what had been accomplished by the small group of volunteers and brave students in saving the start-up ND program from annihilation bonded the group together and set the stage for the many challenges still to be faced. Every step along the way, dedicated individuals who had faith in the Boucher vision made themselves available above and beyond any reasonable expectations to further the goals of the school. Dr. Isis van Loon ND is one of these individuals who volunteered in 2001 to begin planning the teaching clinic that would be needed to train the students and she continues to give endlessly of her time to ensure excellence in clinical education for Boucher students. Dr. Nathalie Desrocher-Allen ND, with charter student Sanjay Mohan Ram, was another who volunteered innumerable hours setting up and managing the tiny BINM library that has since grown to a respectable collection of 5000 items.

It was not unusual to see board members, staff, volunteers and students working side-

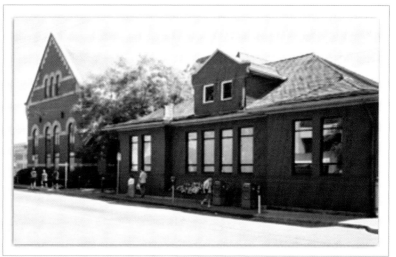

BINM campus

by-side painting walls or moving furniture into a new space the weekend before classes or the new clinic started, or hosting an open house complete with home cooking to inform prospective students and the public alike about naturopathic medicine and our new school. On one occasion, on the way to present our second and successful application for candidacy to the CNME, our board chair at the time, Dr. Heathir Naesgaard ND, Dr. Paiva PhD and Dr. Wolfe ND were required to jump out of a plane whose engine had caught fire. Dr. Nolan ND only partly joked that, in future, no more than two members of the Boucher team should travel together, lest a significant portion of BINM's management, faculty and staff be eliminated in one fell swoop! The CNME presentation went incredibly smoothly in comparison.

There were several instructors who began their tenure with the school in the early years who have continued as core faculty and / or department chairs. These are: Hal Brown, DC ND (Physical Medicine Department Chair), Nathalie Desrocher-Allen ND, Mike Dixon, RMT, Rochelle Heisel, PhD (Associate Dean of Academics), Rowan Hamilton, Isis van Loon ND (Dean of Clinical Studies,) Quinn Rivet ND (Associate Dean of Educational Integration,) Dr. Sarah Beasleigh ND (clinical faculty) and founding board member, Dr. Neil McKinney ND, continues in the

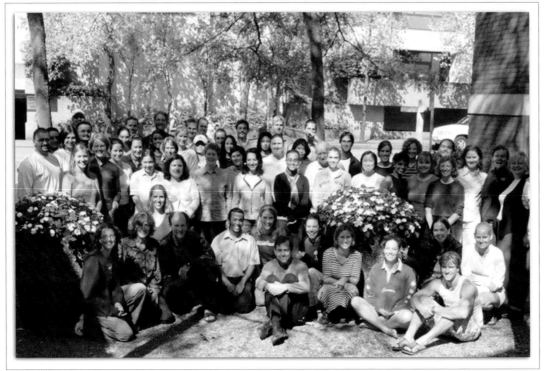

BINM Community

capacity of valued faculty member and past chair of the Traditional Oriental Medicine Department.

In January 2002, Dr. Pat Wolfe ND was asked by the board – and humbly agreed - to serve in the capacity as president and executive director when Dr. Paiva PhD announced that she would be unable to fulfill this role as expected. Dr. Wolfe's main task was to focus on establishing the foundational policies and administrative structures that would enable BINM to eventually achieve accreditation with the Council on Naturopathic Medical Education (CNME), a goal that was realized in December of 2008.

In September 2005, after an incredible series of serendipitous events, BINM purchased its own 46,000 square foot building in New Westminster that also houses a public transit Sky train station. The teaching clinic, under Dr. van Loon's watchful direction, has grown from three treatment rooms and a closet in those early years to 12 rooms in a spacious new clinic that is serving an average of 600+ patients per month by a full cohort of senior students under the tutelage of 22 supervising doctors. Dr. Scotten ND continues to lead the faculty in the development of an innovative and integrative curriculum. In June 2008 the fifth class of doctors graduated bringing the total number of graduates as of that date to 73. As of September 2008, enrolment had grown to capacity for the first time with 140 enrolled students and due to growing demand, we are about to implement our new 6 year part-time program in January 2009.

BINM has made incredible strides in a very short time and we are now ready to position ourself as an established and credible institution with the overwhelming support and respect of the other naturopathic colleagues in the profession. The passion, commitment, faith and sheer perseverance of so many who have made this dream a reality is more than can be described in the limited space available. But I consider it to have been an incredible honour to have had the privilege to work with this amazing group of individuals. In particular, if not for the many brave and dedicated students who took a chance on a venture that many thought would not succeed, who have contributed in uncountable ways to creating our incredibly beautiful Boucher community spirit and who inspired those of us who worked on their behalf, the Boucher Institute of Naturopathic Medicine would not be a reality today. My sincere thanks, appreciation and gratitude goes out to all of them and I know the world will be a better place for their efforts. Dr. Pat Wolfe ND

PART 4

SUPPORTING
THE PROFESSION

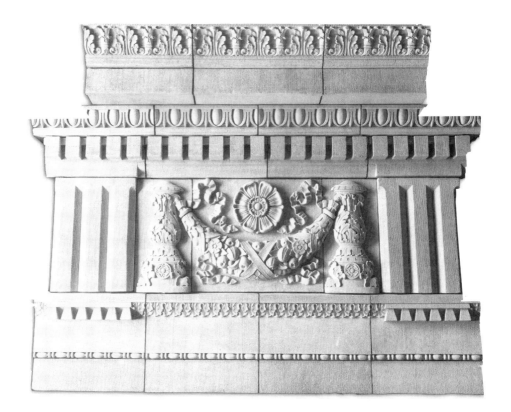

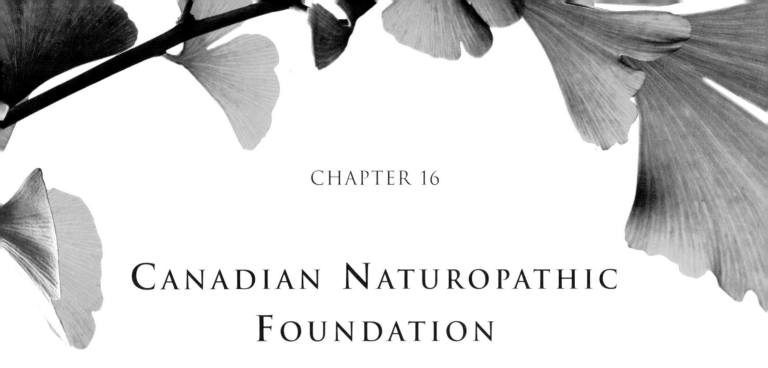

CHAPTER 16

CANADIAN NATUROPATHIC FOUNDATION

Securing funds, whether for education, public affairs or other initiatives, has been a long and continuous challenge. For the most part, naturopathic medicine has been on its own without the support of government grants or assistance. Fundraising for the profession has typically been done at the provincial level or by individual colleges with members and students providing the majority of funds to ensure the ongoing survival of the profession. The profession has also benefited greatly from the ongoing support of naturopathic doctors and the public – especially patients and a few generous supporters. The support has been a testimony to the skill and expertise of naturopathic doctors, and at times instrumental in 'saving' an aspect of the profession.

Start of the Foundation

The dedication and perseverance of many practitioners have been key to the development and establishment of naturopathic medicine. One such individual was Dr. Joseph A. Boucher ND. When he passed away in 1987, at age 70, Dr. Robert "Bob" Fleming ND in concert with his wife Ann and other local doctors established Canadian Naturopathic Education Research Society (CNERS) to commemorate his valuable contribution to the profession.

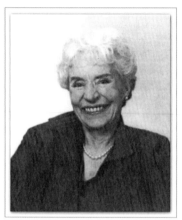

**Ann (Boucher) Fleming
co-founder of Canadian
Naturopathic Education
Research Society**

CNERS was officially incorporated on January 10, 1988 as a charitable organization. The initial board were family members and individuals who had been very close to Dr. Boucher: Tony Boucher, Joe's brother, was president; Madeleine Cleveland, Joe's sister, was Secretary; Ann Fleming, Joe's sister, was Treasurer and Richard Cleveland, Joe's nephew, was the Legal Advisor. These family members were the only ones that could be persuaded to attend meetings at inconvenient times without daring to whine too much! Other elected directors included naturopathic doctors Robert Fleming, Allen Tyler (a long time friend and an important member of the British Columbia association), Susan Hood and David McKeeman.

On April 21st, 1997, CNERS formally changed its name to the Canadian Naturopathic Foundation (CNF) and converted its status to a charitable foundation. This allowed the Foundation much more flexibility in management of revenue and disbursement of funds. The objectives of the Foundation, as set forth in its Constitution, were not changed, and the CNF remains committed to providing scholarships to students at approved colleges, supporting naturopathic research and promoting greater public awareness. In 2007, with the aim of providing a stronger foundation and increased sustainability, the administration of the CNF was brought under the CAND.

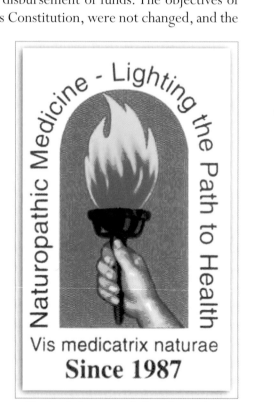

The torch logo was designed as a stamp by Dr. Joseph Boucher ND. The stamps were sold to raise funds for the CNA and the provincial associations, years before CNERS was formed.

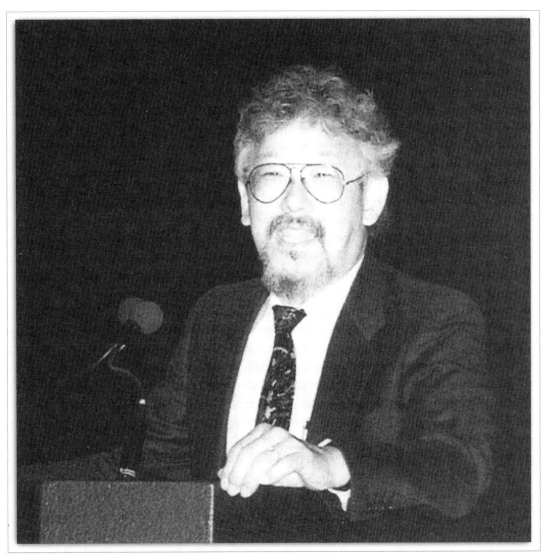

A fundraising dinner, held in 1996, with guest speaker David Suzuki raised over $1 million dollars. This event allowed CCNM to purchase the building at 1255 Sheppard Avenue East in Toronto.

Fundraising Initiatives

CNF has been instrumental in supporting the profession since its inception. It has provided over sixty scholarships, has dispersed funds to different research projects, supported CNME and the opening of Boucher Institute of Naturopathic Medicine (BINM).

In 2007 the CNF launched a bequest program and in 2008 a fundraising program was established to fund a cost-effectiveness study on naturopathic medicine. To find out the details of the bequest program and other initiatives of the CNF visit www.cand.ca

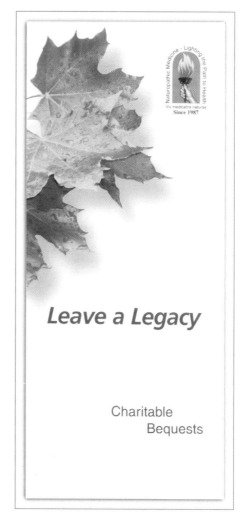

> *"It's a great tribute to the public's common sense that people are looking for alternatives and ready to use them. People know that there's a need for a more holistic framework within which to fashion a healthy way of living."*
>
> Dr. David Suzuki, PhD

CHAMPION:
DR. ROBERT FLEMING ND
Written by Dr. Mona Zarei ND

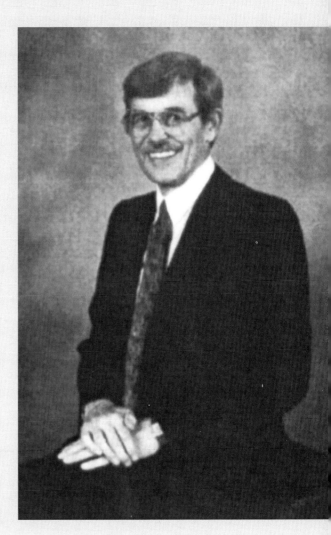

ROBERT (BOB) FLEMING WAS BORN July 27th, 1918 in Alloway, Scotland. His family came to Canada in 1919 and settled in B.C.

Because of the depression years his father's job ended and his family moved from Vancouver to Princeton, B.C. In his early teens it fell upon Bob to keep his family supplied with meat; fishing with a willow stick, string, a plain fish hook and using a grasshopper for bait and by shooting deer and grouse with a 22 rifle and by snaring wild rabbits.

After completing grade eight (in a tiny school house two and half miles away, with a total of nine kids) it was decided he would go to high school in Princeton, boarding with an old friend of the family, a catholic priest, Father Ben Carlyle. When Fr. Carlyle was transferred to Ocean Falls, B.C. in 1935, Robert went with him in order to continue his schooling.

He was very active in the following years: leaving school in 1936 to work in the paper mill; moving to various departments as openings occurred when workers were laid off. He also worked on the town site crew, cutting lawns, sawmill work, finishing room, paper mill, pipe fitting, etc. To be laid off a job, albeit part time, during the 30s was always traumatic. However, it was with some degree of relief that he left Ocean Falls and returned to Princeton.

In the 1940s, the Canadian Armed Forces decided it was time for a mandatory one-month army training for all single men aged 20 to 25 (he was 22). The camp had just opened and construction was being hurried, a number of things were inadequate, such as no water in the barrack huts and no cubicles around the toilets. When water was finally turned on, someone apparently forgot to properly flush out the pipes! The consequence was an epidemic of intestinal distress! An indelible memory of this episode is the line up of 10 to 15 men with anguished faces waiting their turn on the line of toilets (eight in all!) with some returning to the back of the line immediately after completing the front of the line. During that month, more than half the population of the camp was also struck with influenza, including Robert.

After the stint in the army Robert returned to Princeton and worked in the Power Plant for a year or so and then enlisted in the Commonwealth Air Training Plan followed by the RCAF where he initially trained as an aero engine mechanic and then a pilot. In August of 1944 he graduated from pilot training with the promise of an overseas posting. To qualify for the posing he was required to take commando training. (He mentioned that he was puzzled over why a pilot was required to take hand to hand commando training. He remarked if he was not killed or injured, he would hide, not look for someone to beat up!) During the commando training he fell off a swinging rope and dislocated his right elbow. This ended his active career.

Robert married Ann Boucher and a few years later he met his wife's brother, Joseph Boucher. His life soon changed forever. Joe Boucher ND persuaded Bob, coupled with Ann's encouragement, to enroll at Western States College of Chiropractic and Naturopathy. After graduating in 1956 Robert, Ann and their daughter Sharon returned to Vancouver and opened a naturopathic practice with Dr. Charles McKeown ND.

At that time the naturopathic profession was in jeopardy — the medical and pharmaceutical professions had almost eliminated the profession. During the 1920s, 30s, and 40s there had been some 120 naturopathic physicians in B.C., yet when he joined the B.C. association in 1956 there were only six members. He quickly became active in the association and held positions of secretary, treasurer and register. During those years, the BC association might not have survived if it wasn't for the efforts of Ann Fleming. Dr. Robert Fleming ND and Ann were active in the association for over twenty-five consecutive years.

He often recalled those early days in practice. The skepticism and doubt of some and the criticism and fear that medical practitioners imposed on those that inquired about his services. Despite all that, Dr. Flemings practice grew by word of mouth and over time he had patients coming to see him from other provinces and from the United States. For years he spent over 100 hours a week in the office due to the high volume of patient visits that he attracted.

When his brother-in-law Joe Boucher ND passed away in 1987, Dr. Fleming and Ann were responsible for establishing CNERS in Joe's honour. Dr. Fleming stayed active with CNERS until 2000, at which time he also retired. Dr. Robert Fleming wrote the story of his life for the BCNA Bulletin in 2002 and in it he remarked, "I wouldn't trade a minute of my life for a year of anyone else's."

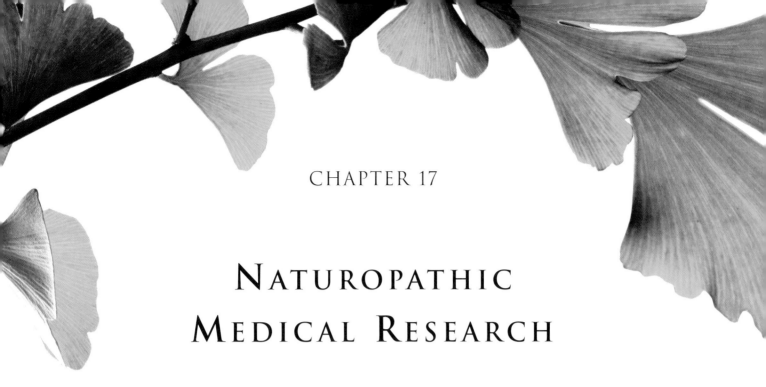

CHAPTER 17

NATUROPATHIC
MEDICAL RESEARCH

THE PRACTICE OF NATUROPATHIC MEDICINE has always been supported by research. In fact, research on nutrition, Chinese medicine, acupuncture, homeopathy and botanical medicine has been conducted and published for over 100 years.

Despite evidence for its effectiveness and safety, naturopathic medicine has historically been accused of not being scientifically based. Some of this concern has recently been alleviated due to the increasing value placed on different forms of research, the acknowledgement of differences in philosophies and practice between conventional medicine and naturopathic medicine, and the increasing opportunities for funding for naturopathic medical research.

Every profession strives to develop a knowledge base that maximizes the effectiveness and safety of its practice and research is the process that is used and it also provides a common language between professionals and aids collaboration and integration.

Research in healthcare is most valuable when the type of research that is conducted closely matches the theories and therapeutic methods being tested. If the aim of research is to test the elements of clinical practice, then the research design must match to how a professional actually practices. There are many ways in which the current scientific method is used and applied appropriately to naturopathic medicine, but there are also

> *"Not only do we have good scientific basis for what we do, but we also use the same scientific literature orthodox MD's use to prove the validity of what we do and to discredit much of current orthodox medical practices."*
>
> JOE PIZZORNO ND

many ways in which this method is neither appropriate nor applicable. With advances in new forms of research there is a greater ability to design effective research studies that address the vitalistic and holistic principles of naturopathic medicine.

Where Research Began

Until the mid-nineteenth century, personal and peer experiences were the primary sources of 'evidence-based' medicine. Over time, 'scientific' research became ingrained in a reductionist and dualistic model and hence, the randomized controlled trial became the 'gold standard'. Yet, difficulties were encountered as practitioners and scientists attempted to explain psychosocial factors in disease causation, how body functions were integrated and the physiological impact of intangible qualities such as thoughts and emotions on health. Debates about vitalism versus mechanism, holism versus reductionism and quantitative versus qualitative approaches occurred between different systems of medicine and have hindered researchers and medical professionals from observing the overall essence of life and maintaining the sense of curiosity and wonder that it holds.

Initially, research included a balance of subjective and objective measurements. However, over time, observations became more objective with less emphasis on the subjective. Research focused on the mechanisms of disease and the impact of therapeutic interventions. Reductionist driven research has provided a great deal of medical knowledge, but has also contributed to a greater separation between physicians and their patients and separation both between the mind and the body, and between humans and their environment.

With increasing knowledge of bodily functions and with new technologies, the practice of research has had to change to meet the needs of the current way of thinking. In the 21st century, we often delude ourselves into thinking that we already have a complete understanding of health and disease, but that is not true. There are still many mysteries about life, health and disease that are not understood. Uncovering these mysteries will require different research methods.

Many of the research methods used in the past seem antiquated and unscientific, yet they served to further the understanding of that particular time period. The question is whether one of the concerns with the current state of the health care system is that the current 'gold standard' used in research - the randomized controlled trial (RCT) - is now antiquated and is impeding the growth and development of our understanding of health and disease.

Differing Philosophies

Theories and methodologies used in healthcare research were primarily developed and created to support the theories and practice of conventional medicine. The challenge is that conventional medicine and naturopathic medicine are two distinct systems of health care. There is some overlap but the theories, principles and philosophies are different. The purpose of comparing naturopathic medicine to mainstream medicine is not to judge one as correct or superior to the other, but to acknowledge that there are differences. The 'gold standard' in research for conventional medicine is not necessarily the 'gold standard' for naturopathic medicine. Appreciation of the differences in philosophy and theory is important to understanding which research methodology is the most appropriate and what outcomes (and variables) the different methods of research are actually testing.

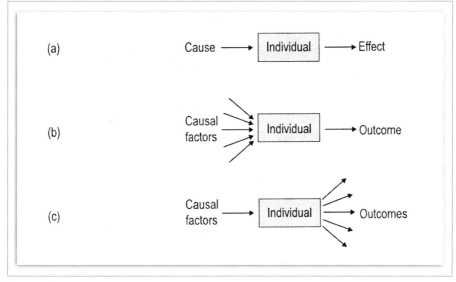

Causality

a) linear causality: there is a direct correlation between cause and effect;

b) mutual causality: a single outcome can be due to the interaction of various factors;

c) mutual causality: a single factor can result in various outcomes.

With permission from Dr. Iva Lloyd ND The Energetics of Health, a Naturopathic Assessment, Elsevier, 2009

> *"The trends of modern medical research and practice in our great colleges and endowed research institutes are almost entirely along combative lines, while the individual, progressive physician learns to work more and more along preventive lines."*
>
> *Henry Lindlahr ND*
>
> *(1862 – 1924)*

The main differences between these two systems is how health and disease are viewed. Conventional medicine is based on reductionist, dualistic, mechanistic and linear causality concepts; naturopathic medicine is based on vitalism, holism and mutual causality concepts. A focus of conventional treatments is to 'kill the bug' or 'kill the disease; the focus of naturopathic medicine is to support the innate healing ability of the body and to address the cause of disease. Naturopathic doctors employ treatments to address 'the bug', but the emphasis of treatment is on supporting the body's innate healing and on identifying the factors that are contributing to a person's susceptibility.

Overview of the Conventional Approach

The *mechanist* view of human health is that the body functions as a machine which obeys fixed laws. From this perspective, only the physical or biological causes and tangible parts are considered. The mechanist approach supports the idea that you can simply remove 'faulty' parts or 'damaged' sections of the human body without it affecting other aspects.

The *reductionist* belief is that the nature of complex things can be explained and broken down into smaller parts: i.e., that is each organ system of the body functions and can be treated in isolation of other organ systems. For example, if an individual has high blood pressure, treatments are often directed at managing the functioning of the heart or blood vessels often with little or no attention paid to psychological or structural factors.

Dualism refers to the separation of mind and body: the belief that a person's thoughts, language and beliefs do not influence the function of the body and that a person's thoughts are not altered by the function of the body.

The assumption of *linear causality* is based on the belief that there is a direct relationship between one cause and one effect see (Causality diagram a)). Thus you can test individual drugs or treatments in isolation. The concern is that many people are on multiple drugs at the same time, as well as different supplements, herbs and dietary and lifestyle habits. Although potential adverse interactions and events are often listed, there is minimal consideration for the overall impact of the drug or treatment on the rest of the body nor the acknowledgement that linear relationships are not indicative of real life.

These theories have been beneficial in explaining many complex processes in the human body have, and continue to save many lives. Yet there are concerns, both within and outside the field of conventional medicine, that this approach has its limitations.

Overview of the Naturopathic Approach

Vitalism refers to the view that life is governed by forces beyond the physical self. Often vitalism is associated with concepts of spirit or soul and the term vitality refers to the inherent capacity of an organism to live, grow, develop and heal.

Holistic or holism means all, entire or total. It is based on the realization that the whole is greater than the sum of the parts. Holism considers the spiritual, psychological, functional and structural aspects of an individual, as well as the interaction of an individual with their environmental, external and social factors. It also acknowledges that every aspect of a person works as an integrated whole, not as individual parts. For example, when a naturopathic practitioner is treating a patient with high blood pressure, they will often provide supportive treatment for the heart, as they address psychological and lifestyle factors, external factors and other environmental factors that may be contributing to the problem.

Mutual causality acknowledges that similar conditions often produce dissimilar results based on external factors and internal feedback influences. For example, it is seldom possible to say that one factor caused a direct change in health; often there are many different factors, with varying degrees of impact. Similarly, a single factor can have many different impacts because of the uniqueness of each person (see Causality diagram b) and c)). Naturopathic medicine recognizes this and realizes there is seldom one treatment for any specific symptom or disease that works for everyone.

To research and validate the theories and therapeutic methods of naturopathic medicine, it is imperative that the research methodology be based on the principles of vitalism, holism and mutual causality. The conventional scientific method may be appropriate for assessing pharmacokinetics or physiological response to specific herbs, nutrients or other treatments. Yet, for many aspects of naturopathic medicine whole system research methodologies are more appropriate as they are more in line with naturopathic principles.

Inherent Challenges

Choosing the correct research methodology and evaluating research across multiple systems of health care has its challenges. For example:

Definitions provide a foundation for how to look at and understand concepts and theories. Although different systems of healthcare use the same words, there is no standardization on key terms, such as the definition of health, disease, healing, etc. Even the terms "root cause" and "prevention" mean different things. For example, the root cause of disease, as defined by naturopathic medicine, relates to the lifestyle, external or environmental factors that created the disruption in health. It does not refer to another symptom or illness. Pubmed, a major reference source of research, uses search terms based on conventional definitions from the National Library of Medicine and therefore, does not adequately represent the differences in terminology used in natural medicine. Conducting or comparing research that encompasses all the various interpretations of medical terms is not plausible.

Subjective experiences. Pain, discomfort, mood and many other human attributes are subjective and often intangible. Naturopathic medicine places a strong emphasis on a patient's subjective experiences and recognizes that there are many health conditions such as arthritis, where the physical findings and the subjective experience do not relate. For example, a patient with arthritis can experience extreme pain with minimal physical changes in the joints; or they can have tremendous joint destruction and experience little or no pain at all. The major challenge or art in addressing health concerns is determining when the physical findings hold more weight than a patient's subjective experience.

Number of research variables. There are a number of variables that impact health, contribute to disease, and influence healing. The validity of research to real-life is questionable when it restricts the number of variables being tested. Research that narrows the criteria to the impact of a single drug on the body without accounting for other variables has limited applicability.

Duration of research. There are always ongoing concerns as to whether research trials are long enough, whether they adequately reflect the safety and health benefits of treatments or whether the safety of chemicals and substances used in our food supply, personal care products and environment are properly assessed. The question is whether or not research that is conducted over a couple of years provides a true reflection of the impact of long-term exposure of drugs, chemicals and heavy metals. Historical data and traditional research in many situations are a better indicator of the long-term impact of different treatments, lifestyle and environment factors.

Research Designs

Research can involve the documentation of a single case, the random analysis of many individuals over a set period of time, the wisdom gained through years of observation and the retrospective look at a number of different research studies. Each form of research has its value and purpose. What is important is understanding the strengths and limitations of each form.

Traditional, Ancient, and Folk Knowledge and Research

Many forms of knowledge and tradition have been inherited and accepted based on historical use over hundreds or thousands of years. The healthcare and disease management components that are based on 'common sense' and traditional wisdom have legitimate value. Some examples include: putting more clothes on when you are cold, resting when you are sick, changing the amount and type of food you eat when you are ill, expressing your emotions in an appropriate and timely manner, taking a deep breath to decrease anxiety, etc. There are traditional forms of health care, such as Chinese Medicine and Ayurvedic Medicine that have

"People who categorize naturopathic medicine as 'non-scientific' are conveniently uninformed. They are using emotionally-loaded terminology to discredit us."

JOE PIZZORNO ND

been around for thousands of years. Conventional medicine has only been around for a few centuries and is the youngest form of medicine. Much wisdom can be gained in studying and learning from the traditional concepts and philosophies and also from fields of medicine that have withstood the test of time.

Many of the principles and therapeutic methods of naturopathic medicine are based on traditional knowledge. Botanicals or herbal medicine are one of the oldest forms of treatment and are used throughout the world. Many uses of botanicals are based on traditional knowledge. Current research methods have assisted in clarifying the potential therapeutic ingredients of specific herbs and the actual physiological reactions and biochemical interactions. However, botanical medicine is still practiced throughout the world primarily using traditional and ancient knowledge.

Quantitative and Qualitative Research

Research studies generate data that is considered quantitative or qualitative in nature. Quantitative results look at objective measurement criteria and provides data that can be counted, quantified, described, measured using statistical methods and reproduced by independent researchers. The aim of quantitative research is to provide a numerical correlation of how one or more variables interact. The vast majority of research done in healthcare is based on this type of research.

Qualitative research is more interested in the quality of information. It takes into account a patient's human and social experience, communication, thoughts, expectations, meaning, attitudes and other processes that affect the validity and nature of the results. This type of data is not used as frequently in "scientific" research as it is more difficult to measure.

Case-studies

A case-study often involves the documentation and study of a individual or small group of individuals with respect to a new treatment or theory. Case-studies observe unusual conditions as well as describe and assess innovative interventions. The value of case-studies is to provide new theories and insight into the complexity of the human condition. They allow for and acknowledge the wisdom that can be obtained by a practitioner testing a new treatment. The challenge is in taking the information conveyed and testing its applicability to larger groups of people.

Scientific Method

Health care research based on the scientific method aims to improve the effectiveness, safety and cost-effectiveness of health services. It follows a sequential and often linear process and is based primarily on quantitative data.

Randomized controlled trials (RCTs) are viewed as the 'gold standard' of conventional scientific research. The intention of RCTs is to statistically prove the efficacy of a given intervention under investigation. One of the principal strengths of the RCT is that it theoretically limits or removes bias. This form of research has provided for a deeper knowledge and understanding of many aspects of physiological function and treatment options.

The scientific method has limitations in that it does not address the complexity and variability within nature and the environment nor the unique psychosocial and physiological capacities of individuals. These factors introduce uncertainty into the interpretation and ability to generalize results. There is more to healthcare than can be tested under the controlled environment required by the scientific method.

Epidemiological Research

The study of epidemiology looks at trends over time and correlates a number of different factors to determine what is affecting health. Epidemiology plays a very important role in health care and in making policy decisions regarding public health. For example, epidemiological studies have provided insight into the correlation of high cancer rates in areas that have done extensive mining or agriculture. It is also epidemiological research that provides insight into the long-term effectiveness, or lack thereof, for different treatment and healthcare strategies, such as specific drugs, antibiotics or vaccinations.

Systemic Reviews and Meta-analyses

A systematic review provides an analysis of the current state of knowledge available on a certain topic. The purpose is to verify and quantify the results of any one treatment method or diagnostic technique being studied. The bias in this type of study is determined by the selection criteria that is used. Systematic reviews are designed to analyze both quantitative and qualitative data.

Whole Systems Research and Pragmatic Studies

Whole systems research, also called a pragmatic study, investigate the effectiveness of a treatment in a real life situation and determine whether an intervention works in terms that matter to a specific patient. A strength of this type of study is that it investigates real life applications hence it is often more applicable to a larger population. In contrast to scientific studies that explore effects within tightly defined populations, pragmatic studies have a broader focus and include the analysis of multiple treatment interventions, as well as lifestyle, psychological, social, external and environmental factors. The placebo effect and the patient-practitioner relationship are not controlled within pragmatic studies and, in fact, play a large role in the findings. This type of study is generally more complex than the typical RCT and more indicative of real life. Consequently it is somewhat more complex to interpret.

Pragmatic studies are more in line with the holistic approach of naturopathic medicine. This form of study does not replace randomized control studies, but provides another depth of research that promises to enhance our understanding of health and to improve disease management and population health management.

Current Initiatives

Research continues to be an important part of naturopathic medicine. It is taught in all accredited naturopathic schools and all schools conduct research and promote the ongoing research of naturopathic medicine. For information on the current research initiatives visit the Canadian College of Naturopathic Medicine (CCNM) website at www.ccnm.edu or the Boucher Institute of Naturopathic Medicine (BINM) website at www.binm.org.

Naturopathic medicine is an eclectic field of medicine with a unique philosophy and a broad scope of practice which includes all aspects of health and disease. As such, there are hundreds of journals providing research that supports the practice of naturopathic medicine. The *Vital Link* is the journal of the Canadian Association of Naturopathic Doctors (CAND). It has developed over time to a peer-reviewed journal that includes articles written by naturopathic doctors. The International Journal of Naturopathic Medicine at www.intjnm.org engages and informs naturopathic physicians and allied health professionals and encourages research and debate within the naturopathic profession. The CAND website at www.cand.ca provides an overview of the research that supports the principles and therapeutic methods of naturopathic medicine and provides a listing of the journals that carry naturopathic research. Your can also subscribe to the CAND's journal, the *Vital Link* on the website. The Canadian Naturopathic Foundation, the national charity institute for the profession, secures funding and does fundraising to promote naturopathic medical research in Canada.

"In this burgeoning field of integrative medicine, research can be a real catalyst for change and allow our profession to have a broader impact on the somewhat dysfunctional health care system and public health overall".

DUGALD SEELY ND, MSc

CHAMPION:
DR. DUGALD SEELY ND, MSc
Written by Dr. Kieran Cooley ND

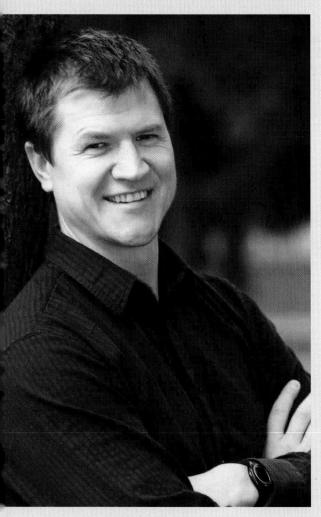

As DIRECTOR OF RESEARCH at the Canadian College of Naturopathic Medicine, Dr. Dugald Seely ND plays an interesting role in the naturopathic profession by advancing the state of knowledge about what it is that is done. Dr. Seely has always been curious — even as a naturopathic student at CCNM he recognized a fundamental need to better understand naturopathic treatments. Whether this is through implementing the scientific method and use of rigorous randomized controlled trials or through a broader examination of how an intervention affects patient care. Dr. Seely recognizes that research can only improve the ability to make treatment decisions and ultimately provide the best care for patients.

Dr. Seely continues to see research as a means to critically examine naturopathic therapies and practices; to establish credibility for those interventions that demonstrate benefit, better understand the context and quality of care that is delivered, and to identify those treatments that may not be beneficial. In a world of medical uncertainty, Dr. Seely uses research to sift through tradition and current knowledge to help identify best practices and highlight treatment gems for the naturopathic profession. He sees research as a noble pursuit if used well; reducing collective bias and objectively examining and expanding the knowledge base.

Currently Dr. Seely is involved in two types of research primarily: synthesis research and clinical research. Synthesis research is collating and summarizing research that has been previously conducted to make it easier and more efficient for the naturopathic physician to access and understand research evidence. In the future he hopes to be able to develop and assess models of integrative medicine for health prevention, promotion and treatment. Additionally he has a keen interest in identifying and researching ways to impact determinants of health, a shift towards prevention of illness and recognition of the role the environment has to play.

Overall, Dr. Duglad Seely sees research as means of breaking down barriers between health care professions as well as an opportunity to undertake collaborative efforts to examine the wealth of knowledge rooted in the experience and philosophy of naturopathic medicine. He greatly hopes that others follow in his footsteps and are able to contribute to this valuable element of our profession.

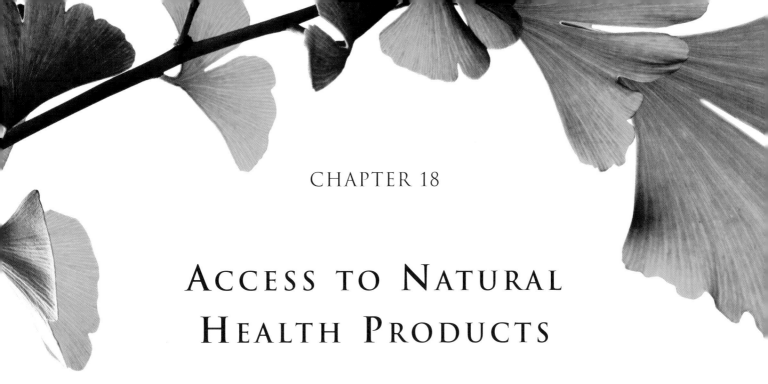

CHAPTER 18

ACCESS TO NATURAL HEALTH PRODUCTS

The primary therapies used by naturopathic doctors are nutraceuticals and herbs and substances that originate in nature. Ensuring the quality and availability of these substances is essential. Naturopathic associations, especially the CAND, work with the government to ensure that patients and the public have access to high quality, safe and effective natural health products.

Historical Uses

The use of individual nutrients is unique to Western medicine. Eastern medicines, such as Ayurvedic and Chinese, primarily use food and herbs, even to this day. If a specific nutrient is desired it is acquired by choosing a herb or food that is high in that specific nutrient. For example, drinking lemon juice or eating oranges to prevent scurvy, a disease caused by a deficiency of Vitamin C.

In the past it was not unusual for naturopathic doctors to plant, cultivate and harvest the plants they needed to prepare their herbal formulas. Raw ingredients could also be sourced from local herbalists or green houses. In the early 19th century there was still the belief that all the vitamins and minerals a person needed could be found in the fruits and vegetables purchased from local farmers or grown in personal gardens. Livestock was healthier as they were allowed to roam free, grazing on land that had yet to be treated with chemical fertilizers and other pesticides. The same cannot be said today.

Homeopathic medicines were one of the first natural remedies, other than herbs, to be mass produced for sale. The initial homeopathic manufacturers started in Europe in the late 1700's. Practitioners in North America often relied on the European homeopathic companies to supply products, sometimes waiting many months for shipments to arrive. It was not until the late 1800's that practitioners in North America had access to homeopathic products from companies on this side of the Atlantic with the opening of Thompson's Homeopathic Supplies Ltd in Toronto in 1868 and Hyland's in Los Angeles in 1903. Today access to high quality homeopathic products from around the world is very accessible.

The use of single nutrients as therapeutic agents started around 1911 with the discovery of Thiamine (B1). Other nutrients, such as Vitamin C were discovered in the 1930s. It was during this time that the mass production and distribution of single nutrients started. Vitamins, minerals, essential fatty acids etc., became readily available commercially in North America after the 1950s. In 1959 NDs on the

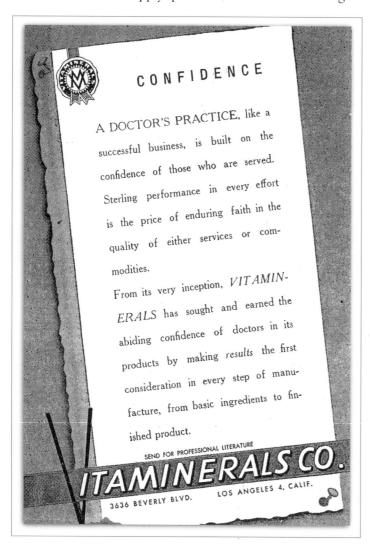

CONFIDENCE

A DOCTOR'S PRACTICE, like a successful business, is built on the confidence of those who are served. Sterling performance in every effort is the price of enduring faith in the quality of either services or commodities.

From its very inception, *VITAMIN-ERALS* has sought and earned the abiding confidence of doctors in its products by making *results* the first consideration in every step of manufacture, from basic ingredients to finished product.

SEND FOR PROFESSIONAL LITERATURE

VITAMINERALS CO.

3636 BEVERLY BLVD.   LOS ANGELES 4, CALIF.

West Coast, frustrated by the lack of quality products available to meet the needs of their patients, created Amo-Vite Health Products, the first company in Canada to sell directly to health care practitioners. As the interest in naturopathic and alternative medicine continued to grow, nutritional companies appeared on the Canadian marketplace, many created by practitioners themselves. An industry that started with less than a dozen manufacturers in the early 70's now numbers in the hundred's and ranges from small "Mom and Pop" to large multinational corporations. Since the very beginning the natural products industry has provided consistent and much needed support to the naturopathic community.

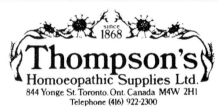

The Specialized Homoeopathic Laboratory for

- Fresh Plant Mother Tinctures (many are made either from selected wildgrown plants or from plants organically grown in our own gardens
- Handmade Hahnemannian Potencies
- High Potencies (Korsakoff)
- LM Potencies

Safe, Quality Products

The preparation of herbs for therapeutic use is an art and a science. Each part of a plant can have different effects on the body. How the plants are grown, harvested and manufactured impacts the therapeutic properties. The same is true for many vitamins and minerals as well as other neutraceutricals. Fish oils, for example, if not manufactured properly become rancid and lose their therapeutic value.

The introduction of, and demand for, vitamins and other natural health products occurred prior to any regulations or standards. As a result, there were some manufacturers and suppliers that were preparing and selling inferior products.

To ensure that naturopathic doctors had access to high quality products that had the correct ingredient levels to deliver a therapeutic effect, a few practitioners and biochemists started to manufacture products referred to

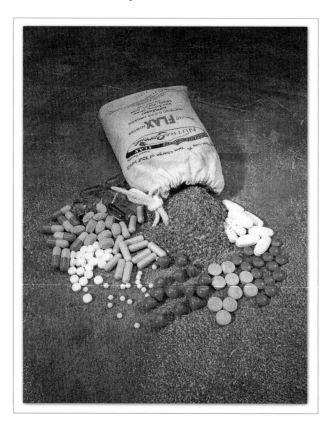

as "professional line products". Typically, even today, professional products are superior in quality compared to over-the-counter consumer products – they have higher doses of specific nutrients or herbs, have fewer fillers and additives, are free from contaminants, are manufactured with quality ingredients that meet or exceeded the Canadian governments Good Manufacturing Practices and are backed by third party assays. That means that a lab, with no connection to the company, has analyzed the ingredients and has verified the amount(s) of the active ingredient(s). Professional line products require the advice and supervision of a qualified health care professional, such as a naturopathic doctor, and are not readily available at retail locations.

Customizing Products

Naturopathic doctors have always created unique formulas for their patients by mixing together various natural ingredients that are backed by traditional and current research. This is known as compounding and continues to be an important part of the practice of naturopathic medicine to this day.

Compounding allows a naturopathic doctor to treat each patient as an individual, developing treatment plans tailored to each patient's specific needs. With the increase in chemical sensitivities, allergies and intolerances that people have it is important for practitioners to create formulas that meet the specific needs of each patient. Naturopathic doctors often use ingredients that are not readily available in the marketplace, are free from preservatives, chemicals and dyes, and compound products in a specific dose, or, dosage form (cream, lotion, gel, capsule, pellets etc). It is for these same reasons that many naturopathic doctors maintain dispensaries in order to have the products their patients need on hand and it allows them to easily address acute conditions. The regulatory boards that govern the profession and that ensure public safety have established policies and procedures for compounding, dispensing and selling products but the naturopathic doctor is ultimately responsible for the safety, effectiveness and quality of the products they compound and prescribe for patients.

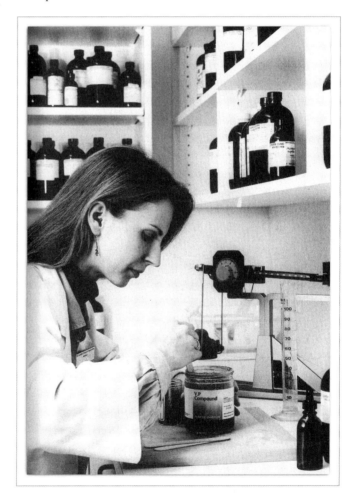

Government Regulations

As the use of natural health products increased so did the concern about their quality, efficacy and safety. Some of the concern was warranted as a few suppliers and manufacturers jumped on this growing market with little regard to quality; other concerns were a result of erroneous research and the government not fully understanding this new field. As a result, Health Canada reacted by moving a number of natural products – including herbs, vitamins and minerals and homeopathic medicines to restricted schedules. This transition has been, and continues to be a contentious issue for the naturopathic profession.

Since the 1970's increasing numbers of products traditionally used by naturopathic doctors have been moved to restricted schedules. As naturopathic doctors currently only have prescribing rights in one jurisdiction in Canada this restriction has denied product access to the very health care professionals who are the experts in their use. Lobbying efforts to acquire prescribing authority for NDs have been ongoing for many years across the country. The challenge is that Health Canada is responsible at the federal level for assessing the risk of products and puts any it considers to be of high risk on restricted schedules; yet since health care is managed at the provincial level, it is provincial Health Ministries that have the authority to grant access to substances on these restricted schedules.

In the 1980's Health Canada initially addressed the standards issue by requesting that manufacturers of natural products, starting with those that contained higher doses of active ingredients, meet the government's standards for drugs and obtain Drug Identification Numbers (DINs) under the Food and Drug Act. The concern was that companies were not allowed to make health claims for the products the way other drug manufacturers could and not all companies were required to comply. This process created havoc for small independent, botanical, homeopathic and supplement companies. The natural health products industry, comprised primarily of small companies at the time, was being strained financially by a process that was designed for large pharmaceutical companies.

In the late 1990's, Health Canada decided to take another look at the way natural health products were regulated. Naturopathic doctors, alternative practitioners, health food retailers and the natural product industry became concerned that more products would disappear from the marketplace if the proposed new regulations were implemented. One of the largest grass roots lobbying campaigns in Canadian history was undertaken. As a result of these efforts the Health Minister withdrew the proposed regulations and agreed to consult with Canadians. At the time, Dr. Pat Wales ND and Dr. Dan Labriola ND had a meeting with representatives from the Food and Drug division of the government to discuss the regulation of natural health products. Dr. Pam Snider ND, around the same time frame, requested that the government meet with natural product stakeholders, as they did on a continual basis with manufacturers and stakeholders of the drug industry. For over a year, Dr. Snider ND worked with government to organize over 25 representatives from the natural health products industry to meet with a similar number of government reps in a first-ever industry / government meeting in 1998. The result was the convening of the Expert Advisory Committee on Natural Health Products by the federal government. This committee undertook in-depth consultations and then tabled 53 recommendations to the House of Commons Standing Committee on Health. All 53 recommendations were accepted and presented to Minister of Health.

On March 26, 1999, the Minister accepted all 53 recommendations. The recommendations included amending the Food and Drugs Act to create a separate category for natural health products recognizing that they were neither drugs or foods; the development of regulations specific to natural health products which took into account the safe history of their use including traditional and scientific uses and a separate regulatory department within Health Canada to oversee the development and implementation of the regulations.

A Transitional Team made up of 17 representatives from government, a consumer advocacy group and a broad range of individuals with expertise in natural health products (including NDs) was formed to move forward with the implementation of the Standing Committee's recommendations. The Office of Natural Health Products (ONHP) was created and Dr. Philip Waddington, a naturopathic doctor and graduate of the Canadian College of Naturopathic Medicine in Toronto was appointed as Executive Director in January of 2000. Upon the completion of the Transition Teams work the ONHP became the Natural Health Products Directorate and Dr. Philip Waddington ND became its first Director General in 2001. The aim of the NHPD is to ensure that all Canadians have ready access to natural health products that are safe, effective and of high quality, while respecting freedom of choice and philosophical and cultural diversity. As of 2008 there are nine naturopathic doctors working at the NHPD in addition to their colleagues working in other departments of Health Canada.

Regulations were drafted, extensive consultations were undertaken across the country and on January 1, 2004 the Natural Health Products Regulations came into effect in Canada. A natural health product must be suitable for self care, safe for self-selection and available over the counter. Natural Health Products (NHPs) are those that are used in: (a) the diagnosis, treatment, mitigation or prevention of a disease, disorder or abnormal physical state or its symptoms in humans; (b) restoring or correcting organic functions in humans; or (c) modifying organic functions in humans, such as modifying those functions in a manner that maintains or promotes health.

Complete details of the regulations including the schedules that set

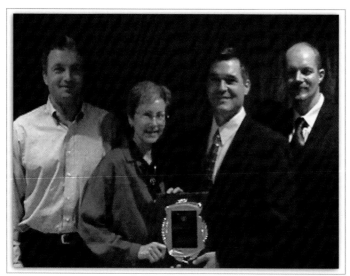

Philip Waddington ND, MBA a passionate proponent of naturopathic medicine. Dr. Waddington utilized his training as an ND and his business background to become the first Director General of the NHPD. In 2002 the CAND presented Dr. Waddington with the Verna Hunt award in recognition of his dedication to the profession.

Naturopathic Doctors Kevin Jackson, Pat Wales, Phil Waddington and Wayne Steinke.

out what is and what is not an NHP can be found on the NHPD website at http://www.hc-sc.gc.ca/dhp-mps/prodnatur/legistlation/index-eng.php. The regulations require site licenses for all Canadian locations involved in manufacturing, labelling, importing, packaging distributing or storing NHPs. Product licenses are required for all products and those that make it through the assessment process are given a Natural Product Number (NPN) or, in the case of homeopathic medicines, a DIN-HM. The NPN or DIN-HM must appear on product labels and ensures the public that the products are of acceptable quality, safe and approved for sale in Canada.

Stakeholders, including representatives from the CAND, continue to consult with government and the NHPD on the full implementation and impact of the regulations. It is only with time that we will see whether the mandate of the NHPD to "ensure that all Canadians have ready access to natural health products that are safe, effective and of high quality, while respecting freedom of choice and philosophical and cultural diversity" is realized.

To make sure the natural product(s) you choose are right for you? Consult with a naturopathic doctor who can assess, diagnose and develop a treatment plan specific to your needs. This is particularly important if you are suffering from a serious or chronic health condition or are on multiple medications. When looking for basic support or prevention, select products that contain natural ingredients and have an NPN on the label. Do your homework and be cautious about purchasing products over the Internet or from vendors at local markets and fairs as you have no guarantee of product quality or effectiveness. If you are unsure whether or not a natural product meets the requirements of the NHP regulations, check the NHPDs product database on its website or consult a naturopathic doctor in your area.

> *Definition:* Natural health products are defined as vitamins and minerals, herbal remedies, homeopathic remedies, traditional medicines such as traditional Chinese medicines, probiotics, and other products like amino acids and essential fatty acids.

PART FIVE

APPENDIX

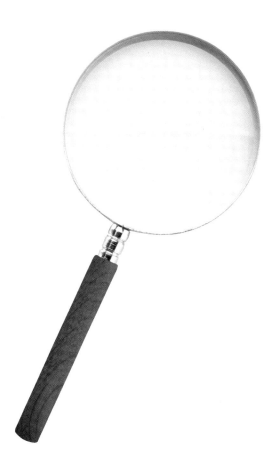

ONTARIO COLLEGE OF NATUROPATHIC DOCTORS
1ST ACCELERATED UNDERGRADUATE CLASS OF 1981

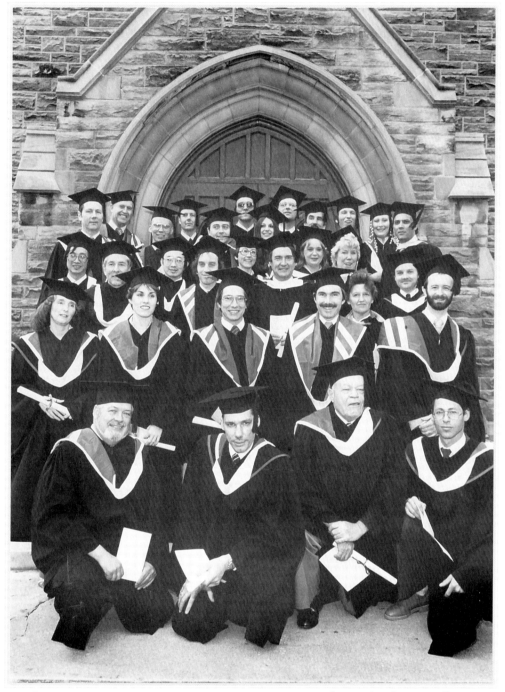

Back row: R.D. Wayne Scott, Leo Roy, Eric Harela, Richard Pragnell, Anton Ingard, Alan Davidson, Elaine Markovitch, Jan Valchar, John McLean, Rob and Sylvia Shackleton, Laurence Grey
3rd row: Steven Cheng, William Sykes, William Cheng, Allan Bortnick, Patricia Wales, Donald Gay, Suzanne Rohn-Szabo, Muriel Grant, Kenneth Dunk
2nd row: Leslie E. Scott, Daria Love, James Wilson, John Cosgrove, Frances Eddleston, David Mann
Front row: William Morris, Eric Shrubb, John LaPlante, G. Asa Hershoff
Not pictured: Edith (Edie) Pett, William Slade Prusin

Ontario College of Naturopathic Doctors
2nd Accelerated Undergraduate Class of 1982

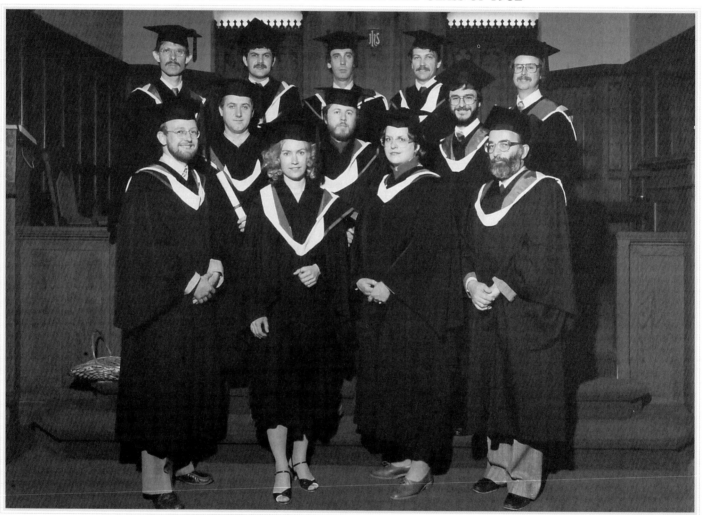

Back row: Ross Andersen, Robert Tripodi, Alexander Wood, John Cadieux, Keith Thomson
Centre row: James McNamara, James O'Neill, Ernest Baustein
Front row: Martin Kura, Eva Mannen, Verna Hunt, Barry Berman
Not pictured: Kim McKenzie, George Roth

ONTARIO COLLEGE OF NATUROPATHIC DOCTORS
3RD ACCELERATED UNDERGRADUATE CLASS OF 1984

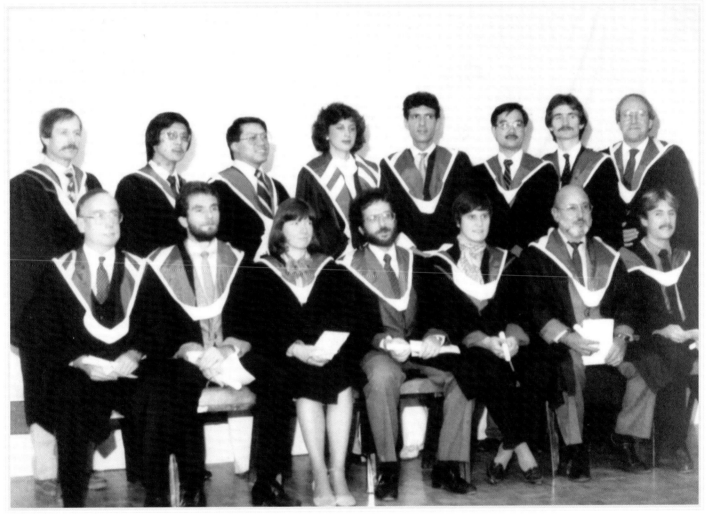

Back row: Richard Putman, David Yu, Allan Chan, Helga Marinzel, Jose DaCosta Reis, Dale Okabe, Fedor Zelina, William Dronyk
Front row: Neall Stedmann, Paul Waunch, Mary Hassard, Joseph Kellerstein, Naide Bruno, Herbert Adirim, Frederick Wilson
Picture provided by Helga Marinzel ND

ONTARIO COLLEGE OF NATUROPATHIC DOCTORS
4TH ACCELERATED UNDERGRADUATE CLASS OF 1986

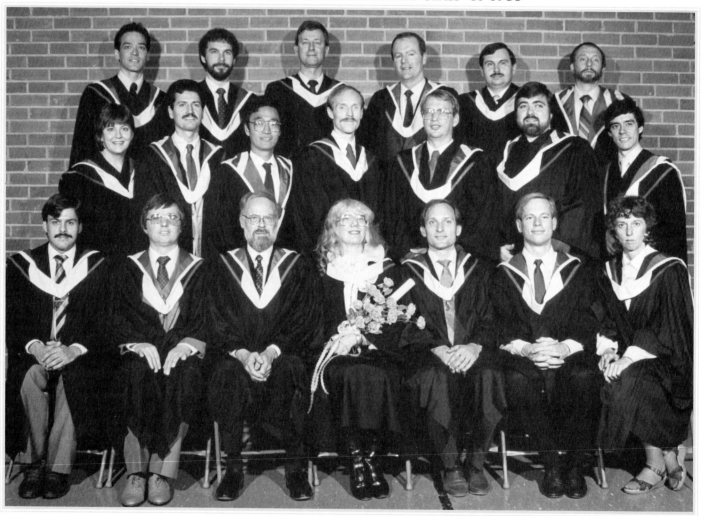

Back row: Timothy Brown, James William Spring, Robert Dronyk, Brian Joseph Nelson, Morris Demborynsky, Jack Hinze
Centre row: Lianne South, Lucas Bozinovski, Alexander Yuan, Gary Hardy, Ronald Levay, Richard David McCrorie, Dennis P. O'Hara
Front row: Frank Amodeo, John Hawrylak, Pieter Taams, Donna Morphy, Howard Levine, Mark Percival, Ingeborg Eibl
Not pictured: Tutti Gould, James Lewer

ONTARIO COLLEGE OF NATUROPATHIC DOCTORS
5TH ACCELERATED UNDERGRADUATE CLASS OF 1987

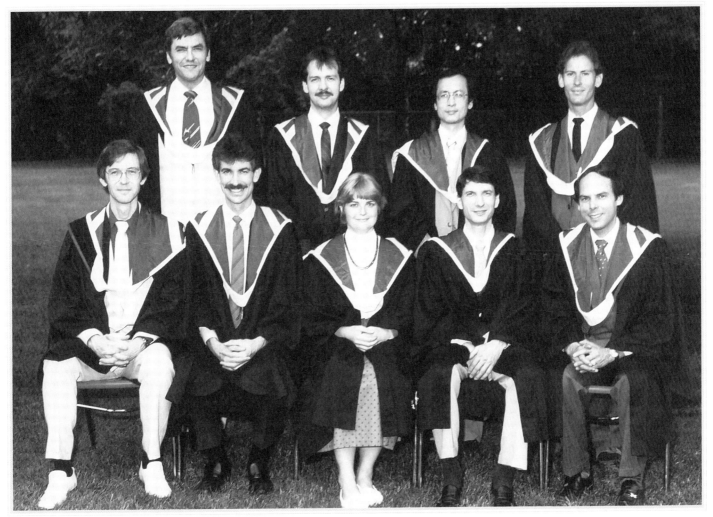

Back row: Anthony R. Toplak, Douglas J. MacLachlan, Isaac Chan, Mark Coates
Front row: Michael V. Miller, George Milne, Daphne Rappard, Avram H. Sussman, Jacob Scheer

ONTARIO COLLEGE OF NATUROPATHIC DOCTORS
1ST UNDERGRADUATE CLASS OF 1987

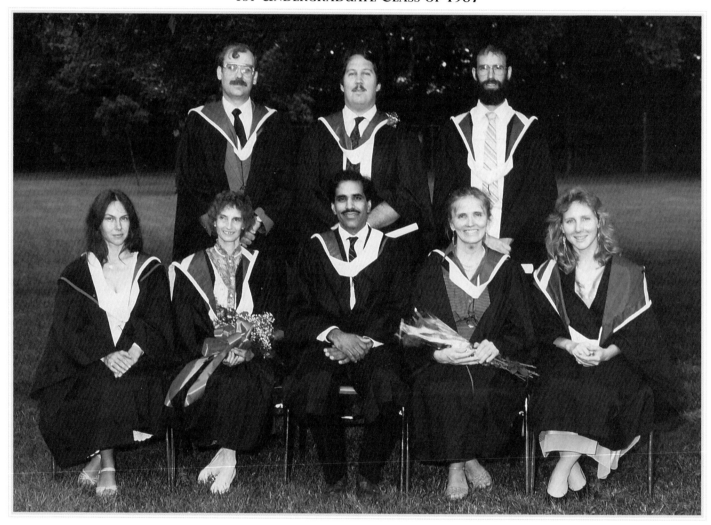

Back row: Robert L. Gatis, Terrance MacIntosh, Richard Tunstall
Front row: Patricia Wolfe, Patricia Roth, Elvis Ali, Lois Hare, Anna Nordin

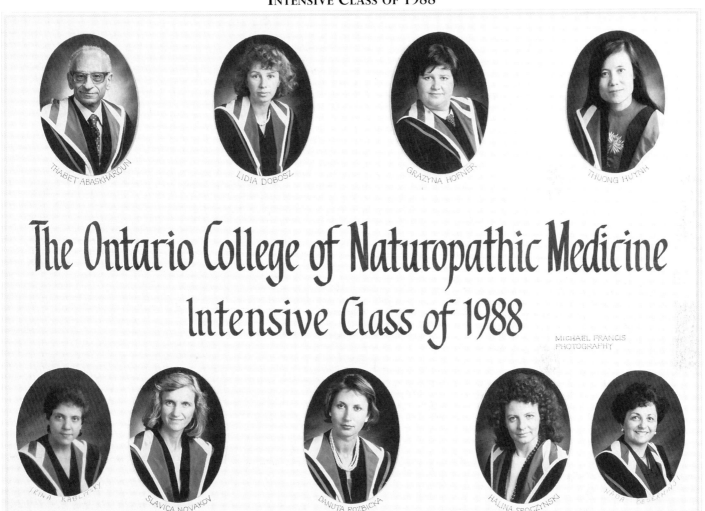

Not pictured: Joseph Kulchyk, Maria L Nurmi, William (Bill) Russell, Alfonso WH Wong

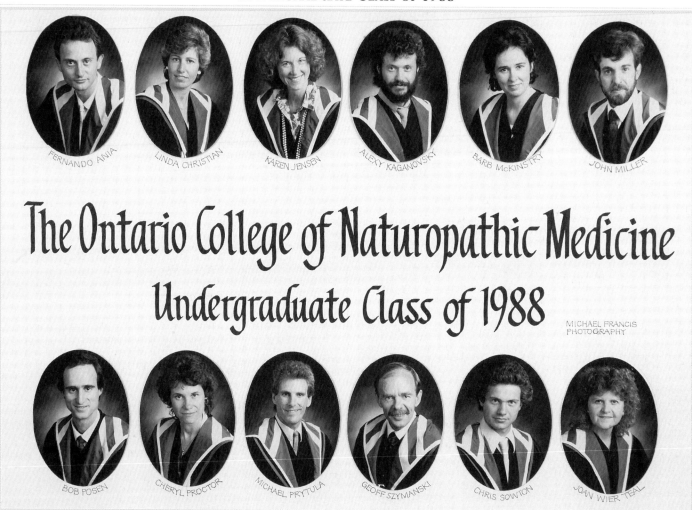

The Ontario College of Naturopathic Medicine Undergraduate Class of 1988

FERNANDO ANIA LINDA CHRISTIAN KAREN JENSEN ALEXY KAGANOVSKY BARB McKINSTRY JOHN MILLER

MICHAEL FRANCIS PHOTOGRAPHY

BOB POSEN CHERYL PROCTOR MICHAEL PRYTULA GEOFF SZYMANSKI CHRIS SOWTON JOAN WIER TEAL

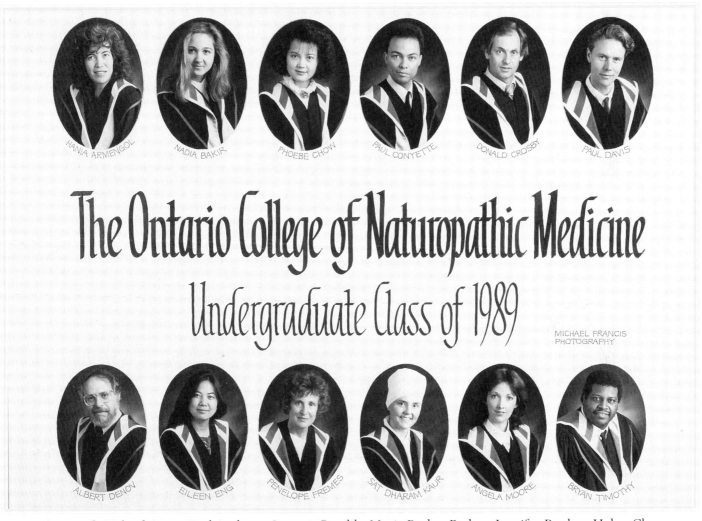

HANIA ARMENGOL   NADIA BAKIR   PHOEBE CHOW   PAUL CONYETTE   DONALD CROSBY   PAUL DAVIS

The Ontario College of Naturopathic Medicine

Undergraduate Class of 1989

MICHAEL FRANCIS
PHOTOGRAPHY

ALBERT DENOV   EILEEN ENG   PENELOPE FREMES   SAT DHARAM KAUR   ANGELA MOORE   BRYAN TIMOTHY

Not pictured: Nabeel Ajina, Paul Anthony, Jaromir Bertlik, Maria Brelny-Radon, Jennifer Booker, Helen Change-Meyers nee Meyers, Nicole Constant, Madeleine F Crnec, Erwin Gemel, Pierre Lemay, Norman F Lewis, Douha Elnachef, Peter George Pooyakkers, Peter Chun-Ting Yam

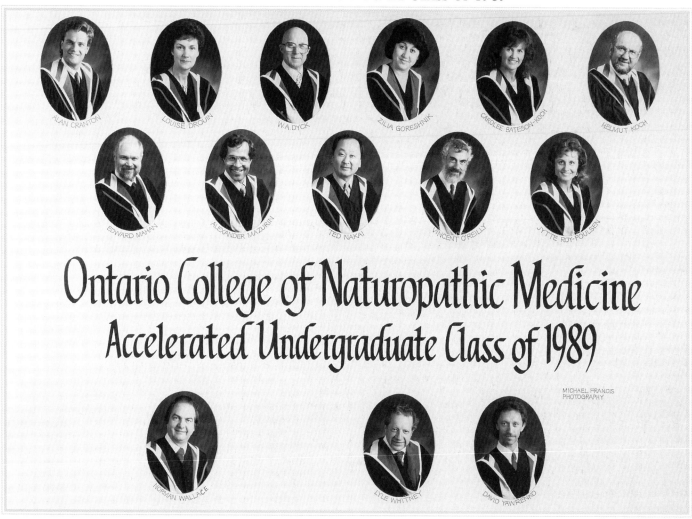

ONTARIO COLLEGE OF NATUROPATHIC MEDICINE
UNDERGRADUATE CLASS OF 1989

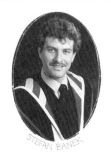
STEFAN BANEK

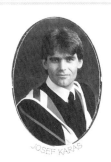
JOSEF KARAS

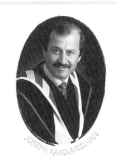
JOSEPH KAYOUMEDJIAN

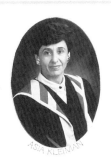
ASIA KLEIMAN

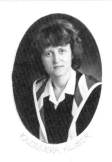
KAZIMIERA KLIBER

The Ontario College of Naturopathic Medicine
Intensive Class of 1989

MICHAEL FRANCIS
PHOTOGRAPHY

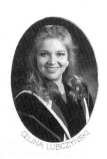
CELINA LUBCZYNSKI

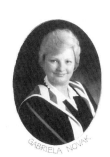
GABRIELA NOVAK

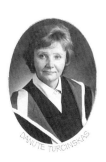
DANUTE TURCINSKAS

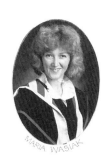
MARIA WASIAK

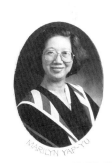
MARILYN YAP-YU

ONTARIO COLLEGE OF NATUROPATHIC MEDICINE
WESTERN ACCELERATED CLASS OF 1989

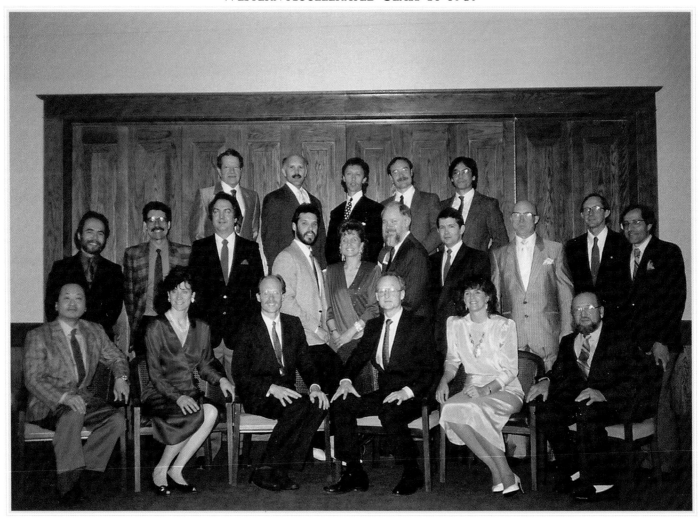

Back row: Tad Nakai, Paula Fainstat, Bruce Adamson, Kenneth Cashion, Carolee Bateson-Koch, Helmut Koch
Middle row: Eric Posen, Harold S (Hal) Brown, Norman Wallace, Ronald Edward Rose, Jytte Roy-Poulson, Edward Mahan, Daryl Robert Bourke, Wiegand A. Dyck, Kevin R Nolan, Alexander Mazurin
Front row: Lyle Whitney, Bill Russell, Dave Yurenko, David E Wasylynko, Lawrence (Larry) Chan,

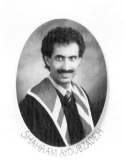

SHAHRAM AYOUBZADEH

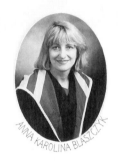

ANNA KAROLINA BLASZCZYK

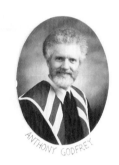

ANTHONY GODFREY

The Ontario College of Naturopathic Medicine
Intensive Class of 1990

MICHAEL FRANCIS
PHOTOGRAPHY

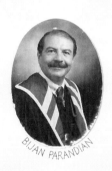

BIJAN PARANDIAN

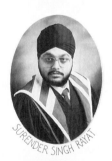

SURENDER SINGH RAYAT

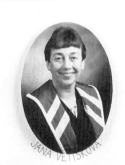

JANA VETISKOVA

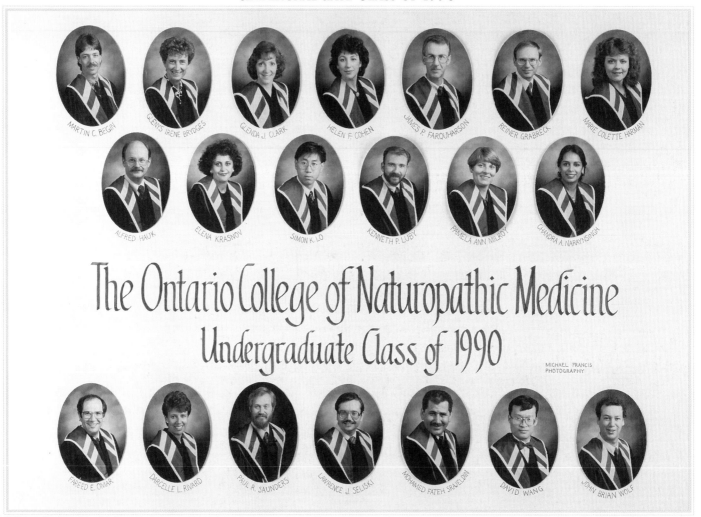

Not pictured: Mervat Bazan, Walter G Blois, Ray Charles, Carl N Greggain, Laurence V Hicks, Cynthia (Cindy) Isles, Urban Albert Hans Edelmalm Nelson, Michael J O'Grady, Mukesh M Patel, Horst Siebert

ONTARIO COLLEGE OF NATUROPATHIC MEDICINE
CLASS OF 1991

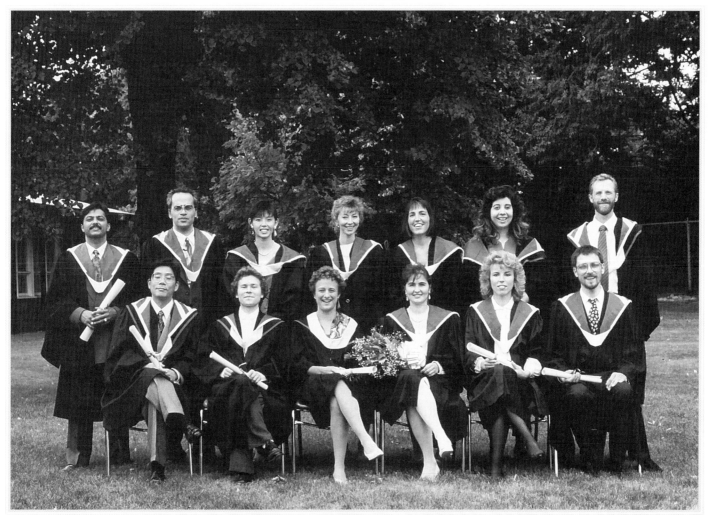

Back row: Harjot Sidhu, Farhad Esfaniari, Joel Lee, Kelly Geddes, Cynthia Bondy, Rena Zambri, Michael Liebscher
Front row: David Oh, Ray Lendvai, Pamela Arychuk, Darlene Gustin, Anke Zimmermann, Robert Medrek

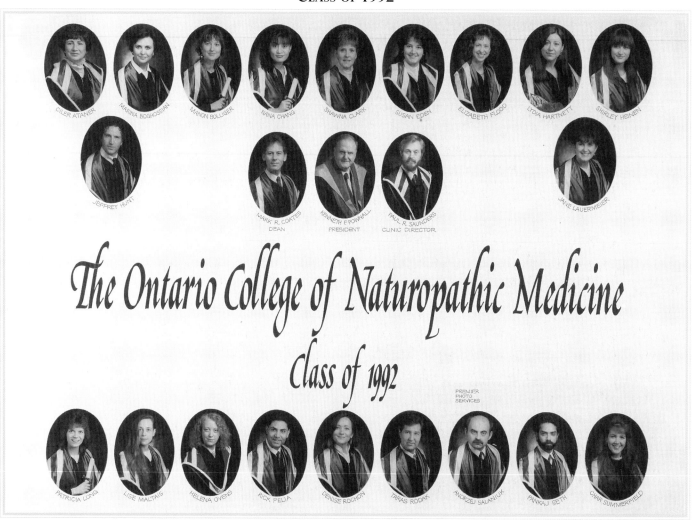

Not pictured: Elizabeth Langdon, Rikninder Singh

CANADIAN COLLEGE OF NATUROPATHIC MEDICINE
CLASS OF 1993

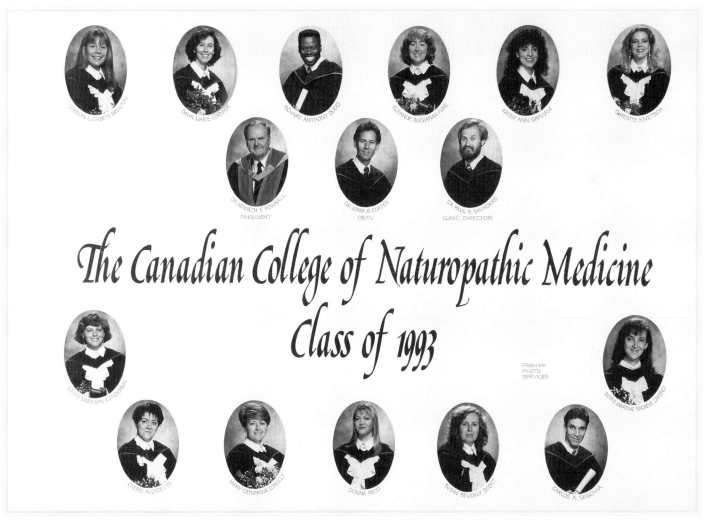

CAROLYN ELIZABETH BRANTON   DAWN MARIE CORMIER   RICHARD ANTHONY DODD   ELEANOR BUCHANAN FUKE   KATHY ANN GRAHAM   CHRISTIE KNETSCH

DR. KENNETH E. POWNALL
PRESIDENT

DR. MARK R. COATES
DEAN

DR. PAUL R. SAUNDERS
CLINIC DIRECTOR

The Canadian College of Naturopathic Medicine
Class of 1993

CATHY MARY ANN KUNDOSZINA

PREMIER
PHOTO
SERVICES

MARIE MARTINE MICHELE LYOND

CHERYL A. LYCELTTE   MARY CATHERINE O'REILLY   DONNA REID   SUSAN BEVERLY SCOTT   CARLOS A. SEGOVIA

CANADIAN COLLEGE OF NATUROPATHIC MEDICINE
CLASS OF 1994

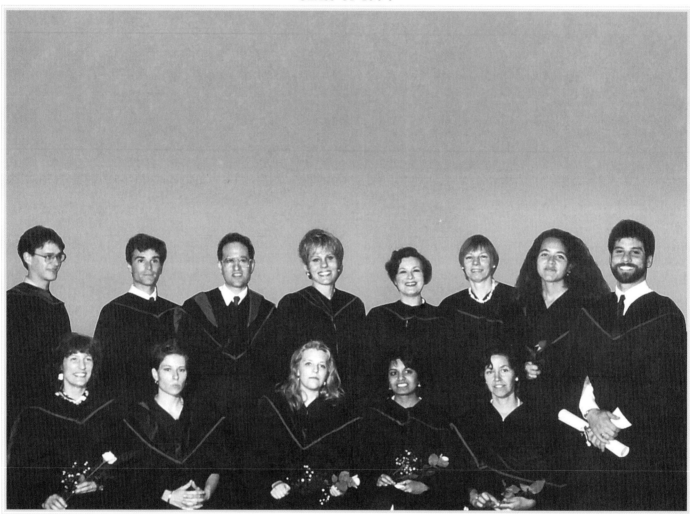

Back row: Terry Vanderheyden, Craig Palmer, Michael Eisenstein, Ruth Anne Baron, Shirley Zabol, Dorothy Roke, Leslie Dewar, Quinn Rivet
Front row: Penny Seth-Smith, Mary Ellen McKenna, Java Exner, Sejal Parikh-Shah, Sussanna Czeranko
Not pictured: Kathleen Morton

CANADIAN COLLEGE OF NATUROPATHIC MEDICINE
CLASS OF 1995

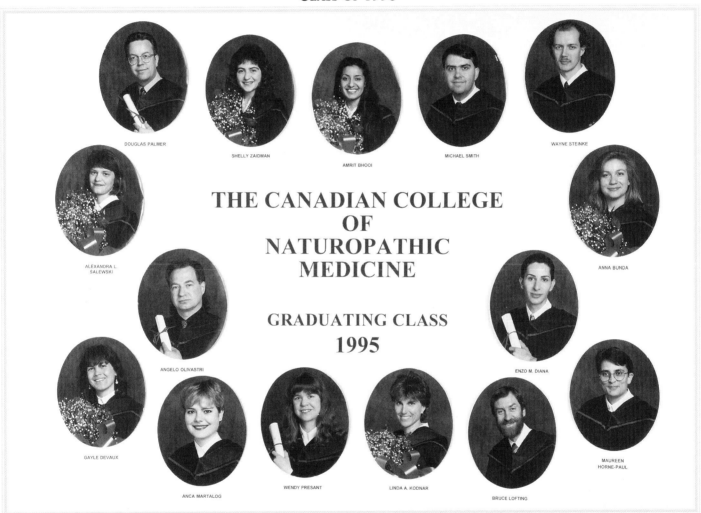

THE CANADIAN COLLEGE
OF
NATUROPATHIC
MEDICINE

GRADUATING CLASS
1995

DOUGLAS PALMER

SHELLY ZAIDMAN

AMRIT BHOOI

MICHAEL SMITH

WAYNE STEINKE

ALEXANDRA L. SALEWSKI

ANNA BUNDA

ANGELO OLIVASTRI

ENZO M. DIANA

GAYLE DEVAUX

ANCA MARTALOG

WENDY PRESANT

LINDA A. KODNAR

BRUCE LOFTING

MAUREEN HORNE-PAUL

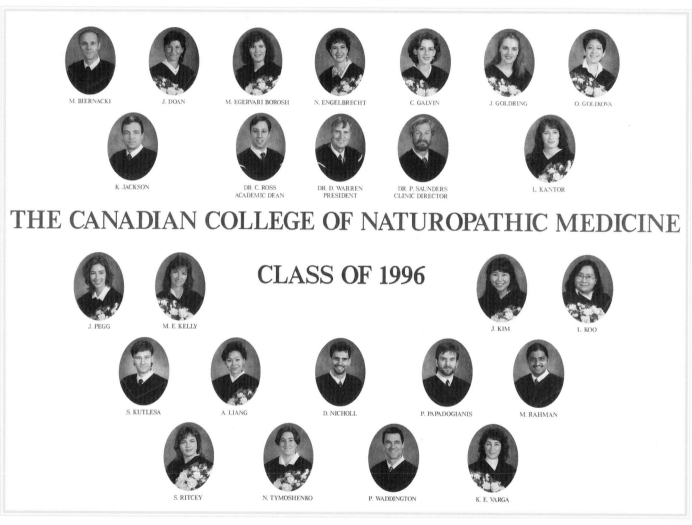

THE CANADIAN COLLEGE OF NATUROPATHIC MEDICINE

CLASS OF 1996

M. BIERNACKI J. DOAN M. EGERVARI BOROSH N. ENGELBRECHT C. GALVIN J. GOLDRING O. GOLIKOVA

K. JACKSON DR. C. ROSS ACADEMIC DEAN DR. D. WARREN PRESIDENT DR. P. SAUNDERS CLINIC DIRECTOR L. KANTOR

J. PEGG M. E. KELLY J. KIM L. KOO

S. KUTLESA A. LIANG D. NICHOLL P. PAPADOGIANIS M. RAHMAN

S. RITCEY N. TYMOSHENKO P. WADDINGTON K. E. VARGA

CANADIAN COLLEGE OF NATUROPATHIC MEDICINE
CLASS OF 1997

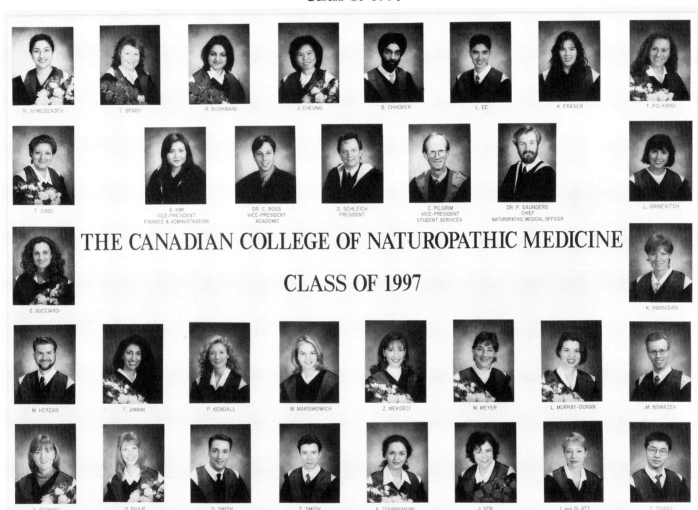

Not pictured and not included in the footer: Carolyn Dean

CANADIAN COLLEGE OF NATUROPATHIC MEDICINE
CLASS OF 1998

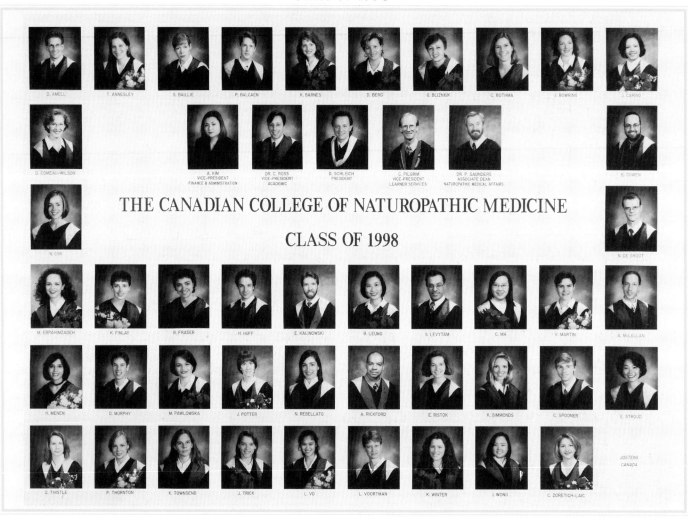

THE CANADIAN COLLEGE OF NATUROPATHIC MEDICINE

CLASS OF 1998

Not pictured and not included in the footer: Michael Friedman, Donna Levesque

CANADIAN COLLEGE OF NATUROPATHIC MEDICINE
CLASS OF 1999

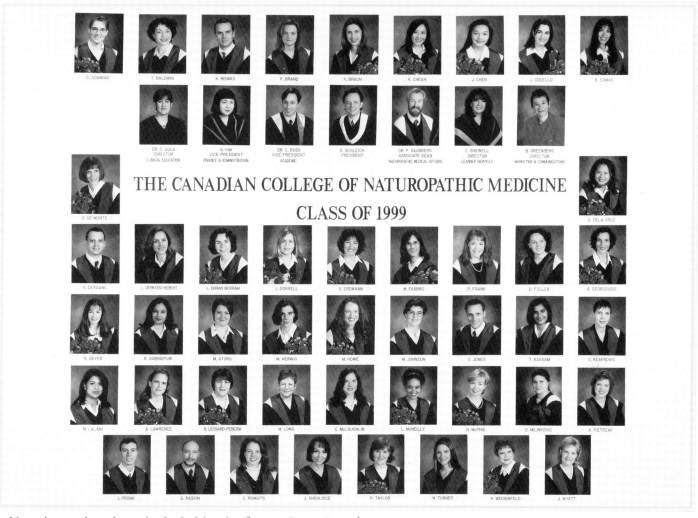

THE CANADIAN COLLEGE OF NATUROPATHIC MEDICINE

CLASS OF 1999

Not pictured and not included in the footer: Susan Benedetti

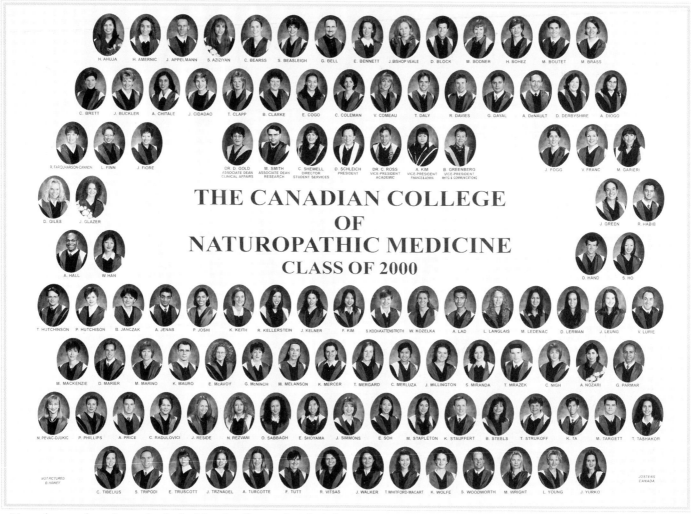

Not pictured and not included in the footer: Leigh A Ipsen

CANADIAN COLLEGE OF NATUROPATHIC MEDICINE
CLASS OF 2001

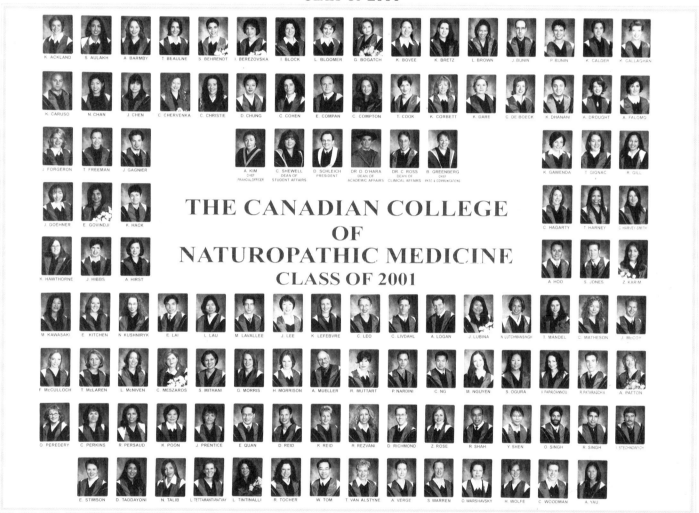

THE CANADIAN COLLEGE
OF
NATUROPATHIC MEDICINE
CLASS OF 2001

Not pictured: Darlene M Ahenakew, Emile J James, Edmond Man Lok Sheehan, Stephanie C Yik

CANADIAN COLLEGE OF NATUROPATHIC MEDICINE
CLASS OF 2002

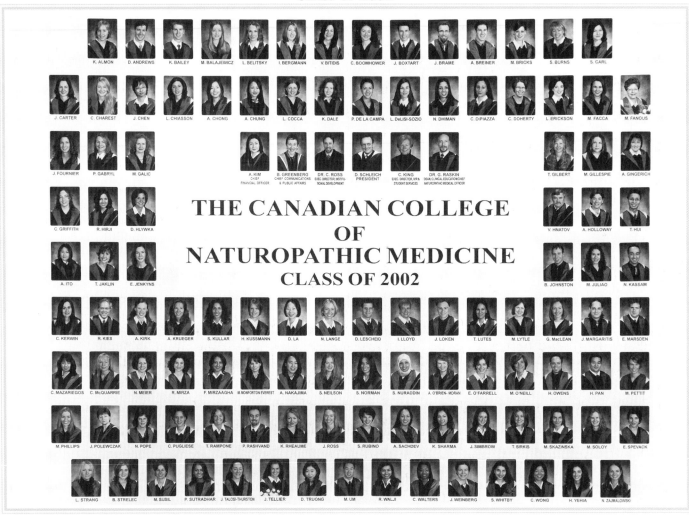

THE CANADIAN COLLEGE OF NATUROPATHIC MEDICINE CLASS OF 2002

Not pictured: Serenity Aberdour, Rob G Ayoup, Karamvir Singh Bains, Parviz Falari-Rashvand, Kira A Frketich, Bonnie J McLachlan, Micheal J Meade, Lilieana Mitrea nee Stadler, Christopher J Neimor, Francis Resinger-Oake, Aaron Samanta, Sandeep Sangra, Jeff Samborski

Canadian College of Naturopathic Medicine
Class of 2003

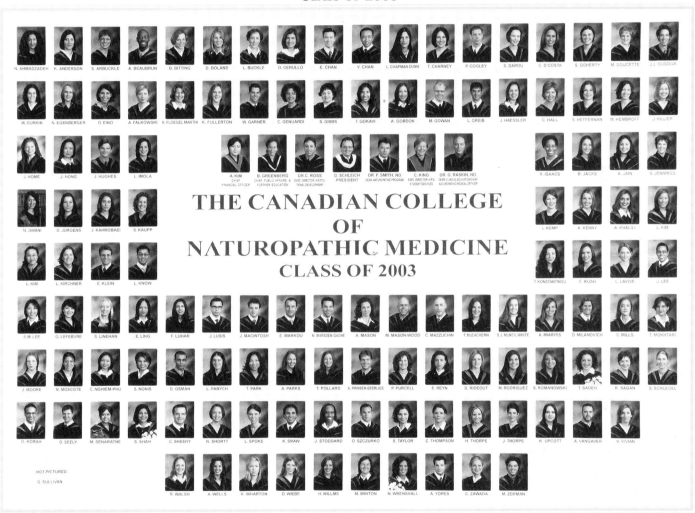

THE CANADIAN COLLEGE
OF
NATUROPATHIC MEDICINE
CLASS OF 2003

Not pictured and not included in the footer: Lucy C Ormerod, Tracey Pike, Rodolfo Adrian (Rod) Santos

CANADIAN COLLEGE OF NATUROPATHIC MEDICINE
CLASS OF 2004

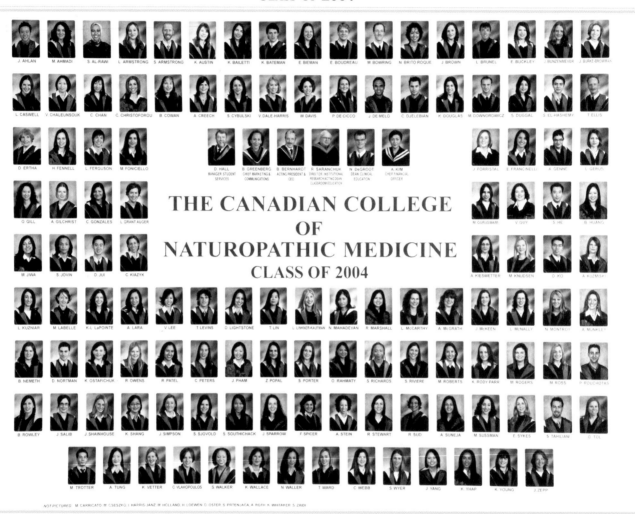

THE CANADIAN COLLEGE
OF
NATUROPATHIC MEDICINE
CLASS OF 2004

BOUCHER INSTITUTE OF NATUROPATHIC MEDICINE
CLASS OF 2004

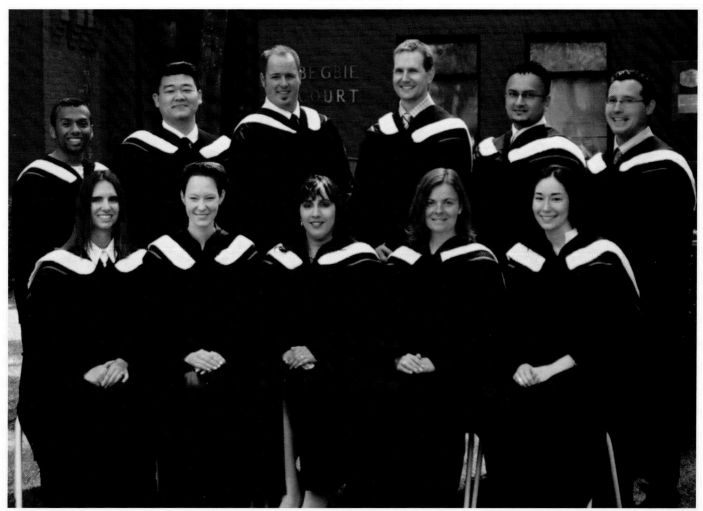

Back row: Sanjay Mohan Ram, Albert M. Kim, Jonas LaForge, Cameron McIntyre, Narbinder (Navi) Badesha, Jamie Gallant
Front row: Alison Vandekerkhove, Andrea Chambers, Sam Sandhu, Shelby Worts, Kelly Fujibayashi

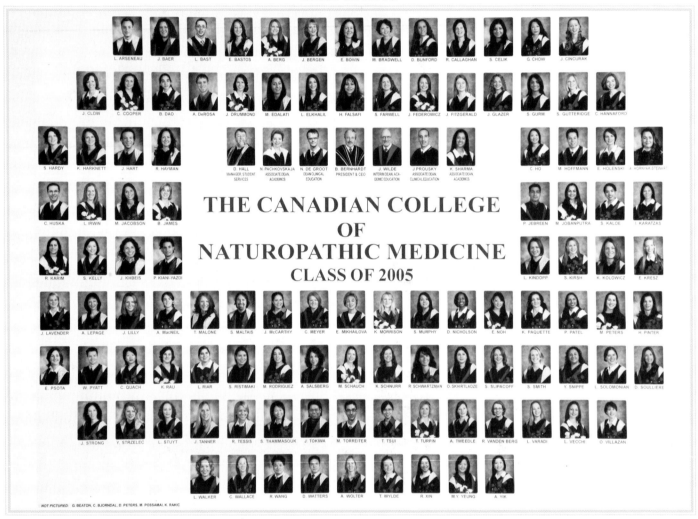

Not pictured and not included in the footer: Olga Cappuccio, Matthew Pyatt, David Chia-Hung Shih, Kathleen van Lierde

BOUCHER INSTITUTE OF NATUROPATHIC MEDICINE
CLASS OF 2005

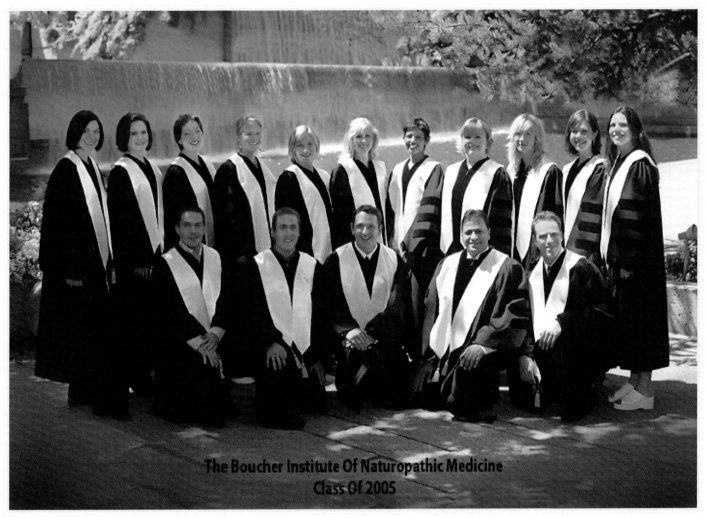

Back row: Sanja Tamburic, Jennifer Moss, Heather Eade, Bryn Hyndman, Marie Zalatan, Anita Bratt, Pushpa Kissun, Cathryn Coe, Melanie Kroeker, Chantelle Mitchell, Jodi Meacher
Front row: Darren Gorrell, Craig Herrington, Ian Brown, Sarge Sandhu, Kris Bentz

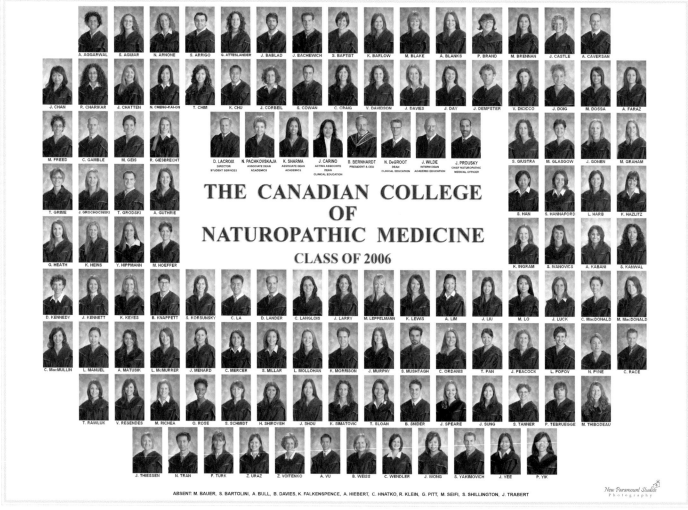

Not pictured and not included in the footer: Marika Jobin, Christopher Sean McConnell

BOUCHER INSTITUTE OF NATUROPATHIC MEDICINE
CLASS OF 2006

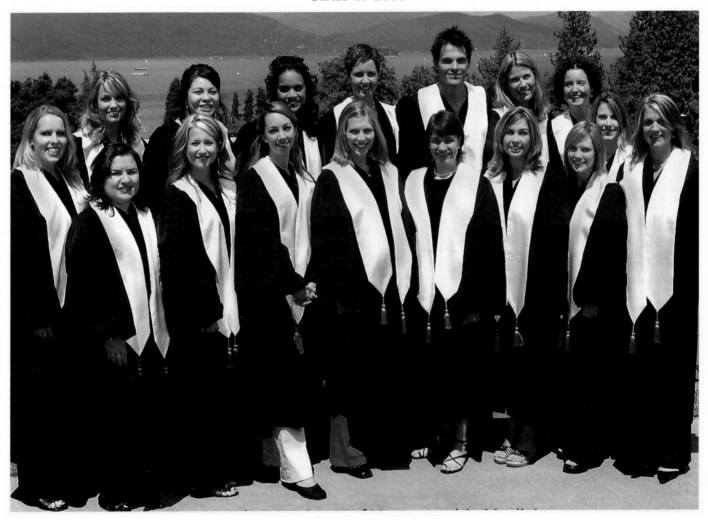

Back row: Karen Solli, Rebecca Hurd, Nicole Robinson, Vicky Radhakrishnan, Michelle Willis, Ryan Oughtred, Corrine Dawson, Karina Wickland

Front row: Rozita Moshtagh, Julie Bowman, Samantha Frey, Heidi Rootes, Rachel Sheehan, Marnie Wachtler, Nicole Duffee, Jennie Weisenburger, Tanja White

CANADIAN COLLEGE OF NATUROPATHIC MEDICINE
CLASS OF 2007

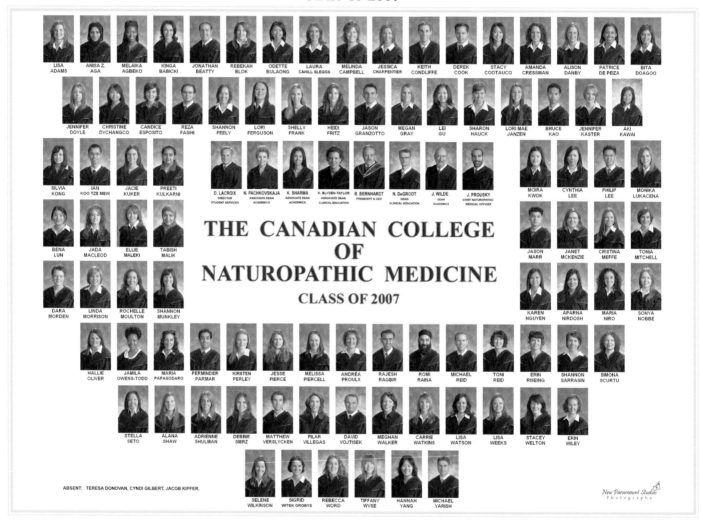

LISA ADAMS | ANISA Z. AGA | MELAIKA AGBEKO | KINGA BABICKI | JONATHAN BEATTY | REBEKAH BLOK | ODETTE BULAONG | LAURA CAHILL SLEGGS | MELINDA CAMPBELL | JESSICA CHARPENTIER | KEITH CONDLIFFE | DEREK COOK | STACY COOTAUCO | AMANDA CRESSMAN | ALISON DANBY | PATRICE DE PEIZA | BITA DOAGOO

JENNIFER DOYLE | CHRISTINE DYCHANGCO | CANDICE ESPOSITO | REZA FASIHI | SHANNON FEELY | LORI FERGUSON | SHELLY FRANK | HEIDI FRITZ | JASON GRANZOTTO | MEGAN GRAY | LEI GU | SHARON HAUCK | LORI MAE JANZEN | BRUCE KAO | JENNIFER KASTER | AKI KAWAI

SILVIA KONG | IAN KOO TZE MEW | JACIE KUKER | PREETI KULKARNI

D. LACROIX — DIRECTOR STUDENT SERVICES | N. PACHKOVSKAJA — ASSOCIATE DEAN ACADEMICS | K. SHARMA — ASSOCIATE DEAN ACADEMICS | K. BLYDEN-TAYLOR — ASSOCIATE DEAN CLINICAL EDUCATION | B. BERNHARDT — PRESIDENT & CEO | N. DeGROOT — DEAN CLINICAL EDUCATION | J. WILDE — DEAN ACADEMICS | J. PROUSKY — CHIEF NATUROPATHIC MEDICAL OFFICER

MOIRA KWOK | CYNTHIA LEE | PHILIP LEE | MONIKA LUKACENA

BENA LUN | JADA MACLEOD | ELLIE MALEKI | TABISH MALIK

THE CANADIAN COLLEGE OF NATUROPATHIC MEDICINE
CLASS OF 2007

JASON MARR | JANET MCKENZIE | CRISTINA MEFFE | TONIA MITCHELL

DARA MORDEN | LINDA MORRISON | ROCHELLE MOULTON | SHANNON MUNKLEY

KAREN NGUYEN | APARNA NIRDOSH | MARIA NIRO | SONYA NOBBE

HALLIE OLIVER | JAMILA OWENS-TODD | MARIA PAPASODARO | PERMINDER PARMAR | KIRSTEN PERLEY | JESSE PIERCE | MELISSA PIERCELL | ANDRÉA PROULX | RAJESH RAGBIR | ROMI RAINA | MICHAEL REID | TONI REID | ERIN RISEING | SHANNON SARRASIN | SIMONA SCURTU

STELLA SETO | ALANA SHAW | ADRIENNE SHULMAN | DEBBIE SMRZ | MATTHEW VERSLYCKEN | PILAR VILLEGAS | DAVID VOJTISEK | MEGHAN WALKER | CARRIE WATKINS | LISA WATSON | LISA WEEKS | STACEY WELTON | ERIN WILEY

ABSENT: TERESA DONOVAN, CYNDI GILBERT, JACOB KIPFER,

SELENE WILKINSON | SIGRID WITEK GROBYS | REBECCA WORD | TIFFANY WYSE | HANNAH YANG | MICHAEL YARISH

New Paramount Studios Photography

BOUCHER INSTITUTE OF NATUROPATHIC MEDICINE
CLASS OF 2007

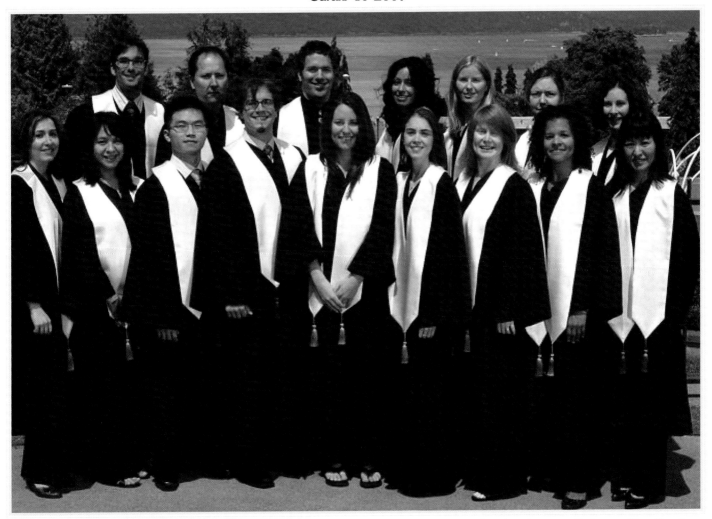

Back row: Justin Lafreniere, Walter Fernyhough, Nicholas Jensen, Sonya Grewal, Rikst Attema, Rebecca Handford, Jese Wiens

Front row: Kathrine Tavakoli, Ana Lopez, Steven Hsu, Brett Phillips, Tina Garrison, Allison Bachlet, Janine Fraser, Natalie Mazurin, Jia Qi Chen

CANADIAN COLLEGE OF NATUROPATHIC MEDICINE
CLASS OF 2008

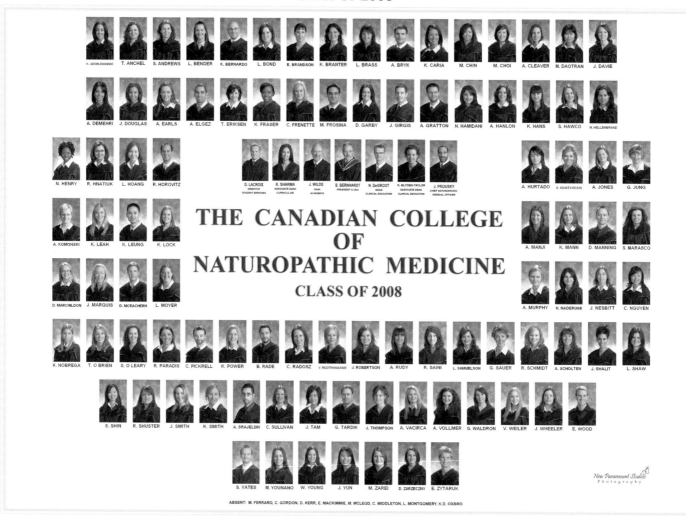

THE CANADIAN COLLEGE
OF
NATUROPATHIC MEDICINE

CLASS OF 2008

New Paramount Studios
Photography

BOUCHER INSTITUTE OF NATUROPATHIC MEDICINE
CLASS OF 2008

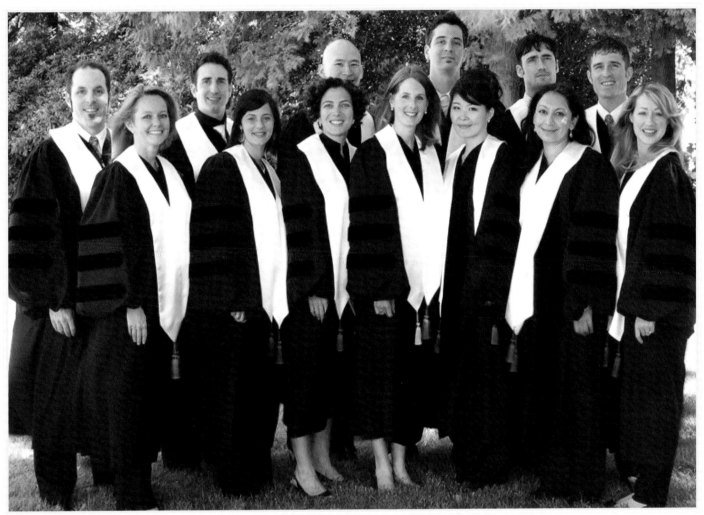

Back row: Jonathan Friz Berghamer, Jordan Atkinson, Adrian Yeong, Rick Santimaw, Elliott Mordy, Martin Gleixner
Front row: Debra Gillott Heald, Stephanie Peltz, Emily Habert, Melanie Marx/McLean, Sooin Lee, Alexina Metha, Lisa Good

STORIES FROM NATUROPATHIC DOCTORS

Dr. Elvis A. Ali ND

Growing up in Trinidad, West Indies, I understood preventative medicine and integrating mind-body medicine to be beneficial in the quest for the overall quality of life. In 1978 during my second year of Pre-Med in Waterloo, I injured my ankle and recovered with acupuncture, Chinese herbs and massage therapy. At this time in my life I began to seek information about complementary medicine and was also intrigued by sports medicine.

In 1981, I met with Dr. Gordon Smith ND and Tom Foster who told me the naturopathic medical school, at 43 Benton Street in Kitchener, was opening up full-time in a few years. I already had my B.Sc. in Biology and they informed me that I could enter the Drugless Therapy (DT) Program, which I did for two years. In 1983 I enrolled in the first full-time undergraduate class at the Ontario College of Naturopathic Medicine and graduated in 1987 with seven other students.

Since my graduation, I have taken post-graduate courses at Harvard Medical School to learn more about mind-body medicine. I have also traveled in Korea, Hong Kong and China to get more education in Chinese medicine. This has helped reinforce my belief in preventative medicine. Indeed the twenty-first century is embracing complementary medicine and I am very proud to teach and educate the public about naturopathic medicine throughout Canada, Asia and the West Indies. I have also had the opportunity to publish articles on stress and five books on natural health topics.

Dr. Pamela Arychuk ND

My practice began near the College, at home in my Etobicoke apartment. I was teaching Biochemistry to the first year students at OCNM at the time. Although Nutrition was always an area of focus in my practice, I have maintained an integrative, comprehensive approach. Homeopathics, Eastern and Western Botanicals, Tissue Salts and Bach Flowers are prescribed whenever indicated. Acupuncture, Manual Lymph Drainage, Colon Hydrothrapy- and Myofascial Trigger Point Release are sometimes required. I attribute the success I have with clients to modalities and to sufficient time spent working at the mental and emotional level; appointments average about 2 hours.

My husband, Michael Liebscher and I ran the Oshawa Naturopathic Clinic until 1998, when we left for Asia in order to faster pay for the Tobago-land-soon-to-be-Spa. I feel honored to teach and very much enjoy practicing naturopathic medicine in The Philippines and in Taiwan. If anyone is interested in helping complete the Tobago project, please contact me!

Dr. Nada Beserminji ND

In September 1986, I passed the Canadian Evaluation Examination for MD and I applied to find a residency in Canada. On Saturday January 3, 1987, Dr. Grazyna Hofner ND told me about the Ontario College of Naturopathic Medicine. She said, "Nada lets go study naturopathic medicine while we are waiting for our medical internship to see how different it is from medicine. We have health problems and maybe the solution is naturopathic medicine." On Monday I spoke to the Dean, Dr. Manolis, and told him my English was poor. He said, "Don't worry, you're a medical doctor, you will pass those few exams." Within five minutes I was already in class as a student of the naturopathic college.

My first exam, physiotherapy, was in March. I didn't understand some words in the exam and so I asked Bob Posen what some words meant. A furious professor came to my desk claiming that I was cheating. "What does cheating mean?" was all I could say. She warned me that she was going to call the police and I didn't understand why. Bob told the professor that my English was very poor, after which she gave me the definition of what I didn't understand. A few exams later, seventeen to be exact, I found out from Dr. Manolis that there were thirty-two exams in total. I want to thank Dr. Manolis for extending the truth.

Today, I have been working twenty years as a naturopathic doctor and I'm grateful for finding the solution to my health problems and the problems of my patients which I couldn't solve medically.

Dr. Cathy Carlson-Rink ND

I have practiced as a naturopathic physician and registered midwife in a family health clinic in Langley, BC since 1996. My focus has been on pregnancy, women's and children's health. I have been an instructor of Obstetrics at the Boucher Institute of Naturopathic Medicine. I also teach continuing education to healthcare professionals in the areas of obstetrics, gynecology and pediatrics.

I graduated with distinction with a Bachelor of Science in Physical Education with a Major in Health and Fitness from the University of Saskatchewan in 1987. I received my degree in naturopathic medicine and Midwifery from Bastyr University in 1995 and 1996 respectfully. I am recognized as the first naturopathic physician in Canada to also work as a licensed midwife and am part of the first group of registered midwives integrated into the hospital setting in British Columbia. To date I have "caught" over 400 babies and helped many others conceive after infertility and miscarriage. Having the opportunity to take care of children since their birth, has allowed me to use the naturopathic tenant of prevention to the fullest extent. The children in my practice are very healthy and there is almost no incidence of chronic disease which is so prevalent in the pediatric population today.

Dr. Nana Chang ND

I believe we are guided…

I earned my black belt at age seventeen. Eager to learn about health and fitness, I graduated in 1989 from the University of Toronto with a B.Sc. in Physiology and Human Biology. There - Destiny called. A stranger, "Gerry" handed me a course calendar for the Ontario College of Naturopathic Medicine (OCNM) with his name and number on it. At the time I was preparing for a career in sports medicine or chiropractic. In the late 1980s, "naturopathy" was unknown or marginalized.

That chance meeting changed my life - I fell in love with the profession. I tried to contact "Gerry" to thank him, but his phone was not in service. Catching a glimpse of him again in second year, I went to speak to him but he had disappeared. No one else had seen him and I discovered that the college had no recruiters. I never saw "Gerry" again.

Graduating OCNM in 1992 I sat on the OAND Board for four years, trying to make a difference. Faced with an uninformed public and an unfriendly medical establishment, I needed to know my treatments were making a difference, and not just placebo. At the time blood markers were primitive at local labs and as naturopathic doctors, we had no lab rights. Blood draws were taught but not allowed in practice.

Desperately wanting proof and benchmarks for patients' progress, I started the Meridian Naturopathic Assessment Centre, providing computerized thermography, EAV testing, BTA, and light microscopy services. Now, we can request lab work and do intravenous injections. We've come a long way baby!

Dr. Wayne J. Chindemi ND

I graduated with a Doctor of Chiropractic degree (DC) from the National College of Chiropractic (Illinois) in 1980 and started my practice in Toronto. By 1984 I felt something was missing and subsequently stumbled onto naturopathic medicine which led me to take an 18 month sabbatical to attend NCNM in Portland, Oregon.

While there, I met fellow Canadian Dr. André Saine and many other wonderful NDs. I wanted to help the naturopathic profession in any way I could so after I graduated from NCNM in 1986 I became involved at OCNM. At that time Tony Manolis was president and Dr. S. Alexander Wood, Dennis O'Hara and James McNamara, among others, were on the OCNM Board. Some distinguished teachers included Dr. Kenneth Dunk, Dr. Eric Shrubb, Dr. Frances Eddleston, and Dr. Leo Roy. At OCNM I taught physical diagnosis to year one students, as well as integrative therapeutics to year four and was clinical director for one year (1986-1987). Between 1986 and 1990, we put out some pretty fine, decent graduates - I was proud to be a part of it.

I practiced in Grimsby, Ontario from 1987-1990, then Vineland, Ontario from 1991-2002. I returned to Grimsby, Ontario where I have an active practice focused on homeotherapy and chiropractic, in addition to teaching part-time at the Toronto School of Homeopathic Medicine (1998-2002) and at the Ontario College of Homeopathic Medicine (Toronto, 2001-2002).

Dr. Shawna Leigh Clark ND

After graduating from university, I considered a career in one of a number of disciplines including nursing, physiotherapy, nutrition and psychology. After speaking with my sister (fellow ND Glenda Clark), who was at the time entering her second year at the Ontario College of Naturopathic Medicine, I realized that the naturopathic profession encompassed many of the things I was considering for further training and then some.

The four years of naturopathic training were filled with political turbulence and uncertainty but also fulfilling friendships that grew out of the experience, the kind that last a lifetime. I taught for a number of years at the college, within the clinic and in the classroom but left in 2002 to focus solely on my practice. I am still practicing after sixteen years, and I am looking forward to continuing in a new way over the next few years with the development of a healing retreat based in naturopathic principles.

Dr. Paul Anthony Conyette ND

In August of 1985 there was a soft chill in the cool Manitoba breeze which exacerbated the excitement I felt as I headed east to a new life in the big city of Toronto. The site of the CN tower reminded me of the time when helicopters hoisted the last pieces onto its summit. At that time, I was only a teenager battling acne and envying Bruce Lee - never once did I know I was going to be a doctor. The Ontario College of Naturopathic Medicine, a small building located on Bay Street in Toronto, was somewhat disappointing. Upon entering however, I was happily surprised to witness all the herbal charts on the walls, as well as friendly and enthusiastic students from all over the world.

As time passed, I learned the science and art of naturopathic medicine. Towards my last year at the college, I became disenchanted with the fact that there were deficiencies in the delivery of naturopathic education – for example, a routine diagnostic lab had not been established on campus. Having obtained permission from Dr. Tony Manolis (Dean of Biochemistry), I asked Mr. Kim Wei (a representative of a large national medical diagnostic laboratory) for assistance in developing the college's menu of lab tests and services. Today, lab services are enjoyed by doctors everywhere.

An internship at the Naturopathic Physicians Clinic with the late Drs. George Kroeker and Lambert Grube, led me to settle in Brandon. The clinic became my primary office, and has since evolved into Canadian Biologics Inc. and expanded to Winnipeg and Arizona, USA.

The past 19 years in Manitoba have been both rewarding and challenging for me. To this day, I have kept my first pay-check. Since I introduced chelation and other intravenous therapies in Manitoba, when the province had no clear regulations or by-laws to govern such practices, my work has been challenged by local authorities. I saw the need and believed that I would be protected as long as my services were required. I am pleased to recently learn that the naturopathic scope of practice is under review for expansion of its services.

Dr. Aloel Cristal ND

I was admitted into CCNM in 1993 as an advanced standing program student together with a few other former medical doctors from Europe and the Middle East. My medical background consisted of working as an orthopedic surgeon after graduating from one of Moscow's medical institutes (analogous to medical schools in Canada). The naturopathic program was consequently slightly shortened, as some of the basic science subjects were credited

even though we still had to go through all of the licensing examinations.

Going back to the schooling process after a few years of practice was a challenge, especially considering the fact that my English was not great then. In addition, I was dealing with some of my own health issues that resulted from the tremendous stress of a very recent immigration process. I remember that all those years I was just studying non-stop, as hard as I could, trying to keep up with the very intense pace.

Nevertheless, I really enjoyed my schooling experience at CCNM. I realized that I had finally discovered for myself the area of medicine that made sense and I felt that I was finally learning how to truly be of use to people.

Since my graduation, the college has grown tremendously, and the naturopathic profession has become an integral part of our health care. This would not be possible without all of our naturopathic doctors contributing to this process of growth and development.

Dr. Arthur William Dennis ND

(Arthur William Dennis was born in 1884. He received his degree as a Chiropractor at Chicago, his Doctor of Natural Science at New York and completed post-graduate study at the college of Sanapractic. He wrote this story in the 1950s)

My practice commenced in Vancouver in the fall of 1919 after some years of delay through the First World War. Looking back this places me among the earliest practicing Naturopathic Doctors in Canada. To myself also fell the honour of calling together the first group to consider the formation of an association for the direction and development of Naturopathy in BC. In this period I was a member of the School Board, and also its Chairman, and in 1922 I had the honour of being elected President of the School of Trustees of BC of which body I am a Life Member.

In the naturopathic organization I held the office of Vice-President, and was also a member of the Credential Committee. Several new doctors came to BC in the early years; some were graduates of the National College, Chicago, others came from the Naturopathic College of New York, and in the following years new members came from the various accredited schools.

The early practitioners were a dedicated group of men and women who pioneered in the face of persecution and prosecution by the medical profession, which for several years resorted to the employment of stool pigeons to secure convictions; a proof of payment had to be made, the charge always reading "Practicing Medicine for the hope of gain or reward." Convictions and fines followed, but some refused to pay, and were sent to prison. This procedure helped us very considerably, and was frowned upon by many medical men, among whom all of us had several good friends.

Yearly, for several years, we presented Bills to the BC Legislature, and as early as 1922 we were only defeated by one vote in the second reading of our Bill. In the year 1922 the Medical Association drafted a Bill called the Drugless Physicians Act, and appointed one of our men, Dr. W. Coates, to sit with a committee of four or five medical men as an examining Board, but Dr. Coates refused to sit on the Board and none of our men presented themselves for examinations, so the Bill died.

On several occasions I was a delegate to Victoria to appear before the House Committee whom we found to be quite sympathetic, but was nevertheless under pressure from the Medical Association, which never failed to have legal representation on such occasions.

In general practice over the years we always found good acceptance by the public at large, and on one occasion we presented a petition bearing 36,000 signatures.

In the face of continuing difficulties our organization maintained its good work of supervising the field, holding monthly discussion groups and lectures, and keeping abreast of all the latest and best methods in Naturopathy for the benefit of our patients. Some had members of the Medical profession come for treatment.

The early years of the thirties presented many problems for all of us, but we continued to press for legislation, and in the mid-thirties we had a good friend in the person of Dr. Weir, who was a member of the Provincial Cabinet, resulting in the passing of the existing Act in the 1936 Sessions, after a very careful survey of the Naturopathic Colleges, legalizing us as Naturopathic Physicians of BC. This measure went through the House with very little opposition. Our men had proved themselves to be competent, reliable, and skilled through the efficient and lengthy training they received.

Dr. Autumn Louise Drouin ND

From my earliest days of veterinary practice, I dabbled in nutrition, herbs, acupuncture, and homeopathy. My fascination with natural therapies eventually led me to the Ontario College of Naturopathic Medicine from which I graduated in 1989.

My fondest memory of OCNM is of walking into an afternoon lecture 20 minutes late and having missed the introduction of the lecturer. Within minutes I realized that everyone seemed in an altered state. This related not so much to the content of the lecture but to the atmosphere created by the kind, relaxed and loving man sharing his wisdom and experience of naturopathic practice. This man was naturopathic doctor John Laplante who was a legend in his time. On the way home I experienced an emotional healing relating to a comment made by Dr. Laplante: "Diabetes affects those who lack sweetness in their early life". I wept and was flooded with love, compassion and understanding for my diabetic father who had lost his mother at the age of 18 months. For the first time I understood why my dad was not affectionate. This also opened up an entire new realm, the connection between physical illness and emotions. It deepened my interest in homeopathy and in 2000 I received my diploma from the Canadian Academy of Homeopathy. Practicing as a naturopathic doctor, whether with people or animals, is a source of great satisfaction for which I am grateful every day.

Dr. Kenneth R. Dunk ND

I was originally educated and trained as a chiropractor and practiced as such for five years before commencing my training as a naturopathic doctor. During my third year at the Canadian Memorial Chiropractic College, a classmate showed me a course calendar from the National College of Naturopathic Medicine in Portland, Oregon. To make a long story short, an instant "love affair" with naturopathic medicine was kindled. I saw in the training and scope of practice, naturopathy was exactly what I needed and wanted to expand my scope of practice in a meaningful and logical manner.

Starting in September of 1978, I began a course of training through the Ontario Naturopathic Association, the forerunner of the Ontario Association of Naturopathic Doctors. Through what was referred to as the Accelerated Post-Graduate Program – a series of three day weekend training sessions every month over the course of 3 ½ years – primary health care practitioners like myself were able to acquire the additional training needed to become naturopathic doctors. My dream of acquiring a naturopathic education turned into reality with this program.

In addition to practicing naturopathic medicine, I went on to serve the profession as secretary treasurer of the ONA for two years and then for over six years with the BDDT-N as secretary treasurer and vice-chairman. To this day, I continue to teach future naturopathic doctors at CCNM and supervise fourth year interns in the Robert Schad Naturopathic Clinic. I love what I do and I have never looked back.

Dr. James (Jim) P. Farquharson ND

Naturopathic medicine was in my DNA and created a profound bias from my earliest recollection. My father (Dr. Bob Farquharson) and my grandfather (Dr. James Farquharson) were dually licensed D.C. / ND practitioners. When the small naturopathic college (OCNM) was initiated in Kitchener, Ontario in 1977, I provided some business expertise, as a pro-term business administrator, trying to empower practitioners to act as astute business people.

In 1984 I sold my business assets to attend Wilfred Laurier University to qualify for entry into the Ontario College of Naturopathic Medicine, convinced that naturopathic health-care was my ultimate calling. In 1990, I graduated and began a family oriented practice in the countryside of Waterloo region. Since 2005, I have developed a growing series of seven humanitarian clinics in the slums of Nairobi which provide first aid care to the residents and which treats HIV/AIDS patients.

Life is very fulfilling as a naturopathic physician. Every day in practice has become a complete pleasure to me. My holistic homeo-pathic orientation, significantly developed watching my father, has produced such tremendous personal satisfaction and has inspired my eldest daughter Rebecca to follow suit. I am reminded daily of the personal sacrifices of the ND's who have gone before us which enable us to stand in such a productive place in health-care. We truly stand on tall shoulders.

Dr. Penelope Ann Fremes ND

Before entering naturopathic college, my education and experience was as professor and counselor in natural healing, nutrition and lifestyle. I also had an extensive background in business and education, including Profession Representative for the H. J. Heinz Company and Home Economics Specialist for the Toronto Board of Education. My interest was, and still is, in teaching people alternative ways to stay well and to be ecologically responsible.

After graduation I opened a private practice in Toronto and was a regular guest on cable TV in a phone-in format. Some topics were: Herbalism in Action, Fathering

Healthy Babies, Pediatric Digestion, The Hyperactive Child, How to Ease Away from Caffeine One Step at a Time, Grief in Recovery, Eat Right for Your Blood Type.

Some publications: Naturopath's Challenge: Quick Fix Methods of Treatment (Toronto Midtown Voice); Burnout-Can Diet Help? (The Creative Edge); Plant Enzymes Fight Candida (The CRIF Newsletter).

When I moved to Los Angeles in 1996 I continued in private practice. Currently I am retired from practice.

Dr. Peter Gleisberg ND

I was born in 1951 in Germany, where I was raised and educated. In 1977 I graduated from the school of naturopathic medicine, and pursued a six month internship with a fellow Naturopath before opening my own office. The therapies used in my clinic included ozone therapy, fresh-cell therapy, and many other modalities.

After starting a family 1981, we relocated to Canada (Saskatchewan) in 1983. I started with a home based office in the Battlefords and expanded from there. In the summer of 2005 we moved to Warman in the Saskatoon area. Resuming my career was a challenge - many of the modalities I practiced in Germany where not allowed or known of in Canada. After opening my mind to different modalities I found new ways to incorporate them into my practice; from then on my clinic started expanding.

Now I am waiting for my son to graduate from CCNM in 2009; he will be joining me in the quest to help improve peoples' health.

Dr. Tutti Timmins Gould ND

I fell in love with naturopathy when I was a chiropractic student in Toronto in 1978. To supplement my income, I was working part-time transcribing lectures on naturopathy for chiropractic interns. The talks were inspiring, and eventually changed the course of my life.

My studying years were wonderful and upon finishing chiropractic college a group of us went on to study naturopathy, after first finishing a required year of drugless therapy training. To complement our naturopathic studies, we had weekend intensives in homeopathy with Robin Murphy, who we invited from NCNM, Portland. After our group graduated from naturopathy, André Saine established a homeopathic fellowship program at OCNM with our support and enthusiasm.

Life was hectic - as it often is for parents with young families and a practice. I took over two practices from colleagues in chiropractic and homeopathy in Toronto, all the while continuing my studies in naturopathic medicine. I eventually returned home to Quebec, in the beautiful mountains of the Eastern Townships, and with three children under four years old, I pursued the homeopathic business I had co-founded with colleague Pamela Snider.

From the beginning in my practice as a naturopathic doctor, I relied on my training in homeopathy to complement - and eventually replace - my chiropractic practice. I remember thinking then that I would probably never see the day where homeopathy would become mainstream or published in popular magazines - it seemed so unconventional.

The 80s and 90s were a period of organization and maturity for the naturopathic profession as well as for the remedies we use. Naturopathic medicine has made it as a recognized profession in Canada, and has come a long way since the late 70s.

Dr. Muriel Grant ND

I graduated from the Canadian Memorial Chiropractic College in May of 1977 and opened my office, Total Life Care, in October of 1977. Several years prior to that date, I had graduated as a Registered Physiotherapist.

Some of my classmates in the chiropractic college wanted to go on to naturopathic colleges, but I felt I could not afford to take time off to go study in the USA. Then I heard of the newly opened Ontario College of Naturopathic Medicine in Kitchener. I hesitated at first, as I was already a graduate of two other healing professions. A classmate of mine Alan Davidson, DC, ND, helped me make the right decision. I have had no regrets. Since then, I was fortunate enough to have had two major mentors for many years -

Dr. Leo Roy and Dr. John McLean.

The three professions, naturopathy, chiropractic, and physiotherapy, blend extremely well – cleansing and nourishing the internal tissues while balancing the structure and relieving pain of the soft tissues.

Dr. Lambert (Bert) Kenneth Grube ND

Dr. Lambert Kenneth Grube was born the youngest of five children to Bertha and August Grube on January 10th 1928 in Steelman, Saskatchewan. Midway through his teens, Bert was struck with a very serious illness called "Brights Disease" – a kidney condition that landed him in bed for more than a year and was believed to have no hope of ever recovering by all the medical doctors around. As he hung onto life by a thread, his parents chose to visit a naturopathic doctor in North Dakota as a last resort. Their hope restored, Lambert ultimately made a wonderful and miraculous recovery, vowing that he himself would someday become a naturopathic physician.

Lambert attended National College in Chicago, Illinois - his older brothers and sisters helped their parents by contributing funds to see his dreams come through. Upon graduation he returned to Estevan (Saskatchewan), with a wife (Betty Kohler) and young daughter (Claudia) to set up practice. Bert had patients come from many towns, provinces and states for treatment. He believed strongly in holistic medicine and treated the bodies, minds and spirits of his patients. He spent many hours with each patient, taking the time to listen, counsel and advise. He was later joined by Dr. George Kroeker ND and for many years worked with naturopathic friends to have the Saskatchewan government pass the Naturopathic Act.

Suddenly, in June of 1988 after forty years of practice in Saskatchewan, Alberta and then in Brandon Manitoba, Dr. Grube passed away of a heart attack. To this day, Bert's children and grandchildren still meet people who were past patients of his. They are always so excited when they speak of him and are very willing to relay stories of how "Dr. Grube was such an amazing doctor, how he helped when no one else could and how they miss him!" His family agrees!

Dr. David Charles Hann ND

I truly appreciate the opportunity to have studied and used naturopathic medicine in my practice of helping people. It was really after using the knowledge and applying what I had been taught that I realized this profession truly used "healing" principles. To be able to diagnose and treat, when others could not, was so rewarding. It has been a wonderful experience.

Dr. Lois Hare ND

My interest in naturopathic medicine began as a child gathering "flowers" for my Great Aunt Nell, a lay midwife who used traditional herbs. When I first heard about the curriculum at the Ontario College of Naturopathic Medicine, I knew I had found my vocation - one that resonated with my beliefs in treating the whole person and respecting the healing power of nature. I was accepted into the first full time class at OCNM and graduated in 1987.

Our class was often referred to as the pioneers or guinea pigs, which we hope referred to our enterprising, hard working and flexible natures. Along with the thumps and bumps of a new school, our daughter was born at the end of my third year. This brought Brian and I great joy, and some complications, as we balanced breast feeding and parenting with the stresses of school life.

After graduation, our family headed back to our Nova Scotia home where I set up practice as the first naturopathic doctor in the province. It was a lonely time made easier with the support of my mentors, Drs. Pat Wales, Verna Hunt, and Carolyn Dean. I found that people were open to this non-invasive and respectful form of healing - above all they needed to be listened to.

It has been very important to me to live my life according to naturopathic principles. It has been difficult at times being considered "odd" but over the last twenty one years there has been an amazing change in attitudes, culminating in the proclamation of title protection legislation in Nova Scotia in July 2008.

I realize now that finishing naturopathic college was just the beginning of my education. I continue to learn daily from my patients, my family, and my community, about the beauty and harmony of the human body and spirit.

Dr. Gregory Asa Hershoff ND

In 1978, six intrepid souls founded the Ontario College of Naturopathic Medicine (later to be renamed the Canadian College of Naturopathic Medicine). These six consisted of three veteran practitioners and long time mainstays of the profession in Ontario and Canada as a whole: Dr. John LaPlante, Dr. William Morris and Dr. Robert Farquarson. The three "youngsters" were myself, Dr. Eric Shrubb and Dr. Gordon Smith. I had just graduated from the Canadian Memorial Chiropractic College, but from the start, this was merely a stepping stone for me, as naturopathic medicine was my goal. My inspiration, from day one, was Dr. John LaPlante, who I met in 1969. It was not long after that I decided I wanted to follow in his footsteps in every sense. He was an extraordinarily skilled healer, and what today would be called a "medical intuitive." Here was a being of immense psychic power, but also of profound compassion and of expansive consciousness. Indeed, I stayed in Toronto (my hometown) for the next 16 years, largely to work with John, both personally and in the grand project we had started.

In 1974, the ONA had exactly twenty members, and had not had a single new member in almost twenty years! I know this is so, because I became secretary of the ONA, and for the next five years, was part of the small group of newcomers that set out to save and revive naturopathic medicine in Canada. Over the next five years, I poured every ounce of energy and intelligence into making this a reality - the result is what we see today. This is the power of an idea. It would be difficult, and very arduous to describe the steps and stutters of going from zero to having a functional college. Our first stage however, was to create new naturopathic doctors, so that we would have a basis for everything that would follow. To this end we created a postgraduate course, designed specifically for chiropractors, but welcoming medical doctors and some dentists, to receive adequate hours to take exams and become licensed naturopaths in Ontario. One of the most interesting (and anachronistic) efforts at the time, was to keep unlicensed, "holistic" healers of every stripe from running rampant. Those were the early days of the resurgence of natural health and the first glimmerings of untrained and unqualified people hanging out their shingle with no degree or license whatsoever. We met with the Ministry of Health to try and have such individuals certified and overseen by the naturopathic profession, who were the only ones with the expertise and knowledge to qualify such health workers. Of course, we were rebuffed, and the avalanche of "everything-ists" began.

After five or so years as secretary of both the ONA and CNA (two years) and director of the college, a new generation of inspired individuals, graduates of the postgraduate courses, began to emerge, including Dr. Frances Shrubb, Dr. John Cosgrove and many others. Though at that time, I was offered the deanship of the school, I felt it was time to refocus on my own life and allow the school to grow and expand in the hands of its successors. Others were less fortunate and eventually the original young founders were pushed out by political machinations.

Without the work of six dedicated individuals, and the Herculean labors of the "troops on the ground," the profession would have truly died out. Of the three soldiers of the day, myself, Gordon Smith and Eric Shrubb, none of us made a single dime of profit out of creating the college and reviving the associations. I trust in the future generations to carry forth the unflinching principles of the founders, in spite of whatever obstacles and enticements they meet. For myself, I will always have the deepest gratitude of my many mentors, teachers and yes, gurus, who transformed my life personally. Every day I try to pass on this level of brilliance and power to patients, readers, students of every sort.

Dr. Ronald Anton Ingard, DC ND

I graduated from the Canadian Memorial Chiropractic College in 1967 with DC and DT qualifications. Philosophically when we graduated we had an image of holistic Chiropractic being a viable alternative to standard Allopathic Medical practice. Many graduates from the 50's and early 60's had both Chiropractic and Naturopathic diplomas. It was a time of great change in the profession. Political negotiations were underway and Chiropractic was included in OHMSIP (later called OHIP).

Over time the Chiropractic profession became divided into "straights" and "mixers". "Mixers" were those who practiced as holistic (Naturopathic) Chiropractors (in the US in some states "Chiropractic Physicians") and the "straights" were the followers of D.D. Palmer's son B.J. Palmer who promoted adjusting the Atlas only (HIO – "Hole-in-one" Palmer upper cervical technique). In the mid 60's Dr. Himes from the Palmer College became dean of CMCC and the shift away from "mixer" chiropractic really moved ahead. By the mid 70's the chiropractors were easily "manipulated" into dropping the naturopathic part of their charter in order to complete the negotiations for the new Chiropractic Art. And it should be remembered that those who saw this as a major loss of scope got together and started OCNM.

My first practice was in Timmins with branch offices in Iroquois Falls and Matheson. In the north the demand for the alternatives, that a holistic approach provided, were high. By 1975 I moved to Orillia, as a compromise with a Toronto born wife. That marriage soon failed coincidentally as the first classes started at OCNM. After graduating in 1981 as part of the first grad class I developed colon hydrotherapy as a major part of my practice and in the later 80's taught this procedure at the Burl Street Campus and as a post grad course in BC for the college. During the 80's I was director on the college board and was vice president of the Ontario Naturopathic Association. I became "burned out" by the early 90's. I consider my training in naturopathic practice started at CMCC; was completed at OCNM; led to some 40 years to date providing an integrated approach to naturopathic health care in this province.

Dr. Alexey Kaganovsky ND

My love for natural medicine was inspired early in life as I often assisted my mother, a pharmacist in a European pharmacy specializing in herbal medicine. I began my medical career as a paramedic in Kiev, Ukraine at the prestigious "Kiev Central Ambulance Station," well known all over Europe.

Upon moving to Canada in 1979, I began studying to fulfill the prerequisites to enter the naturopathic college. I became the first naturopathic doctor to open a practice in Mississauga Ontario, in 1988. As a great lover of yoga, I studied at the Mount Madonna Center for Creative Arts in California, and became a certified yoga teacher in 1987. In 1990, I continued studies in acupuncture and received a degree from the Ontario Association of Traditional Chinese Medicine. I continued on to study bowen therapy - a technique used for treating muscles, joints and ligaments and a treatment used by the Australian Olympic Team. Additionally, in 1993 I became a certified hypnotherapist at the OMNI Hypnosis Center in Florida.

From 1995 to 2008 I studied with many renowned doctors and healers worldwide. Some of those courses include acutonics, A.R.T., family constellation therapy, biological medicine, homotoxicology, and E.A.V. testing. I have served on the boards for the Ontario Association of Naturopathic Doctors and the Ontario Association of the Traditional Chinese Medicine. Now, I continue to teach yoga, homeopathy, and acutonics for professionals and for the general public.

Dr. Sat Dharam Kaur ND

Our small 1989 graduating class of naturopathic doctors endured four years of growing pains and personal transformation during our time together at the college. When I first intended to become a naturopathic doctor, it was unclear whether the profession would survive as it had only existed for a few years in its current incarnation at OCNM.

We started in several classrooms on the second floor of a building on Bay Street just north of Bloor, initially with no library and few resources other than the notes our teachers provided. We bonded and helped one another through personal crises, through the death of a classmate from testicular cancer and through our studies. For several classes we researched the topic ourselves and taught one another when teachers were scarce or spread too thin. Jim MacNamara, as dean, was a guiding light for many of us and his classes were an exciting journey into the mind-body connection, self-reflection and experimentation. Dr. Leo Roy was a goldmine of information in providing tools for detoxification and therapies for cancer patients.

I was challenged personally when my daughter was born in June of my third year and I was unsure if I could complete my fourth year. Luckily, a daycare next to the school in the Etobicoke location, and a supportive husband who spent many hours at the college while I was working in the clinic, made it all possible. I am thrilled with the growth and acceptance of naturopathic medicine today and am very grateful to the pioneers who laid the foundation for us.

Dr. Antonin Kodet ND

My career began when treating high level athletes and the severely injured in the best sport rehabilitation program in Prague. I attained my first doctoral degree, with honors, from Charles University in Prague, one of the oldest universities in the world. Concurrent with my Pedagogicae Doctris degree, I completed training in kinesiology, coaching and sport rehabilitation.

After moving to Vancouver, British Columbia, I established a very successful rehabilitation practice that introduced new approaches and standards to the treatment of severe injuries. Several years later I completed my Doctor of Naturopathic Medicine degree at NCNM in Portland, Oregon. Subsequently, I established Integrative Medical Care Inc. in Calgary, Alberta, specializing in the treatment of children and adults with chronic illnesses/conditions and providing supportive cancer treatments.

Over the years I have enjoyed studying at leading European universities and Asian institutions as well as treating patients in Nepal, Burma, Thailand, Latin and Central America. Time permitting, I have taught and developed courses at the University of Calgary, Calgary's Mount Royal College (MRC), Calgary College of Traditional Chinese Medicine and Vancouver Community College - courses including pathology, internal medicine, pharmacology, kinesiology, rehabilitation, nutrition, herbal medicine, homeopathy and others. I played a key role in establishing the Herbal Therapist diploma program at MRC. I was the first kinesiologist, and later naturopathic doctor, qualified as an expert witness by the courts of law of both British Columbia and Alberta. Having competed in several sports, I became two-time Champion of the Czech Republic and had the opportunity to coach many top level athletes. I have been a guest on many radio and television shows, and have published numerous articles and a book titled Cook Your Way to Health and Vitality.

Dr. Gabrielle Kropp ND

I was born in Germany and there earned a degree in Naturopathic Medicine, Lymphedema Therapy and Massage Therapy. I had my own practice until I immigrated, in May 1996, to Pictou Waterside and made Nova Scotia my new home. I was the first ND in the region and it was hard work to open minds, but over time people recognized that there are more ways to better health.

I use a variety of therapies like pain and stress management, anti-aging medicine, Chinese medicine and lymph therapy. I created the Caribou River Retreat, for workshops, fasting and detoxification, where people are able to stay overnight. I also work out of the East River Wellness Center, my clinic in New Glasgow.

Dr. Fred W. Loffler ND

Eighty-six-year-old naturopathic doctor Fred Loffler has been known to kill time before a talk by standing on his head. It's not hard to imagine as the ex-wrestling champion and Olympic Marathon contender strides to the stage. He's wiry, bald and throws his arms out to punctuate his words.

He's attempted to retire twice, but his 50 years of experience and success have made him a popular man. He still agrees to consult with some patients and give talks, like the one Health Action Network Society (HANS) sponsored last October. Loffler remembers the exact day he decided to become a health practitioner. It was February 5, 1937.

"I was in a hospital in Victoria, waiting for my dad to die after 20 years of ulcers, operations and drugs," he said. At this time the options for naturopathic school in North America were limited. He went to visit Western States University in Oregon in the US and was unimpressed.

"It didn't look much like a college—It was a dump," he said with a smile. But he put aside his hesitation and went on to graduate from the school, which was far more credible than its shabby exterior had led him to believe. During this time he met and married his first wife, who completed her studies at the same school, and he began his lengthy practice. Over the years he has seen the acceptance of naturopathy grow and the number of schools increase, including a Naturopathic College opening in Western Canada.

Dr. Loffler was a firm believer in food combining. It is only natural that when asked to reflect on his career, he passes out detailed sheets with columns of foods and the best matches. And when the floor opens to questions, his answers always come back to food combining and when you eat what.

For example, in the morning it's fruit—maybe grapefruit juice with garlic and vitamin E. In the evening, it's vitamin B-complex and blood builders. He has theories on common ailments–like his peanut theory. He says peanuts are the worst thing for kids, contributing to bronchial infections and excessive mucus.

He also has little patience for people who won't help themselves by changing their lifestyles or diets. The force and conviction with which he speaks and his infectious energy is all the convincing his audience needs. People tend to listen to a man who did a 40 kilometre overnight hike at Garabaldi when he was 85!

Looking forward, Loffler sees chlorella as the natural substance that may prove to be the answer to cancer in the next millennium, particularly in its ability to help build hemoglobin. What he thinks is the next immediate breakthrough, though, is B vitamins and folic acid for Alzheimer's.

"You heard it here first," he said to the audience. Although Loffler's experience is firmly rooted in the 20th century, he seems to have every intention of using it to explore the boundaries of health in the 21st.

Dr. Daria P. Love ND

The words of Adele Davis ("You are what you eat.") echoed through my teenage years. My family had a health food store, my father treated us with herbs for our various ailments, we gardened, composted (and thought this was most disgusting), raised chickens, and basically led a life swimming upstream within the defines of small town Ontario.

My eldest brother enticed me to go to chiropractic college saying it would offer a real alternative health perspective; so in 1973 I headed off to the Canadian Memorial Chiropractic College. By my second year there I realized that this was not what I had envisioned. I was not alone. A number of my CMCC classmates and myself became the first graduates of the Ontario College of Naturopathic Medicine in 1981. OCNM was initiated as a school without walls; the Chelsea Inn, downtown Toronto, was our classroom and many of our classmates were also our teachers. Most of us were chiropractors, some were medical doctors and there was a dentist or two.

We had found our calling, or perhaps our calling had found us. I will always remember our enthusiasm and dedication to naturopathic medicine. Some amongst us have passed on, while others of us have served as leaders in our profession; in education, on our national and provincial associations and regulatory boards, as leaders in the naturopathic industry, but especially as the pioneers of naturopathic health care in Canada. We were the Renaissance of naturopathic medicine in Canada. We are now its elders. I have felt privileged to be a naturopathic doctor and have come to recognize that naturopathic medicine is not simply what I do, it is who I have become.

Dr. Heather Marinaccio ND

I grew up in Pennsylvania and developed

an interest in natural medicine early on as my mother and grandmother were interested in organic gardening and vitamin therapy. I immigrated to Canada after falling in love with a Canadian longshoreman.

When I first joined my colleagues in B.C. we were a small group - there were only about 24 members and I was the only woman. The members were very gracious and encouraging and they immediately accepted me as an equal. I started my practice in Courtenay (Vancouver Island) during the fall of 1981 in my home, with a 6-month-old baby. Dr. Allen Tyler became my mentor by phone. I was so starved for naturopathic companionship that I started attending the monthly board meetings in Vancouver along with Joe Boucher, Allen Tyler, Doug Kirkbride, Bob Fleming, and Gerald Farnsworth- a core group who wore many hats.

Every year as more doctors joined there was excitement at the growing membership. Yet, there was often uncertainty at the survival of our profession in B.C. as numerous crises came and went where the government would threaten to dismantle our Act or restrict access to medicines for our pharmacies.

Over my career, I lectured in 12 communities as I was the only one accessible to patients in the north of Vancouver Island and Powell River on the mainland. Now I enjoy the kinship of six other naturopathic doctors in my area. Soon it will be my thirtieth year since graduation. I have

seen more change and acceptance of our profession than I ever expected to see in my lifetime. It continues to be a very rewarding life's work.

Dr. Marilyn May ND

My decision to practice alternative medicine came while I was traveling in South America from, 1976-1979. When people got sick around me I would be there to help them get well. After studying music of the Andes in Bolivia I decided that I had absorbed enough of the culture and needed to give something back. I returned to Canada to continue my studies.

A friend, Rebecca Sugarman, told me about naturopathic medicine. It seemed to be the perfect next step and was the most thorough of any alternative medical education.

I went to Vancouver Island, worked at Malaspina teaching ESL (English as a second language) to save money for school. In 1981 I enrolled at National College of Naturopathic Medicine, Portland, Oregon. I had all of my prerequisites through my Bachelor of Physical Health and Education from Lakehead University.

Portland and NCNM were great. I was vice president of the student body during my third year. We organized "Run a Volcano" a 10K run over Mount Taber. We used the proceeds to help the school put a polyurethane finish on the newly built but not protected clinic. There was always the question of whether the school would survive or go bankrupt, so the students helped whereever they could. We were in a small school in the suburbs, similar to CCNM at 60 Berl Avenue.

During my third year several students from the closed California school joined us, including Paul Mittman. Most of their forth year students went to John Bastyr.

After graduation, summer 1985, Joan Laurence and I went back packing in the Wallawa mountains. There we met a professor from Washington State University doing field research during the summer session. On the way down from Glacier Lake we explained to him what Naturopathic Medicine was. His name was Paul Saunders.

Paul was accepted at CCNM and as I had family in Ontario we moved back to set up a practice in Dundas, Ontario, in 1987 with Jim Spring and have been there ever since.

I was on the OAND (ONA) board in 1987. In 1988 I was elected to the CCNM (OCNM) board by INER but was removed by the other members of the OCNM Board upon questioning the school administration's honesty; inside source "deep throat," Paul Saunders. This infuriated myself and Pam Snider so we became the requisitionist to restore CCNM. I returned to the Board of CCNM as Vice-Chair after the requisitionist were successful, resigning in 1991 when Paul Saunders was hired by OCNM.

I taught nutrition and endocrinology at CCNM through the late 1990s. Now I divide my attention between Naturopathic Medicine, gardening, piano, and traveling. We enjoy living in the country near Ancaster.

Dr. Neil Mckinney ND

I was born in Vancouver, BC, in 1952 and graduated in Biosciences from Simon Fraser University in 1975. I worked several years in cancer research in the field of radiation biophysics. I attended the University of Waterloo in the field of Kinesiology and Health Studies and the Ontario College of Naturopathic Medicine in 1981. I graduated from National College of Naturopathic Medicine in 1985 and concurrently did three years at the Oregon College of Oriental Medicine.

I practiced about 16 years in Vernon, BC and moved to Victoria in 2001, shifting my practice focus to oncology. I am member of the Oncology Academy of Naturopathic Physicians. I have served many years on college boards, was registrar of CNPBC for five years, an evaluator for CNME, and had many other roles as inspector, mediator and leader. I have had many teaching roles, from microbiology lab instructor at the University of Victoria and at NCNM, to professor at schools of traditional Chinese medicine, massage therapy, and finally at BINM.

I was a founder of the BC Naturopathic Association and of the Boucher Institute of Naturopathic

Medicine. I authored the book, Naturally There's Hope - A Handbook for the Naturopathic Care of Cancer Patients, and many other publications.

Dr. Pamela Ann Milroy ND

I entered OCNM in 1986 when it was on Berl Avenue in Etobicoke. I car pooled most days with Paul Saunders and occasionally with Olga Pulido, our professor for Anatomy and Physiology. In fourth year I was our class representative for the student council (NSA - which was started by one of my classmates David Wang), as well as president. In my last year I initiated the standardized patients from McMaster University. I helped Pam Snider do a lot of work in the area for political thrust to get naturopathic medicine under the RHPA (which was unsuccessful the first time). I, also with Paul Saunders and other ND's like Pat Wales and Pam Snider and Verna Hunt, helped to get information on the college's current administration for the OCNM board. That administration used up the John LaPlante Endowment Fund. It was then that Robert Schad graciously stepped up to the plate for the profession. Because of the political sensitivity at the time it was decided by the new Board not to litigate - which I believe was a mistake. I was valedictorian, along with Jim Farquharson, upon graduation. That year I also won the Golden Guinea Pig award.

After graduation, I continued at the college on the board as secretary and then as chair of admissions. It was then that we started to incorporate what McMaster used as their admissions model for students. After four years I left the OCNM board to go to the ONA and I served there for four or five years being president for two years. I received the Naturopath of the Year Award in 1998.

I set up private practice in Ancaster where I have practiced since 1990. My practice is fairly eclectic and I see a wide variety of patients. I have stepped back from working for the profession to helping the community through Rotary. I now also dedicate time for family especially my two grandchildren.

Dr. Kevin R. Nolan ND

I entered the Accelerated Post-Graduate Program at OCNM after I realized that the course was covering all that I had been teaching myself. I had been practicing as a holistic medical doctor since 1971. Upon graduation (1989) I continued under my MD (BC) license, since declaration of an ND affiliation would have rendered me as a target of orthodoxy.

I assisted the naturopathic profession by joining the board of Canadian Naturopathic Foundation, as treasurer for three years. I was the treasurer for the newly formed College of Naturopathic Physicians BC for three years, guiding it through some tempestuous times. I then assisted a small group of naturopathic doctors to rescue a private naturopathic college, which became the Boucher Institute of Naturopathic Medicine. As treasurer of the BINM board and school I had intimate knowledge of the extreme fragility of the new school in its first few years. I continue to practice as an MD and teach at BINM.

At this time naturopathic physicians are greatly needed in Canada to balance the increasing loss of primary care MD's. The profession needs to strive not to be co-opted in the orthodox field through grants and financial enticements. It is hoped that ND's will continue to work in partnership alongside other practitioners, but maintain private billing with the ability to spend adequate time with each patient. The naturopathic profession in North America can be a model for the rest of the world.

Dr. Steven Olsen ND

I practiced classical homeopathy from 1988 to 2000 in the Maple Ridge area, then moved just south of the border to Snohomish, Washington where I continued to see patients, conduct research on new homeopathic remedies and teach at Boucher Institute of Naturopathic Medicine.

My grandparents were ahead of their time and I was lucky enough to receive their gifts plus an intuition tempered with training and discipline. My great grandmother was a tuberculosis nurse in London back in the 1880s, she was a very compassionate person with many friends and an amazing ability to listen to intently. My mother also had this trait. From my grandfather I inherited the love of nature and ability to see the connectedness in all things. He was a farmer who knew what was 'sustainable' in the big picture.

I estimate that in twenty years I have completed over 35,000 patient visits. For each I have tried to see the patient as a complete individual and used my intuition to help them find their own way to heal. The anecdotal stories I could tell are endless. I have been called to treat people who had been given their 'last rights' at the hospital and yet are still alive today - his kidney and liver had stopped functioning, he was in a coma - lets hear it for Curduus marianus 30C. There were those who called me on the way to commit suicide and who, after Aurum metallicum, changed so much within a week that their regained happiness and appreciation of life is unbelievable.

The most beautiful cures I have seen are with single remedies. Of course, there were cases I never solved and that is why I continue to do research, as each new remedy has its potential. I have tried to pass on what I have learned by teaching at various colleges and through publication. The most rewarding experience has been to do research on new homeopathic remedies and be able to use them successfully in practice - the book Arbor Medica is the culmination of this work. With the advances in epigenetics and hormesis-dose-response research I think homeopathy is on the verge of more scientific validation.

It has been an honor and privilege to serve our profession.

Dr. Edie Pett ND

My naturopathic journey began in 1981 with a personal consultation with one of our professions pioneers – Dr. Leo Roy. I had recently graduated from Chiropractic College and was feeling a desire to work at a deeper foundational level of healing. Dr. Roy informed me about the accelerated naturopathic program soon to begin in Kitchener at what was then the Ontario College of Naturopathic Medicine. It's been an adventure ever since.

I've found many kindred spirits within our profession and they have made my life and my practice rich with heart and soul and wisdom. Pamela Snider and I spent endless hours in the early days (1984-85) scheduling appointments with Members of Parliament, attending Liberal events, and working closely with our beloved Pat Wales toward attaining regulatory status. Looking back, it was the beginning of a long road. That gauntlet has been passed several times to bring us closer to our regulatory goals. My dear friend, Verna Hunt, was often behind the scenes with a voice of wisdom and a deep love for our profession – always guiding – a true mentor.

My memories are of exploration, sharing laughter and connection. Having a Watsu treatment from Glenys Brydges, in the pool at The Briars on Lake Simcoe. One of the most intimate and memorable naturopathic conventions for me was thanks to the talents and efforts of Angela Moore. And nobody dances with such abandon as my fellow naturopaths!

So now I find myself as one of the elders in our profession coming full circle after twenty five years in practice – after the many seminars and conferences, so much studying and integration, and the immense joy of helping someone. At the beginning of yet another spiral, I feel the depth and breadth of our history as healers and what it truly means to serve. I will always remember my naturopathic roots as I look forward to the next twenty five years.

Dr. Ingrid Pincott ND

I was the first female ND to practice in Vancouver proper in 1985. Myself and Drs. Stefan Kuprowksy, Kelly Farnsworth, Kerry McGuiness and Donal Sabourin put together the first pamphlet on naturopathic medicine in BC to use as a promotion for our practices. I served on the BC board during these early years (new grads have more time to volunteer).

I started in Dr. Joseph Boucher's office. He worked six am until noon and I worked noon until six pm, Monday to Friday - and he made half of what I made. For about eight months this worked very well, but after the local CIBC bank gave me a personal unsecured line of credit Dr.

Stefan Kuprowsky told me of a 500 square foot office for rent in a medical building at 1541 West Broadway - the rest is history!

I also served on the CAND board and was the one who speared headed Naturopathic Medicine Week (NMW) week. I began teaching Practice Management at BINM in 2005 and started selling my Practice Management and Office Manual sets in 2002.

I have been writing a health column for the local paper in Campbell River called MidWeek since 2000, all of which are archived on my very extensive website which is managed by my husband Grant Skinner. My passion is education; not only do I educate my patients but my students as well, in the "art of success" in their health and their practices.

Dr. William Slade Prusin ND

I was originally born in Brooklyn, New York. At the age of three, my family moved to Chicago, where I was raised and educated. I had my oral surgery training in New York and Boston and master's fellowship year at the Boston University School of Graduate Dentistry and Medicine. I was an oral maxillofacial surgeon in the United States Army, part of the NATO forces stationed in Germany from 1963 to 1965 and practiced in Boston from 1965 to 1968. I came to Canada in 1968 for a special program for my deaf son and have stayed since.

I was part of the first accelerated program at OCNM for professionals who already had a doctorate degree. I was motivated towards naturopathic medicine and wellness for myself, family and friends. I started studying health when it was not as fashionable, back in the 1960s and 1970s. I took numerous courses and eventually signed up for the entire naturopathic course.

I have lectured at the naturopathic college & elsewhere. I have been head of oral & maxillofacial surgery at the Rouge Valley Health Centre Centenary Site since 1968 and currently run an oral and maxillofacial private surgical practice with a staff of eight (including dental assistants and registered nurses). I receive referrals for my expertise on surgical care for infections and problems in the jaws. My medical, surgical, naturopathic background has been sought after by individuals from the Golden Horseshoe as well as different parts of Ontario, Canada, and the United States. I manage craniofacial pain, TMJ problems, and have trained in sacro-occipital therapy cranial osteopathy.

Dr. Raj-Inder Rakhra ND

In 1964 I received my degree in Ayurvedic medicine from the Faculty of Ayurvedic and Unani Systems of Medicine, Amritsar, Punjab. Following graduation I took the position of medical officer for various civil Ayurvedic clinics in the Punjab Health Service. Eventually a fellow GAMS colleague and I opened a private practice in my home town of Moga, Punjab. My family and I emigrated from India to Canada in 1974, living in Vancouver and then finally settling in Calgary.

The naturopathic and holistic community in Calgary was very welcoming. I was encouraged to write the naturopathic board exams and then joined the AANP in 1989, which I have supported fully these many years. Early on I had the opportunity to work with Dr. Pat Ranch ND, and then take over his family practice at the Calgary Naturopathic Clinic. My education has continued in order to widen the scope of my practice. For the last twenty years I have used intravenous therapies that include chelation, vitamins, minerals, ozone, and hydrogen peroxide as well as homeopathic intramuscular treatments. My clinic also offers a variety of Ayurvedic, homeopathic and naturopathic supplements, therapeutics and testing to assist the patient with chronic or acute conditions.

Dr. Leo Roy ND

Dr. Roy passed away in Kelowna on March 3, 2001, after a brief illness and a stroke. Dr. Roy was an ND and a MD. Like his father before him, Dr. Roy was originally educated as a medical doctor and graduated from the University of Montreal.

After practicing mainstream medicine for several years, he became discouraged with the poor progress his patients made on drug therapies. It led him to research natural methods of healing, and ultimately he converted his Toronto practice to naturopathic medicine. He was one of the first doctors in Canada to treat cancer with natural remedies. Subsequently he was persecuted for it by the medical establishment.

Dr. Roy, who would never be discouraged, spent much of his time and energy on extensive studies over many years, culminating in his book on cancer. He was a seeker after truth, and a great teacher and lecturer. As a prolific writer he created a whole series of booklets dealing with individual health issues and problems, as a means of educating his patients.

He was a generous to a fault in his willingness to share. Being light years ahead in his holistic approach to healing, his written materials showed quantum leaps in original thought on various health problems. So did his diagnostic method.

In order to determine the cause and treatment for each condition, he had developed a computerized diagnostic system, comprising thousands of questions in a health questionnaire for the most in-depth analysis. His death is a very great loss to the naturopathic profession, as well as to his many students, patients and friends.

He was one of the great pioneers in that profession and broke the hardest ground for those who follow in helping humanity.

Dr. William (Bill) Russell ND

I graduated from Canadian Memorial Chiropractic College in Toronto, Ontario, in 1981 after which I moved back to Vancouver, British Columbia to set up practice. In 1985, I entered the Accelerated Post Graduate Program at

Ontario College of Naturopathic Medicine and graduated as a Doctor of Naturopathic Medicine. It was in White Rock, British Columbia that my naturopathic practice began in 1989. Currently, White Rock is home to the multi-disciplinary clinic I practice in, and to my wife and three children.

Dr. Garry Schafer ND

In 1973 while studying massage therapy in Toronto, I attended a lecture by Dr. Leo Roy. Although he was the first and only naturopathic doctor I had encountered, I knew immediately that naturopathic medicine was what I wanted to study. I contacted someone in Seattle, Washington who queried me on my educational background and experience, she also recommended that I get prerequisites in chemistry and remain in contact with her. It had not yet been finalized whether the naturopathic program (NCNM) would be taught out of Seattle, Corvalis or Wichita. I eventually enrolled in Wichita (1975), spending two years studying basic sciences there before moving to the old postal building in Portland, Oregon for two years of clinical sciences and clinical experience. In those years the average "Joe public" could not even pronounce "naturopathy," nor did they know anything about our profession. However, the tenacious commitment of such elders as: Drs. John Bastyr, Joseph Boucher, Gerald and Earl Farnsworth,

Doug Kirkbride, Robert Fleming, Fred Loeffler, etc., kept the profession alive and prospering.

I graduated from NCNM in 1979 and set up a practice in Victoria, B.C., where I practiced with two other naturopaths until July 1994. My partner and I were numbers 11 and 12 in the BCNA.

In the summer of 1994, our family moved back to Saskatchewan (our place of birth) and set up practice within my father's health food centre from July 1994 to November 2000. In those years, many people came to know of naturopathic medicine. The demand for our services increased greatly. Our clinic was always booked three to four months in advance and many folks would travel eight to twelve hours for an appointment. With such conviction about health and healing many, many people regained or improved their health. The value of naturopathic health care and its benefits has spread incredibly fast by word of mouth.

In November 2000 our family made another move. This time we settled in Sherwood Park, Alberta. My wife and I set up a small clinic and continue to serve people from all across North America. We have a waiting list of four to five months at anytime continuously. The demand for naturopathic care continues to be huge and increasing still. Even with the increased numbers of practicing naturopathic doctors the needs of the public increase continuously.

In the past thirty years I have seen our

profession shift from relative obscurity, to an accepted flourishing profession. Our educational institutions have shifted as well. They are now based in "scientifically" accepted information as are allopathic schools of medicine. We must be vigilant, therefore, in maintaining focus on our philosophy of the healing power of nature. We must treat the cause of any imbalance, treat the whole person and focus on wellness, as apposed to illness. I have seen many young doctors, with impressive amounts of intellectual information, who struggle to find a "system" or way to focus all their information.

Our profession has a very bright future because a large part of the populace wants to take responsibility for personal healthcare and find answers to healing themselves rather than mere symptom relief.

Dr. Eric F. Shrubb ND

I graduated from the CMCC in May of 1964, summa cum laude. After serving as X-ray lab and clinic supervisor I also taught most of the clinical subjects over the next seven years and became co-clinic director and X-ray department head, as well as Co-Chairman, Department of Clinical Sciences. Specialty status was achieved in May 1971 as a Chiropractic Radiologist.

Interest in natural medicine and especially in clinical nutrition was stimulated by Dr. Frances (Eddleston) Shrubb and she suggested I look into naturopathic medicine. I joined the ONA in 1971 and was immedi-

ately asked to testify before the Kreeuer Commission on Health Care (Ontario) chaired by Mr. Horage B. Kreeuer.

My strength and passion is to get things off the ground and over the years I was fortunate to be a founder and active participation in the start-up of many initiatives including: co-founder of the Council on Nutrition of the American Chiropractic Association in 1974, Vice-President of the ONA and the President in 1976, co-founder of OCNM in 1978, co-founder of CNME, among other positions.

I coordinated and directed the initial accelerated program of OCNM and had the opportunity to work with a number of other naturopathic doctors such as Sandy Wood, John Cosgrove, Murial Grant, Susan Rohn and Frances (Eddleston) Shrubb. During those years I taught radiology, nutrition and some jurisprudence. Drs. Farguharson and LaPlante taught homeopathic medicine. Drs. Morris and David Lam taught acupuncture. Drs. Hershoff and Smith presented lectures in herbology, homeopathy and nutrition. There were also a number of presenters such as Dr. Plog from Germany, Drs, Jeffery Bland, Joe Pizzorno and Ronald Hoye.

This was indeed an exciting time. I continued to teach radiology and jurisprudence in the undergraduate program until 1988 and also Chaired the BDDT-N from 1984-1988.

We have seen, by the grace of God, the birth of a College. OCNM has now become CCNM, a truly Canadian College. I have watched a group of twenty practitioners in Ontario become a profession of over 900 in the last thirty years. This indeed is the stuff that life is made of.

Dr. Gordon Smith ND

After graduating from NCNM in 1976, I moved back to Ontario and started a practice in Waterloo while further studying with Dr. Arno Koegler. Recognizing the need for naturopathic education in Canada, I joined forces with a few colleagues and became involved teaching our post-grad course.

I am one of the co-founders, as well as inaugural dean, of the Ontario College of Naturopathic Medicine (OCNM). I have served as an OCNM board member and helped formulate the college's first prospectus. I was also Chair of the Botanical Medicine faculty at OCNM. In addition, I was vice-president of the Ontario Naturopathic Association for a few years.

I initiated, along with Asa Hershoff, a public education advocacy group entitled "Friends of Naturopathy" (FON), which helped to raise the profession's profile via a regular series of public health talks, plant medicine walks, seminars and courses. Membership in FON included a quarterly naturopathic journal, The Healing Crisis, which was co-edited by Asa Hershoff and myself.

I have had the opportunity to study and practice in various First Nations communities for over 14 years. At Georgian College (Barrie, Ontario) I co-taught a course entitled Holistic Health and Healing as part of their Native Family and Social Development programs.

Currently, I live and work in Whitehorse, Yukon Territory and I am a proud parent of five and grandfather of four.

Dr. Mohamed Fateh Srajeldin ND

The choice to join the naturopathic medicine movement probably was the best choice I have ever made in my life second to choosing my wife Rowayda 35 years ago. Being a naturopathic doctor had distinguished my treatments in contrast with pharmaceuticals. It placed me in the right place at the right time. I was commissioned to treat a Crown Royal Princess of the Royal Saudi family who introduced me to many members of her family for treatment. Naturopathic philosophy made me the choice of the President of Yemen for treatment of him and his family's concerns. My successful approach granted me a hospital position in Saudi Arabia from 2002 to 2004.

I began my naturopathic studies in 1985. I have traveled to many conferences all over the USA and Europe to see the point of views of other practitioners in the naturopathic and in the medical field. Of course, I attended numerous medical conferences to understand the rationale behind diagnoses, therapies and medications. This clarified why certain medical treatments failed even though the medical doctor did his best.

I traveled to study skin endpoint titration, parenteral therapy, ozone-oxygen therapies, live blood cell analysis, and advanced procedures in treating cancer. My main focus of treatment is allergies, hepatitis, asthma, digestive tracts, candida and related illnesses through the use of diet, enzymes, amino acids, IV therapy, vitamins and minerals.

I am currently the clinical director of a Naturopathic and Allergy Clinic, which is one of the largest naturopathic clinics of its kind in North America.

Dr. Fran Storch ND

Well!!! Who would have thought that a girl from New Jersey in the US would wind up in Atlantic Canada? Not me, but that's what happened! It used to be that Newfoundland was just someplace I'd heard about; then it was a Canadian province that used to be a country; then it was the place where the plane hangs a right on the way to London. Then...it became the home of my then beloved!!!

I'd always wanted to be a doctor. Told the guy in my interview for Yale, where I never wound up going; ended up at Rutgers, the State University of New Jersey. Four years later found me eventually in the pharmaceutical industry...getting really familiar with RATS. Eventually, that's what I said everyday about my job...RATS. One day I said that's enough! I really needed to make a switch. So, I did what all left-leaning, hippy-ish 20-somethings do in the US...I planned to go West! And that I did, after rediscovering my desire to practice medicine. Only...I could do it in a much more sensible, holistic way...the way of the Healing Power of Nature! Off to the National College of Naturopathic Medicine I went.

Well, in August of 1996 I drove back across the country with my then-beloved, Bill...and saw the great terrain of the US in the reverse order ...somewhat to my chagrin. I was going to be a pioneer! The very first naturopathic physician to practice in the province Newfoundland. I made my home in the city of St. John's, the capital.

Well, it's a very interesting place. Especially for a Jewish girl from New York and New Jersey. It's very stark there; very intense weather, not far from where the warm Gulf Stream meets the cold Labrador current. The trees closest to the water are bent over sideways from all the wind. I really liked that when you walk down the street in Newfoundland, people not only say hello, they mention something about the weather...and if you're standing by yourself looking at Quidi Vidi Lake, someone will come over to you and strike up a conversation.

So practicing in Newfoundland. Let's see...it was a non-licensed jurisdiction, so I was left to do the things only naturopathic practitioners can do and NOT the things M.D.'s can do. I had the good fortune to become a permanent resident of

Canada, because I was the only person volunteering to do a job that no other Canadian wanted to do at that time! Gordon Higgins, M.D., the owner of the Wellness Center on Bonaventure Avenue in St. John's, took me on and vouched for me; and off I went to practice there for a couple of years. But eventually the economic depression was too much for me and I moved my practice to Halifax.

As marvelous as the experience of Newfoundland was, I was happier in Halifax. The climate was not as harsh and it was easier to visit home and family in New Jersey. I had a great friend in Lois Hare, to this day one of the premier naturopathic doctors in Nova Scotia, Canada, the World, and the Universe. I do miss her and hope to visit with her before too long... There were regular meetings of the Nova Scotia Naturopathic Doctors association. I didn't feel so alone. I also found it somewhat easier to maintain a practice; Halifax is generally more prosperous than Newfoundland. In 1998 I made the decision to return to the US...and one of the places I sent my resume was...to Mystic, Connecticut. I had an easier time getting on television in Halifax than on the radio. Duane Lowe had me on her show a couple of times; I also made it onto Women's Television Network. I was a national television star!

Over the next few years I worked at a number of different places in the United States and eventually found my way to Willimantic and Mansfield, Connecticut,

where I am happily settled. My current practice is terrific; 3.5 miles from my home. I am remarried to a wonderful man and his son. I have rediscovered the bicycle, and in the summer ride anywhere from 1-200 miles/week. I have great friends and a great community. I have a radio show now for 5 years on WHUS, the local University of Connecticut radio station. My practice is better than ever and growing in leaps and bounds! We are licensed here in Connecticut and I am able to accept insurance. I must say...life is good!

Pioneering naturopathic medicine in Canada was a wonderful experience; it taught me to think independently, and to take charge when necessary. It gave me a lot of confidence, and made it so that I don't mind being one of few naturopathic physicians in a large area. I also fell in love with Canada, so much so that after 3 ½ years I made the decision to become a citizen even though I was leaving! I am very proud to be Canadian.

Dr. Albert J. Thut ND

Dr. Albert Thut had an active practice in Guelph, Ontario for 70 years until three months before his death. He was born in Oberentfelden, Switzerland in 1903, and immigrated to Canada in 1923. As a child, I remember passing by the big blue and white house with the writing "Swiss Alps Herbal Remedies", just down the street from my parents home, often seeing the large black cars driven by the Mennonites parked in front of his door. Later, as a naturopathic student, he kindly allowed me to write a biography about him for a class assignment, and on several occasions we would talk about the many benefits of natural medicines and the use of various herbs. His primary treatment modality was botanical medicine, and he collected and manufactured most of the medicines he used in treatment.

Albert Thut was a graduate of the National Association of Medical Herbalists college in England, the Naturopathic Institute of California, and the Nashville College of Naturopathic Medicine. He was awarded a research fellowship by the department of Rational Therapeutics at Emerson University, given a prestigious award for medicine in Cuba, and recognized by the Canadian Naturopathic Association as a Life member in 1998. He contributed to the education of naturopathic doctors in the early days of the Ontario College of naturopathic medicine, and was a past President of the Ontario Naturopathic Association in the early years. He treated thousands of patients, and would often make house calls, driving many miles to visit a patient. He had a number of stories to tell of patients close to death or given a terminal prognosis who he helped back to health. Through his life's work, Dr. Thut forged one of the first links on our chain of naturopathic medicine. He was a valued contributor to the

profession, and his patients and we will miss him.

Dr. A. Scott Tyler ND

My career as a physician seemed to be sealed from birth. My father (Allen Tyler) had trained as an MD, then a chiropractor and naturopath after WWII, and my Great Grandfather, Tanner was an MD with his own hospital in upstate Minnesota. My mother's colourful nursing career further instilled in me a deep desire to help others with their health-care needs.

After realizing that there was more to "medicine" than antibiotics, tranquilizers and pain pills, I embarked on an adventure to discover the truth of the healing arts. At the time (1982) my only option was to travel to the west coast and study at NCNM (Portland), or Bastyr (Seattle). At NCNM, I met the most wonderful and sincere group of teachers and healers. I was nurtured and encouraged, until finally the day came to leave and enter practice. Dad established a booming clinic in Langley (British Columbia) that had room for me to work during the "off" days. Soon was busy enough to open a clinic of my own. Somewhere in there Dad and I found the time to collaborate on a book, A Pound of Prevention.

I can't believe that twenty two years have passed so quickly. It hasn't all been a bed of roses, but I wouldn't trade any of those days away. I have met many wonderful patients who have taught me countless lessons. Taking care of them "one at a time" has been the best advice I was given. Some days now I wish it would slow down, and I contemplate retirement. Then I think, whatever could I do that would be so profoundly fulfilling as the practice of naturopathic medicine? I guess I will just keep on going, like dad, and so many of my predecessors. What a wonderful life!

Dr. Audrey Ure ND and Sherry Ure ND

Audrey Ure was diagnosed with lupus in the 70's and was greatly helped by complementary medicine. After the loss of her youngest son, she decided she needed to do something different with her life. Meanwhile, in 1981, Sherry was attending Okanagan College in Penticton and found a catalog for the National College of Naturopathic Medicine (Craig Wagstaff, ND had placed catalog at all the OK College satellites campuses in the Okanagan), this inspired Audrey to get moving. Her husband, David, was totally supportive and encouraged Audrey to take the challenge.

After attending college to fulfill the necessary prerequisites Audrey and Karen Jensen headed off to NCNM in 1984. Two years later Sherry joined Audrey in Portland where they shared an apartment and were able to take some courses together until Audrey graduated in 1988.

Audrey felt that she would never have survived the early days of her practice without the guidance and support of Dr. Wagstaff and always gives him much of the credit for her early success. Sherry joined the practice after graduating from NCNM in 1990, giving the South Okanagan Naturopathic Clinic a much more eclectic approach. Sherry continues to expand her scope of practice and Audrey, while retired, continues to consult with Sherry. They both give God the glory for His guidance and direction and for the dedicated staff they have had the privilege of working with.

Dr. Jan Scott Valchar ND

The seventies represented the fifth wave of the health care re-revolution. People were beginning to feel medical deficiencies and information about nutrition, herbals, and mental health cures were getting press. As a young chiropractor I felt that there was more to natural medicine.

Dr. Eric Shrubb suggested that I join the naturopathic course, which was in its infancy, in Toronto. Along with friends, Dr. Asa Hershoff, Dr. Larry Grey, and Dr. Bill Morris I attended the post graduate course for almost fours years at OCNM. We passed our exams and became naturopathic doctors in 1982.

My first actual case was a patient with tonsillitis. He was in exceptional pain and I had just acquired a group of twelve alterative herbs so I mixed up some Hydrastis,

Baptisia, Echinacea Equisetum and Taraxacum. Thankfully the patient took the combination and returned the next day remarkably better. My career as a naturopathic doctor was launched and it has just gotten better as the years pass by. Every manner of ailment afflicting mankind has passed through our doors and, looking back, the vast majority has been helped by our approach.

The political side of activities started in 1985 when the College of Physicians and Surgeons started raiding naturopathic offices to collect evidence for licensing infringements on the doctor title. At the same time, the Ontario Legislature was cooperating with them and wanted to strike down the Drugless Practitioners Act as it applied to naturopathy. I decided that this was the time to act in Eastern Ontario and delivered a host of media presentations on behalf of our profession. Since there were no other registrants east of Oshawa the field was definitely rough ground and uncut forests.

Dr. David Wang ND

I started the Naturopathic Students' Association at OCNM before it became CCNM back in 1987 to 1988. Dr. Leo Roy, MD, ND, recruited me to British Columbia after graduation in 1990. In 1992, I opened up one of the first multidisciplinary clinics in B.C. Between 1993 and 1995, I served on the regulatory board called the ANPBC, now the CNPBC. During that time, around 1993, I was successful in adding ozone therapy and the very first IV therapy into our scope of practice in B.C. I then served on the BCNA board in 1996 and was president from 1997 to 2002. In 2001, I was one of the individuals involved in the West Coast College of Massage Therapy starting up a for-profit naturopathic college. Today, it is the Boucher Institute of Naturopathic Medicine. I was on the board of governors at BINM and served as chair for three of my last years between 2001 and 2007. Today I still serve on various committees for both the CNPBC and BCNA.

Dr. Katherine Schad-Byers Willow ND

I graduated from the National College of Naturopathic Medicine in 1983 and have live and worked in Ontario ever since. I taught at CCNM in its beginning years and was its first clinic director with a budget of zero dollars! In addition, I was secretary for the OAND for a few years in the 80s.

Now I run a healing centre – Carp Ridge EcoWellness Centre – in the rural part of Ottawa and am developing a holistic inpatient program. Most importantly, I am preparing to be a grandmother this September 2008.

Dr. Patricia Wolfe ND

I was among the twelve students who graduated in 1987 from the first full-time class of the Ontario College of

Naturopathic Medicine in Toronto, Ontario. The four years at OCNM were life altering! We were all mature students who were so intensely passionate about naturopathic medicine that we persevered through chaos, uncertainty and the many challenges that had nothing to do with the stringent curriculum. The invaluable lessons we learned about self-responsibility, problem-solving, deep soul-searching and friendship were a function of being in the first small class in a tenuous new school.

Upon graduation, I opened my practice in the small town of Bancroft, Ontario, where I focused on core modalities: hydrotherapy, homeopathy, botanical medicine, lifestyle counseling and gentle hands-on techniques such as cranio-sacral technique. I had developed a fascination and respect for the meaning of illness on a deep psycho-spiritual level and was honored to have many of my patients allow me to join them on the often scary journey of uncovering deeply unconscious sources of illness.

Dr. Alfonso W. H. Wong ND

I have been residing and practicing naturopathy in Hong Kong, China for the last ten years. Besides consulting patients I regularly deliver naturopathic lectures to audiences throughout the Asian countries, including Hong Kong, Japan, Malaysia, and Singapore. Often I address audiences ranging from a few hundred to ten thousand participants, and from corporations to the public alike.

Since 1999, I have been managing the Asia College of Naturopathy (ACN). The professional naturopathic medical program boasts 4,000 hours of lectures and graduates approximately 100 students annually – we are proud to have over one thousand alumni. The ACN does joint-research with a number of state universities and has published in the "International Journal of Molecular Medicine". Within the next two years, the college plans to merge with the University of Hong Kong. Additionally, our College joined the Chinese Ministry of Health and is moving into China to deliver naturopathic lectures. The ACN is also an international representative of the Chinese government for those applying to practice medicine in China.

It is our hope that naturopathic medicine be regulated in China & Hong Kong in the near future and I have worked to push regulation of naturopathy in Hong Kong, Malaysia and China. Of course, the Asia College of Naturopathy aspires to be accredited by the Canadian College of Naturopathic Medicine and the Canadian Association of Naturopathic Doctors as a branch college in order to continue promoting naturopathic medicine in Asia.

My vision is that all who are continuously suffering from discomforts under the care of conventional medicine, be relieved and cured by true medicine - naturopathic medicine.

LISTING OF
CANADIAN PRACTITIONERS

Abaskharoun, Thabet A.M., 1988, OCNM, NS, Egypt
Abbadessa, Joseph, c1981, ON
Abbott, Lareina, 2005, SCNM, AB
Aberdour, Serenity S., 2002, CCNM, BC
Abt, Thomas M., c1953, ON
Abt, William Leon , c1944, ON, CA
Ackland, Katherine L. M., 2001, CCNM, ON
Adamiak, Dorothy, 1999, CCNM, ON
Adams, Lisa Eva Maria, 2007, CCNM, ON
Adams, Mikhael, 1981, NCNM, ON
Adamson, Bruce, 1989, OCNM, BC
Adatya, Tasnim, 1996, NCNM, BC
Adirim, Herbert J., 1984, OCNM, ON
Ador-Dionisio, Kara, 2008, CCNM, ON
Aesoph, Lauri, 1987, Bastyr, BC
Aga, Anisa Z., 2007, CCNM
Agbeko, Melaika, 2007, CCNM, BC, Tobago, West Indies
Aggarwal, Ameet, 2006, CCNM, BC
Aguiar, Shelley Loura, 2006, CCNM, ON
Ahenakew, Darlene M., 2001, CCNM, ON
Ahlan, Jason Chia, 2004, CCNM, AB
Ahmadi, Martha Mariam, 2004, CCNM, ON
Ahmadzadeh, Nasreen, 2003, CCNM, ON
Ahmedzadeh, Nahid, 1997, CCNM, ON
Ahuja, Harminder K. (Minda), 2000, CCNM, ON
Aikens, Violet May, c1953, ON
Ailsworth, Charles E., c1953, ON
Ajina, Nabeel, 1989, OCNM, BC
Al- Rawi, Sara N., 2004, CCNM, MI
Alberti, Otto Heinz, c1953, ON
Albin, Jeanne M. see Paul
Albin, Stephen, 1977, NCNM, BC
Albin, Sydney John, c1953, ON
Alexander, Alexina see Metha

Ali, Elvis Azad, 1987, OCNM, ON
Alibhai, Tasreen, 2000, Bastyr, BC
Allan, Kenneth J., c1953, ON
Allen, Nathalie D. nee Desrochers, 1997, NCNM, BC
Almon, Kirsten M., 2002, CCNM, ON
Alsberg, Charles E., 1983, NCNM, BC
Amell, Douglas, 1998, CCNM, SK
Amernic, Heidi J. P., 2000, CCNM, ON
Ames, Herbert M., c1953, MI
Amodeo, Frank, 1986, OCNM, ON
Amos, Margaret J., 2001, CCNM, ON
Amsden, c1954, AB
Amsden, Frank E., 1962, NCNM, MB
Anchel, Tara, 2008, CCNM, ON
Andersen, Ross Kent, c1976, 1982, OCNM, ON, BC
Anderson, A. C., c1953, ON
Anderson, Arnold C., c1953, ON
Anderson, Harley Clayton, 1924, PC, BC
Anderson, Howard A., 1951, CMCC*, ON
Anderson, J.C. Marshall, 1953, ON
Anderson, Katherine E., 2003, CCNM, OK
Anderson, N. D., c1959, BC
Anderson, Thomas D., c1953, ON
Andrews, Douglas A., 2002, CCNM, ON
Andrews, Hilary, 2000, NCNM, AB
Andrews, Stephanie, 2008, CCNM, Nicaragua
Andrichuk, Stephan, c1922, ON
Ania, Fernando, 1988, OCNM, ON
Annesley, Tara Lee, 1998, CCNM, ON
Anousaya, Chanpheng, c1983, ON
Anthony, Paul, 1989, OCNM
Appelmann, Jeffrey S., 2000, CCNM, ON
Arbuckle, Sarah-Dash, 2003, CCNM, AB
Ariss, L. H. George, 1953, CMCC*, ON

Ariss, W.H.D., c1926, ON
Arkell, Bessie M., c1926, ON
Armengol, Hania, 1989, OCNM, ON
Armstrong, Heidi see Kussmann
Armstrong, Lara Naiomi, 2004, CCNM, ON
Armstrong, Sean Daniel, 2004, CCNM, ON
Arnet, Werner J., 1955, CMCC*, ON
Arnone, Nadia Rosa, 2006, CCNM, ON
Arrata, Eric S., 1995, Bastyr, AB
Arrigo, Salvatore Anthony (Sam), 2006, CCNM, ON
Arseneau, Leigh, 2005, CCNM, ON
Aruncois de Jules, Robert, c1968, ON
Arvidson, Steven K., 1994, NCNM, BC
Arychuk, Pamela K., 1991, OCNM, Taiwan
Asada, Paul K., 1950, CMCC*, ON
Ashfield, Nicholas Walter, 1975, CMCC*, SK, ON
Ataner, Ciler, 1992, OCNM, ON
Atkinson, Angus N., c1953, ON
Atkinson, Jordan, 2008, BINM, BC
Attema, Rikst, 2007, BINM, BC
Atteslander, Galia Irene, 2006, CCNM, ON
Audrichuk, Stephan, c1953, ON.
Aulakh, Safina, 2001, CCNM, ON
Austin, Kelly Marie, 2004, CCNM, ON
Austin, Liza K., 1996, Bastyr, BC
Avonde, Henri E., c1953, ON
Aylward, Harry A., c1953, ON
Ayoubzadeh, Shahram, 1990, OCNM, ON
Ayoup, Rob G., 2002, CCNM, ON
Aziziyan, Soodabeh, 2000, CCNM, ON
Azzopardi, Lisa Ann (Analisa), 1993, Bastyr, CA, BC
Babicki, Kinga, 2007, CCNM, ON
Bablad, Jonathan R., 2006, CCNM, SK
Bachewich, Jason, 2006, CCNM, MB
Bachlet, Allison, 2007, BINM, BC
Badesha, Narbinder (Navi), 2004, BINM, BC
Baer, Jennifer Leigh, 2005, CCNM, ON
Baile, Marcia Louise, 2000, NCNM, BC
Bailetti, Maria Katia, 2004, CCNM, ON
Bailey, Ace Leonard, c1952, ON
Bailey, Edna nee MacInnis, c1953, ON
Bailey, Kent, 2002, CCNM, SK

Baillie, Sarah Elizabeth, 1998, CCNM, NS
Bain, Grant E., c1953, ON
Bains, Karamvir Singh, 2002, CCNM, ON
Baker, A.T., c1926, NS
Baker, Arden, 2005, NCNM, AB
Baker, Royce G., 1962, NCNM, MB
Bakir, Nadia, 1989, OCNM, ON
Balajewicz, Malgorzata E. (Maggie), 2002, CCNM, ON
Balcaen, Philip, 1998, CCNM, ON, BC
Baldwin, Tanya, 1999, CCNM, CA
Ball, Albrair H., c1953, ON
Ballew, Taraneh nee Tashakor, 2000, CCNM, CA
Banek, Stefan, 1989, OCNM, Poland
Banga, Margaret Joy nee Graham, 2006, CCNM, ON
Banks, Herbert J., c1926, ON
Baptist, Summer, 2006, CCNM, HI
Barbeau, Raymond J., c1968, QC
Barlow, Kerry Elizabeth, 2006, CCNM, ON
Barmby, Alana L., 2001, CCNM, SK
Barnes, Karen E., 1998, CCNM, ON
Baron, Ruth Anne, 1994, CCNM, ON
Barron, Dorothy F., c1953, ON
Bartolini, Suzanne, 2006, CCNM, QC
Barton, Dana S., 1996, Bastyr, BC
Basham, Kenneth D. A., c1976, ON
Bast, Lindsay R., 2005, CCNM, ON
Bastos, Elizabeth M., 2005, CCNM, ON
Bateman, Kenneth Charles, 2004, CCNM, ON
Bateson-Koch, Carolee, 1989, OCNM, YT
Bathie, Austin C. A., 1950, CMCC*, ON
Bathie, Helen Marie. c1953, ON
Batience, W. W., c1953, ON
Bauer, Meghan Elizabeth, 2006, CCNM, ON
Baum, Simone Sophie, 2004, Bastyr, BC
Baumann, Pauline nee Crouch, 1985, NCNM, OR
Baustein, Ernest J., 1982, OCNM, ON
Baustein, Michael, c1981, ON
Bayley, David, 1986, NCNM, BC
Bayley, Wendy, 1986, NCNM, BC
Bayrock, Roman, 1984, NCNM, AB
Bazan, Mervat, 1990, OCNM
Beales, Margery, AB

Bearss, Caroline L., 2000, CCNM, ON

Beasleigh, Sarah J., 2000, CCNM, BC

Beaton, Graham E., 2005, CCNM, ON

Beatty, A. C., NS

Beatty, Jonathan, 2007, CCNM, ON

Beaubrun, Andrea nee Kenny, 2003, CCNM, AB

Beaubrun, Arnel Josue, 2003, CCNM, AB

Beaulne, Tracey Michelle, 2001, CCNM, ON

Beazer, Lynn M., c1953, ON

Begin, Martin C., 1990, OCNM, ON

Behrendt, Sharon R., 2001, CCNM, ON

Belitsky, Lorraine E., 2002, CCNM, ON

Bell, Allan J. 1951, CMCC*, ON

Bell, George K., c1926, NB

Bell, Glen M., 2000, CCNM, ON

Bender, John W., 1979, NCNM, ON

Bender, Leanne, 2008, CCNM, ON

Benedetti, Susan, 1999, CCNM,

Bennett, Elaine M., 2000, CCNM, ON

Bennett, Peter W., 1987, Bastyr, BC

Bentz, Kris., 2005, BINM, BC

Berezovska, Iryna, 2001, CCNM

Berg, Alana, 2005, CCNM, BC

Berg, Deborah, 1998, CCNM, ON

Bergen, Angela Jill, 2005, CCNM, BC

Berghamer, Jonathon Friz, 2008, BINM, BC

Bergmann, Irena H., 2002, CCNM, ON

Berman, Barry, 1982, OCNM, ON

Bernardo, Kevin, 2008, CCNM, ON

Berni, Marika Ann nee Maksimowich, 1997, CCNM, ON

Bertlik, Jaromir, 1989, OCNM, ON

Beserminji, Nada, 1988, OCNM, ON

Bexton, William H., 1978, NCNM, BC

Bhooi, Amrit see Devgun

Bickram, Louise, 1999, CCNM, ON

Bielny-Radon, Maria, 1989, OCNM

Bieman, Erin Anne, 2004, CCNM, ON

Biernacki, Miroslaw, 1996, CCNM, Poland

Billotte, Louis C., c1955, MA

Birzneck, Judy, c1958, BC

Bishop-Veale, Jyl, 2000, CCNM, NS

Bisswanger, Gordan L., c1948, AB

Biswas, Dilip Kumar, 1999, CCNM, NS

Bitidis, Via M., 2002, CCNM, ON

Bitting, Blossom Diana, 2003, CCNM, NB

Bizios, Vivian nee Papaioannou, 2001, CCNM, ON

Bjarnson, Prart, c1981, ON

Bjorndal, Christina, 2005, CCNM, AB

Bjornson, Grant E., 1974, CMCC*, ON

Black, Jennie M., c1953, ON

Blackmore, Walter W., c1953, MI

Blackwell, George A., c1926, SK

Blake, Melissa Frances, 2006, CCNM, NB

Bland, Mary C., c1953, ON

Blanks, Alexis, 2006, CCNM, BC

Blaszczyk, Anna Karolina, 1990, OCNM, ON

Bleything, Martin, c1955, OR

Blizniuk, Galina, 1998, CCNM, ON

Block, Ilana C., 2001, CCNM, QC

Block, Moshe Daniel, 2000, CCNM, QC

Blois, Walter G., 1990, OCNM, ON

Blok, Rebekah C., 2007, CCNM, ON

Blondiau, Julis Felix, c1959, SC, AB

Bloomer, Lisa A., 2001, CCNM, ON

Blyden-Taylor, Kimberlee, nee Pietrzak, 1999, CCNM, ON

Bodewein, J. A. Henry, c1921, NB

Bodgener, Lawrence (Larry), 1951, CMCC*, ON

Bodner, Laura M. nee Kantor, 1996, CCNM, ON

Bodner, Michelle B., 2000, CCNM, ON

Bogatch, Galina, 2001, CCNM, BC.

Boghossian, Marina D., 1992, OCNM, ON

Bohemier, Guy, c1983, QC

Bohez, Heather A., 2000, CCNM, ON

Boisvert, Hervé, c1970, QC

Boivin, Erin E., 2005, CCNM, ON

Boland, Darya Rebecca, 2003, CCNM, CA

Bolliger, Manon, 1992, OCNM, NS, AB, BC

Bond, Lyndsay, 2008, CCNM, ON

Bondy, Cynthia Ann, 1991, OCNM, ON

Bonter, Natalie nee Engelbrecht, 1996, CCNM, ON

Bonyun, Gerald Langford, 1951, CMCC*, FL

Booker, Jennifer, 1989, OCNM, WA

Boomhower, Cherylann (Cher), 2002, CCNM, BC

Boorman, Maria nee Payne, 1999, Bastyr, BC

Boothe, W.C., c1926, ON

Borgen, E.R., c1926, SK

Born, Grant E., c1934, MI

Bortnick, Allan, 1977, CMCC*, 1981, OCNM, ON

Bothma, Cobi, 1998, CCNM, BC

Boucher, Joseph Aime, 1953, WSC, OR, BC

Boudreau, Erik Daniel, 2004, CCNM, ON

Bourgon, Roberta, 1996, Bastyr, MT

Bourke, Daryl Robert, 1989, OCNM, BC, AB

Boutet, Marc, 2000, CCNM, BC

Boutet, Samantha nee Geyer, 1999, CCNM, BC

Bovee, Kristen M., 2001, CCNM, BC

Bowman, Julie see Durnan

Bowring, Janine, 1998, CCNM, ON

Bowring, Marc Stefan, 2004, CCNM, ON

Boxtart, Jason E., 2002, CCNM, BC

Boyer, Ernest A., c1926, AB

Boyer, Hoover S.D., c1926, AB

Boyle, Wade, 1983, NCNM, ON

Bozinovski, Lucas, 1977, CMCC*, 1986, OCNM, ON

Bradwell, Melissa, 2005, CCNM, BC

Brady-Srpova, Miroslava Teresa, 1997, CCNM, ON

Brain, J.W., c1926, ON

Brame, Joel E., 2002, CCNM, AZ

Brand, Patricia, 2006, CCNM, AB

Brand, Penelope see Wilks

Brandson, Erin see Broadfoot

Brant, William Terry, c1981, AL, FL

Branter, Katie, 2008, CCNM, ON

Brass, Laura, 2008, CCNM, AU

Brass, Molly Elizabeth, 2000, CCNM, ON

Bratt, Anita, 2005, NCNM, Bastyr, BINM, BC

Braun, Krista Michelle, 1999, CCNM, ON

Breiner, Adam B., 2002, CCNM, CT

Brennan, Marissa Diva, 2006, CCNM, ON

Brereton, Trent Q., 1997, NCNM, BC

Brett, Cory V., 2000, CCNM, NB

Bretz, Kim D., 2001, CCNM, ON

Bricks, Miriam R., 2002, CCNM, ON

Brito Roque, Nadia C., 2004, CCNM, Mozainbique

Brkich, Lawrence (Larry), 1994, NCNM, BC

Brnings, Bilton, c1953, ON

Broadfoot, Erin nee Brandson, 2008, CCNM, ON

Brooks, Kristina nee Power 2008, CCNM, ON

Brooks, Robert J., 1950, CMCC*, ON

Brouwer, Peter, 1954, CMCC*, BC

Browett, Roger W., 1952, CMCC*, ON

Browett, Wilmot Bright, 1940, NCNM, ON

Brown, Arthur W., c1953, ON.

Brown, B. G., c1936, BC

Brown, George McIntyre, BC

Brown, Harold (Hal S.), 1989, OCNM, BC

Brown, Ian, 2005, BINM, BC

Brown, Jodi Lee, 2004, CCNM, NS

Brown, Joseph W, c1953, ON.

Brown, Kristen, 2004, Bastyr, BC

Brown, Linda Louise, 2001, CCNM, ON

Brown, Stanley E., c1953, ON

Brown, Timothy M. see Taneda-Brown

Brown, William Allin, c1953, ON

Browne, Baptist Gamble, 1926, CCN, BC

Browne, Tamara J., 1996, Bastyr, BC

Brownlee, Harold E. W., c1953, ON

Bruce, K. H., c1953, ON

Bruce, Malcolm Douglas, 1973, CMCC*, ON

Brunarski, David John, 1977, CMCC*, ON

Brunel, Ludovic, 2004, CCNM, AB

Brunet, Jean-Marc, 1968, LCNPS, QC

Brunings, Bilton, c1944, CA

Bruno, Zenaide (Naide), c1981, 1984, OCNM, ON

Brunton, Carolyn Elizabeth see Kaganovsky

Bryant, James Alfred, BC

Brydges, Glenys Irene, 1990, OCNM, ON

Bryk, Andrew, 2008, CCNM, ON

Buckle, Laura Kathleen see Margaritis

Buckler, Jane Alison see O'Malley

Buckley, Erika Danielle, 2004, CCNM, ON

Budd, Ruth Else, c1948, AB

Budden, William A., c1954, AB

Budhwani, Rehana see Kassam

Budnick, William John, 1933, NWC, BC

Bulaong, Odette Isidro, 2007, CCNM, ON

Bull, Andrea, 2007, CCNM, ON

Bullis, Edmund J., c1953, ON

Bullock, Wiebert C., c1953, ON
Bulman, Ronald J., 1954, CMCC*, ON
Bunda, Anna Margaret, 1995, CCNM, ON
Bunford, Deborah, 2005, CCNM, AU
Bunin, Judah S., 2001, CCNM, NB
Bunin, Parissa I., 2001, CCNM, NB
Bunzenmeyer, Jennifer Candace, 2004, CCNM, AB
Burgess, Stanley, c1926, ON
Burgess, Gordon S. J., 1960, CMCC*, ON
Burke-Brownman, Jessica Nicole, 2004, CCNM, ON
Burlinguette, Donald Charles, 1966, CMCC*, SK
Burns, Elsie A., c1953, ON
Burns, Shelley A., 2002, CCNM, ON
Byers, Karen Schad see Willow, Katherine
Bzowy, Joseph D., 1949, NCNM, MB
Cadieux, John Allan, 1975, CMCC*, 1982, OCNM, ON
Caetman, Charles F., c1953, ON
Cahill Sleggs, Laura, 2007, CCNM, NY
Caird, David Baxter, BC
Caird, see Thompson, Emma
Caitcher, F. Wm., c1973, ON
Calder, Kimberly see McQueen
Callaghan, Robyn L., 2005, CCNM, ON
Callaghan-Fleck, Kim Noelle, 2001, CCNM, ON
Calville, Robert A., c1953, ON
Cameron, Carla Danielle nee Mills, 2003, CCNM, ON
Campbell, Donald, 1920, LACC, BC
Campbell, John McPherson, c1943, BC
Campbell, Lauri D., c1985, TX
Campbell, Melinda P. (Mindy), 2007, CCNM, ON
Campbell, Sheree Lynn, 1989, Bastyr
Canning, Ethyle L. "Jimmy", 1951, CMCC*, ON
Cannon, Rebecca D. nee Farquharson, 2000, CCNM, ON
Cappuccio, Olga, 2005, CCNM, ON
Cardinal, Lucien J. B., c1976, ON
Caria, Kristin, 2008, CCNM, ON
Carino, Jasmine, 1998, CCNM, ON
Carlson-Rink, Cathy, 1995, Bastyr, BC
Carl-Sotomayor, Sonya T., 2002, CCNM, ON
Carricato, Mitchell Todd, 2004, CCNM, ON
Carson, W.R., c1926, PE
Carter, Jennifer A., 2002, CCNM, NS

Carthy, Wm. C., c1953, ON
Cartier, H. St. Nicholas, c1953, ON
Caruso, Kevin M., 2001, CCNM, ON
Caruso, Lorraine A. nee Cocca, 2002, CCNM, ON
Carveth, Fred T., c1926, BC
Cashion, Kenneth, 1989, OCNM, BC
Cass, Malcolm E., c1983, BC
Castes, W., c1920, BC
Castle, Jennifer Lynne, 2006, CCNM, ON
Caswell, Lisa Jennifer, 2004, CCNM, ON
Cathoi, George L., c1953, ON
Caversan, Amauri, 2006, CCNM, ON
Cawfield, Norman Charles, 1974, CMCC*, ON
Ceaser, Sean, 1999, NCNM, MB
Celik, Sara, 2005, CCNM, ON
Cerullo, Debbie K.L., 2003, CCNM, ON
Chaleunsouk, Vongdeuan, 2004, CCNM, ON
Chambers, Andrea, 2004, BINM, BC
Chambers, Dennis, c1977, ON
Chan, Allan Wai Kin, 1984, OCNM, China
Chan, Charlene Sih-Lian, 2004, CCNM, BC
Chan, Chun Sing, 1989, Bastyr, BC
Chan, Eric, 2003, CCNM, BC
Chan, Isaac, 1987, OCNM, China
Chan, Jimmy Chun Sing, 1989, Bastyr, BC
Chan, Julie Sook-Man, 2006, CCNM, ON
Chan, Lawrence (Larry), 1989, OCNM, BC
Chan, Natalie M., 2001, CCNM, ON
Chan, Victor Wai - Tak, 2003, CCNM, BC
Chana, Harpreet
Chandra, Pushpa nee Kissun, 2005, BINM, BC
Chang Alloy, Kimberly
Chang, Nana (Bell), 1992, OCNM, ON
Chang, Helen, nee Meyers, 1989, OCNM, ON
Chapell, Sheree, 1991, Bastyr, BC
Chapman, Lanalle Victoria see Dunn
Chapmann, Elizabeth, BC
Charest, Crystal M., 2002, CCNM, NB
Charikar, Ramona, 2006, CCNM, AB
Charles, Ray, 1990, OCNM, AZ
Charles, Ray, c1981, ON
Charlton, William Edward, c1922, ON

Charney, Thalia, 2003, CCNM, ON

Charpentier, Jessica, 2007, CCNM, AB

Charron, Jennifer Suzanne, nee Speare, 2006, CCNM, ON

Chartten, William E., c1953, ON

Chatten, Jayne-Ann, 2006, CCNM, ON

Chattoe, E.J., c1926, ON

Cheah, Katherine, 1999, CCNM, SK

Cheifetz, Nathan, 1978, NCNM, ON

Chen, Jennifer, 1999, CCNM, ON

Chen, Jia Qi, 2007, BINM, BC

Chen, Julie ZhuYan, 2001, CCNM, ON

Chen, Sherry Jui-Lien, 2002, CCNM, ON

Chen, Zhi-Hao, 1996, Bastyr, ON

Cheng, Steven, c1977, 1981, OCNM, ON

Cheng, William, c1977, 1981, OCNM, ON

Cheng-Kai-On, Natalie, 2006, CCNM, ON

Chervenka, Cindy, 2001, CCNM, AB

Cheung, Jennie, 1997, CCNM, ON

Chevalier, E.J., c1926, ON

Chhoker, Baljinder Singh, 1997, CCNM, ON

Chiasson, Lynn, 2002, CCNM, SK

Chim, Trudy, 2006, CCNM, AB

Chin, Michelle, 2008, CCNM, ON

Chindemi, Wayne J., 1986, NCNM, ON

Chitale, Angeli, 2000, CCNM, ON

Chiverton, Maurice Lee, c1953, ON

Choi, Mary, 2008, CCNM, ON

Choi, Moonsang, 2007, UBCNM, BC

Cholewa, Ireneus Jan (Ian), 1999, Bastyr, HI

Chong, Astrid C., 2002, CCNM, ON

Chow, Gabriella K., 2005, CCNM, ON

Chow, Phoebe Po-Wah, 1989, OCNM, BC

Christian, Linda Diane, 1988, OCNM, ON

Christie, Christina M. (Tina), 2001, CCNM, ON

Christoforou, Christina, 2004, CCNM, ON

Chu, Kenneth J., 2006, CCNM, AB

Chu, Raymond Y. K., 1970, CMCC*, ON, Hong Kong

Chung, Ainee, 2002, CCNM, ON

Chung, Diane Carol, 2001, CCNM, ON

Cidadao, Judy, 2000, CCNM, ON

Cincurak, Jennifer L. M., 2005, CCNM, ON

Clack, Gregory Scott, 1997, Bastyr, BC, ON

Clancy, Lloyd D., c1959, AB

Clapp, Tara N., 2000, CCNM, ON

Clark, A. L., c1953, ON

Clark, Glenda J., 1990, OCNM, ON

Clark, Romy L. nee Giesbrecht, 2006, CCNM, ON

Clark, Shawna Leigh, 1992, OCNM, ON

Clarke, Belinda M., 2000, CCNM, ON

Clarke, Malburn R., c1953, ON

Cleaver, Andrea nee Klubal, 2008, CCNM, ON

Clemmer, Cecil G., c1953, PCC, ON

Clow, Jennifer see Pyatt

Clubine, Frederick L., c1953, ON

Coates, Mark R., 1987, OCNM, ON, Singapore

Cocca, Lorraine A. see Caruso

Coe, Cathryn, 2005, BINM, BC

Cogan, Elizabeth Lisa, 2001, Bastyr, US

Coggins, E.P., c1926, BC

Cogo, Elise, 2000, CCNM, ON

Cohen, Cindi Lee, 2001, CCNM, ON

Cohen, Helen, 1990, OCNM, ON

Colclough, W. H., 1938, NCDP, BC

Colello, Jacqueline, 1999, CCNM, ON

Coleman, Cathleen see MacDonald

Colett, J.D., c1926, BC

Collins, David M., PE

Collins, Harry M., c1953, ON

Coltman, Charles Franklin, c1926, ON

Comas, Beatriz, 1999, CCNM, ON

Comeau, Vicki Rochelle, 2000, CCNM, ON

Comeau-Wilson, Danielle see Wilson

Compan, Emile J., 2001, CCNM, ON

Compton, Christina A., 2001, CCNM, AZ

Condliffe, Keith Douglas, 2007, CCNM, BC

Connoly, Lisa M., 1987, NCNM, BC

Constant, Nicole, 1989, OCNM, ON

Conyette, Paul Anthony, 1989, OCNM, MB

Cook, Derek Robert, 2007, CCNM, ON

Cook, Tracy L., 2001, CCNM, ON

Cooley, Patrick Kieran, 2003, CCNM, ON

Cooper, Cheryl L., 2005, CCNM, QC, ON

Cooper, Donald, 1996, NCNM, BC

Cooper, Ernest, c1953, ON
Cooper, R.G.C., c1918, NS
Cooper, Scott
Cooper, William H., c1953, ON
Cootauco, Stacy Ellaine, 2007, CCNM, ON
Copsey, W. G., c1962, MB
Corbeil, Jennifer L., 2006, CCNM, BC
Corbett, Kimber-Lee Anne (Kim), 2001, CCNM, QC
Cormier-Hazen, Dawn Marie, 1993, CCNM, ON
Cosgrove, John Michael, 1981, OCNM, ON
Cottingham, George Edward, 1933, NWCC, BC
Coulter, Susan M., c2004, ON
Cousins, Mark, 1987, NCNM, BC
Coutcher, Frank William, 1947, NCDP, FL
Cowan, Barbara Lynn, 2004, CCNM, ON
Cowan, Shane J., 2006, CCNM, ON
Cowen, Eytan Michael, 1998, CCNM, NY
Craig, Christine, 1997, NCNM, BC
Craig, Clare, 2006, CCNM, BC
Craig, Ingeborg Laura, c1940, BC
Cranton, Alan George, 1989, OCNM, ON
Craren, Andrew E., c1953, ON
Craven, Andrew E., c1961, ON
Creech, Allison D., 2004, CCNM, ON
Cressman, Amanda Sue, 2007, CCNM, ON
Cristal, Aloel nee Golikova, Olga, 1996, CCNM, ON
Crnec, Madeline F., 1989, OCNM, ON
Cronyn, Maria A., nee Herod, 1999, SCNM, ON
Crosby, Donald N., 1989, OCNM, ON
Cross, Frank, c1953, ON
Crouch, Pauline see Baumann
Cseszko, Mark, 2004, CCNM, AB
Cullen, Austin, 1938, WSC, 1952, NCNM, BC
Cullin, F. A., c1956, OR, BC
Currier, George A., c1953, ON
Curtis, Lloyd W., c1953, ON
Cutter, Walter L., 1926, NCDP, ON
Cybulski, Sheryl Elizabeth Rose see Richardson
Cyr, Nadine, 1998, CCNM, ON
Czeranko, Sussanna, 1994, CCNM, ON, QC
DaCosta Reis, Jose, 1984, OCNM, ON
Dacyshyn, Janice, 2005, Bastyr, AB

D'Adamo, James L., 1957, ASN, ON
D'Adamo, Peter, c1987, ON
Dagenais, Linda, 1999, Bastyr, WA
Dahl, Nicole Terase, 2002, Bastyr, BC
Dale, Katherine S., 2002, CCNM, ON
Dale-Harris, Victoria A., 2004, CCNM, ON
Dalen, Corinne, 1992, NCNM, AB, BC
Dalphond, G. C., c1958, FL, BC
Dalson, E. Dean, c1953, ON
Daly, Thomas W. (Tom), 2000, CCNM, ON
Danby, Alison, 2007, CCNM, ON
Dancer, Rosemary, 1996, NCNM, MB
Dangerfield, Elizabeth, c1926, SK
Dangerfield, F.W., c1926, SK
Dann (Donn), Oswald, c1953, ON
Danner, Suzanne, 1997, NCNM, MB
Dao, Barbara P., 2005, CCNM, ON
Daotran, Mary (Hung), 2008, CCNM, ON
Dare, Kimberley M., 2001, CCNM, ON
Darou, Shawna A., 2003, CCNM, ON
Darvish, Nooshin see Khoshkhosal
Davidson, Alan L., 1981, OCNM, ON
Davidson, Victoria-Lee, 2006, CCNM
Davie, Janice, 2008, CCNM, ON
Davies, Alexander B., c1953, ON
Davies, Brian, 2006, CCNM, BC
Davies, Jacqueline, 2006, CCNM, BC
Davies, John Edward, c1948, AB
Davies, Richard, 2000, CCNM, AB
Davis, Paul J., 1989, OCNM, ON
Davis, Wendy E., 2004, CCNM, ON
Dawson, Corrine, 2006, BINM, BC
Dawson, Loreen, 1997, NCNM, BC
Day, Joanne, 2006, CCNM, AB
Dayal, Gurinder, 2000, CCNM, BC
D'Costa, Cheryl Christine, 2003, CCNM, ON
Dean, Carolyn, 1997, CCNM, US, Costa Rica
DeBoeck, Courtney T., 2001, CCNM, ON
DeCicco, Paola, 2004, CCNM, QC
DeGroot, Nicholas James, 1998, CCNM, ON
Dela Cruz, Grace, 1999, CCNM, BC
DeLaCampa, Paulina see Zettel

DeLisi-Sozio, Linda see Sozio

DeMarco, A.V., c1958, FL, BC

Demborynsky, Morris, 1986, OCNM, ON

Demehri, Afrouz, 2008, CCNM, ON

deMelo, Jaime E., 2004, CCNM, BC

DeMent, Gene A., c1962, IA, AB

DeMonte, Denise, 1999, CCNM, BC

Dempster, John, 2006, CCNM, ON

DeNault, Alain Joseph Leo, 2000, CCNM, AB

Dennis, Arthur William, 1919, ASN, BC

Denov, Albert S. (Al), 1989, OCNM, ON

dePeiza, Patrice Marla, 2007, CCNM, ON

Derbyshire, Debra A., 2000, CCNM, ON

Derganc, Gerard M. (Gerry), 1999, CCNM, ON

Derksen-Hiebert, Loral, 1999, CCNM, ON

DeRosa, Aaron M., 2005, CCNM, ON

DesLauriers, Francine

Desrocher, Nathalie see Allen

Devaux, Gayle Maria see Segovia

Devgan, Ravi, c1976, ON

Devgun, Amrit nee Bhooi, 1995, CCNM, MI

Dewab, Ernest R., c1953, ON

Dewar, Leslie, 1994, CCNM

D'Gogossian, Marina, c1993

Dhanani, Karim, 2001, CCNM, ON

Dhillon, Vinnie, 2003, Bastyr, BC

Dhiman, Neetu, 2002, CCNM, BC

Diana, Lorenzo M. (Enzo), 1995, CCNM, ON

DiCicco, Vanessa K., 2006, CCNM, SK

Diogo Ferraioli, Ana Cristina, 2000, CCNM, ON

DiPiazza, Claudia, 2002, CCNM, ON

Djelebian, Christopher Steven, 2004, CCNM, ON

Doagoo, Bita, 2007, CCNM, ON

Doan, Jennifer Louise, 1996, CCNM, BC

Doan, Robert, c1953, ON

Dobosz, Lidia nee Pawlowska, 1988, OCNM, ON

Dodd, Richard Anthony, 1993, CCNM, ON

Dodds, Cameron R., 1993, Bastyr, BC, MB

Dodds, Robert J., c1953, ON

Doherty, Carissa E., 2002, CCNM, ON

Doherty, Christine, 1998, Bastyr, NH

Doherty, Sonya Marie, 2003, CCNM, ON

Doholis, Stephen John, 1977, CMCC*, ON

Dohring, Grace H., c1953, MI

Doig, Jeannie, 2006, CCNM, BC

Dolson, Edgar Dean, c1935, NCNM, CA

Donovan, Teresa, 2007, CCNM, NS

Doran, Lisa Marie nee Murray, 1997, CCNM, ON

Dorchester, Frank Edwin, 1920, ASN, BC

Dorrell, Jan Melissa, 1999, CCNM, ON

Dossa, Meera, 2006, CCNM, ON

Doucette, Melissa Rayne, 2003, CCNM, ON

Douglas, Jane, 2008, CCNM, ON

Douglas, Karen Debra, 2004, CCNM, ON

Downie, William John

Downorowicz, Martin, 2004, CCNM, ON

Doxsee, George W., c1953, ON

Doyle, Jennifer H., 2007, CCNM, NS

Drescher, Harold J., 1949, PCN, ON

Drobot, Chantelle, 2000, NCNM, AB

Drobot, Jeoffrey, 2001, NCNM, AB

Dronyk, Robert J., 1986, OCNM, ON

Dronyk, William Michael, 1974, CMCC*, 1984, OCNM, ON

Drought, Alison Catherine, 2001, CCNM, AB

Drouin, Autumn Louise, 1989, OCNM, US, ON

Drummond, Jennifer K., 2005, CCNM, ON

Duffee, Nicole, 2006, BINM, AB, BC

Duggal, Sherry, 2004, CCNM, ON

Dugoua, Jean-Jacques (Dr. JJ), 2003, CCNM, ON

Dumouchelle, Annie W., c1953, ON

Dunk, Kenneth Richard, 1981, OCNM, ON

Dunkeld, William L., c1953, ON

Dunn, Lanalle Victoria nee Chapman, 2003, CCNM, Dubai

Dunn, Oswald, 1951, CMCC*, ON

Duong, Trang, 2000, Bastyr, BC

Dupont, Joseph Ubald, c1953, ON

Durant, Susan Marie, nee Eden, 1992, OCNM, ON

Durham, James V., c1926, ON

Durham, Lena M., c1926, ON

Durkin, Michelle Teresa, 2003, CCNM, ON

Durnan, Julie nee Bowman, 2006, BINM, BC

Durward, Dorothea (Thea), 1992, Bastyr, BC

DuVal, Augustus R., c1953, ON

Duvgun, Amrit nee Bhooi, 1995, CCNM, Minnesota

Dychangco, Christine, 2007, CCNM, ON

Dyck, George J., c1953, ON

Dyck, Weigant Abram, 1989, OCNM

Dyson, G.W., c1926, QC

Dyszuk, Michael R., 1952, CMCC*, ON

Eade, Heather, 2005, BINM, BC, Saudi Arabia

Earls, Aoife, 2008, CCNM, ON

Ebbett, Claude E., c1953, ON

Ebranhimzadeh, Mojgan, 1998, CCNM, TX

Edalati, Mandana, 2005, CCNM, BC

Eddleston, Frances Margaret nee Shrubb, c1976, 1981, OCNM, ON

Eden, Martin, c1953, ON

Eden, Susan, see Durant

Edgar, Martan W., c1953, ON

Edwards, Norman W., c1953, ON

Edwards, William, c1954, BC

Ee Yan Wan, Leslie, 1997, CCNM, ON

Egenberger, Nicole Phyllis Katalin, 2003, CCNM, NY

Egervari Borosh, Maria, 1996, CCNM, ON

Eibl, Ingeborg, 1986, OCNM, NY

Eidt, Carl, J., c1953, ON

Eino, Dina N., 2003, CCNM, ON

Eisenstein, Michael, 1994, CCNM, ON

Elnachef, Douha, c1988, ON

Elgez, Aviad, 2008, CCNM, ON

El-hashemy, Shehab, 2004, CCNM, ON

Elkhalil, Lamise, 2005, CCNM, BC

Elliott, J. Carl, c1953, MI

Ellis, Thomas William, 2004, CCNM, ON

Ellison, Anna C., c1953, ON

Ellison, James Wm., c1953, ON

Ellsworth, Eleanor H., c1953, ON

Elnachef, Douha, 1989, OCNM, ON

Eng Khalsa, Eileen, 1989, OCNM, ON

Engelbrecht, Natalie see Bonter

Entner, Shelby, 2002, NCNM, BC

Erbeck, Alvin C., c1962, Ohio, AB

Erdmann, Uwaya, 1999, CCNM, ON

Erickson, Liane P., 2002, CCNM, ON, Yukon, Alaska

Eriksen, Tamara, 2008, CCNM, AB

Ertha, Elsie Darlene Hardy, 2004, CCNM, MA

Esfaniari, Farhad Ali Mohammad, 1991, OCNM, Italy

Esposito, Candice Marie, 2007, CCNM, ON

Etherington, Robert M., c1953, ON

Everest, Michelle M., nee Monforton, 2002, CCNM, ON

Ewing, Robert, 1993, Bastyr, BC

Exner, Jana, 1994, CCNM, AB

Fabbro, Maria A., 1999, CCNM, BC

Facca, Melanie L., 2002, CCNM, ON

Fainstat, Paula, 1989, OCNM, BC

Fairley, Dorothy A., 1996, NCNM, BC

Fairman-Young, Karrin, 2004, CCNM, BC

Falari Rashvand, Parviz, 2002, CCNM, Dubai

Falkenspence, Karen, 2006, CCNM, BC

Falkowski, Anna M., 2003, CCNM, ON

Falomo, Alene, 2001, CCNM, ON

Falsafi, Hamideh, 2005, CCNM, ON

Fanous, Mireille, 2002, CCNM, ON

Faraz, Atousa, 2006, CCNM, ON

Farina, Valerie, 1997, Bastyr, BC

Farlane, James E., c1953, ON

Farmer, Arthur B., c1953, ON

Farmer, H., c1926, ON

Farnsworth, Earl W., 1956, WSC, BC

Farnsworth, Gerald Ross (Gerry), 1950, NCDP, BC

Farnsworth, Kelly D., 1981, NCNM, BC

Farnsworth, Todd, 1994, NCNM, BC

Farquharson, James P. (Jim), 1990, OCNM, ON

Farquharson, James R., 1922, National, ON

Farquharson, Robert Bowden, 1947, National, ON

Farquharson-Cannon, Rebecca see Cannon

Farr, Alice Elba, c1953, ON

Farwell, Stephanie M., 2005, CCNM, ON

Fasihi, Reza, 2007, CCNM, ON

Fatijewski, F.

Faulkner, William J., c1953, ON

Federowicz, Jennifer, 2005, CCNM, CA

Feegel, Eric D., c1953, ON

Feely, Shannon, 2007, CCNM, England

Fennell, Holly (Heather), 2004, CCNM, ON

Fenner, Rochelle nee Moulton, 2007, CCNM, BC

Ferguson, Charles, c1983, AL

Ferguson, Kellie, 2005, Bastyr, BC
Ferguson, Leshia, 2004, CCNM, SK
Ferguson, Lori, 2007, CCNM, BC
Fernyhough, Walter, 2007, BINM, BC
Ferraro, Michelle, 2008, CCNM, ON
Ferris, Amanda J. see Roth
Finlay, Kathleen, 1998, CCNM, ON
Finley, Richard Mac, 1973, NCNM, ON
Finn, Linda M., 2000, CCNM, ON
Fiore, Judith P., 2000, CCNM, ON
Fish, J.C., c1926, BC
Fish, J.M., c1926, BC
Fitzgerald Eagan, Jennifer M., 2005, CCNM, ON
Fleming, Dora H. see Stewart
Fleming, Robert (Bob), 1956, NCNM, BC
Fleury, Jacqueline L. (Jacqui), 1998, Bastyr, SK, AB
Floegel, Katrine see Martin
Flood, Elizabeth Clare, 1992, OCNM, BC
Flynn, Dawn, 1999, Bastyr, WA
Fogg, Julia Anne, 2000, CCNM, ON
Foisy, Roger, c1988, QC.
Foley, Stacy Elizabeth nee Riviere, 2004, CCNM, ON
Folkard, Tracey Ann, 1997, CCNM, ON.
Foniciello, Mary Lynda, 2004, CCNM, ON
Foord, Wilfred H., 1950, NAA, AB
Ford, John H., c1953, ON
Ford, Stewart, c1953, ON
Forgeron, Jennifer Tara Maria, 2001, CCNM, ON
Forgie, David, 1979, CMCC*, NB
Forman, Stephen E., c1959, AB
Forristal, Jennifer Ann, 2004, CCNM, ON
Fountain, Julia nee Trick, 1998, CCNM, TX, ON
Fournier, Julie C, 2002, CCNM, ON
Fox, Bruce W., c1953, ON
Fox, J. A., c1953, ON
Franc, Valerie H., 2000, CCNM, ON
Francinelli, Elmira, 2004, CCNM, ON
Frank, Pamela, 1999, CCNM, ON
Frank, Shelly, 2007, CCNM, ON
Franks, Olivia, 2007, Bastyr, US
Fraser, Janine, 2007, BINM, BC
Fraser, Karen Lise, 1997, CCNM, BC

Fraser, Kelly, 2008, CCNM
Fraser, Robyn, 1998, CCNM, ON
Frederick, Chelsea, 2004, Bastyr, AB
Freed, Mahalia Nandi, 2006, CCNM, ON
Freeman, Tamsyn Danielle Gow, 2001, CCNM, AB
Fremes, Penelope A., 1989, OCNM, ON, CA
French, Sydney H., c1953, ON
Frenette, Celeste, 2008, CCNM, ON
Frey, Samantha, 2006, BINM, AB
Fridleifson, Erikur Julius, 1936, WSC, BC
Friedman, Michael, 1998, CCNM, VT
Fritz, Heidi M., 2007, CCNM, ON
Frketich, Kira A., 2002, CCNM, BC
Frosina, Michael, 2008, CCNM, ON
Fruden, Wm. H., c1953, NY
Fry, Edwin G., c1953, ON
Fujibayashi, Kelly, 2004, BINM, BC, Australia
Fuke, Eleanor Buchanan, 1993, CCNM, ON
Fuller, Denise, 1999, CCNM, ON
Fuller, George M., c1953, ON
Fullerton, Kerri Lynne, 2003, CCNM, ON
Fulton, Lynne, 2001, NCNM, BC
Fulton, Verdean Duclos, c1954, AB
Gabryl, Patricia Teresa, 2002, CCNM, ON.
Gagnier, Joel J., 2001, CCNM, ON.
Gagnon, Andree, c1988, QC
Gagnon, Henri-Louis, c1988, QC
Gagnon, Michel, c1991, QC
Galic, Mary, 2002, CCNM, ON
Gallagher, Naihaniel T., c1953, ON
Gallagher, Paula Jane, 2002, Bastyr, BC
Gallant, Jamie, 2004, BINM, BC
Galvin, Carolin A., 1996, CCNM, NB
Gamble, Christopher, 2006, CCNM
Gammage, Amanda Jane, 1998, Bastyr, BC
Garby, Danika, 2008, CCNM, MA
Gardner, Steven, 1994, NCNM, OR
Garieri, Michelle J., 2000, CCNM, ON
Garner, A. H., c1959, QC
Garner, Kevan, c1970, AB
Garner, William G., 2003, CCNM, ON
Garrison, Tina, 2007, BINM, BC

Gaskell, Maria Nicole, 2001, CCNM, NS

Gatis, Robert L., 1987, OCNM, ON

Gauthier, Charles E., c1953, ON

Gaudet, Jean M., 1928, LCC, QC

Gaul, Allissa K., 1998, Bastyr, AB

Gaumann, Richard, c1971, ON

Gaw, Thomas, E.A., c1981, ON

Gawenda, Karie Michelle, 2001, CCNM, ON

Gawronski, Michael M., 1953, CMCC*, ON

Gay, Donald A., 1981, OCNM, ON

Gdanski, Stanley A., c1953, ON, SK

Geddes, Kelly Renee Teresa, 1991, OCNM, ON

Geerligs, Adam see Prinsen

Geis, Marika, 2006, CCNM, BC

Gelleta, J., c1961, ON

Gemel, Erwin, 1989, OCNM, ON

Genné, Anne - Hélène, 2004, CCNM, QC

Genuardi, Cinzia A., 2003, CCNM, ON

Georgousis, Alexia, 1999, CCNM, ON

Gerbracht, John Wesley, c1953, ON

German, G. G., c1953, ON

Gerow, Richard J., c1971, NY

Gerus, Liudmyla, 2004, CCNM, ON

Gervais, Roger R., 1993, Bastyr, BC

Geyer, Samantha see Boutet

Ghazali, Johan, 2000, Bastyr, BC

Ghazali, Norlinda, 1999, Bastyr, BC

Ghodsian, Juliet Magdalena, 2004, Bastyr, BC

Gibb, Frauk M., MB

Gibbs, Shelley Elizabeth, 2003, CCNM, ON

Giesbrecht, Romy see Clark

Gignac, Tara Lynn, 2001, CCNM, ON

Gilbert, Cyndi S., 2007, CCNM, ON

Gilbert, Tracy Kristen, 2002, CCNM, ON

Gilchrist, Amy Victoria, 2004, CCNM, BC

Giles, Dianna M., 2000, CCNM, ON

Gill, Brenda, 1996, NCNM, BC

Gill, Odessa Cortes, 2004, CCNM, ON

Gill, Ravinder, 2001, CCNM, ON

Gillespie, Michelle, 2002, CCNM, ON

Gindi, Tabaseem Yassa, 1997, CCNM, ON

Gingerich, Andrea M., 2002, CCNM, BC

Girgis, John, 2008, CCNM, ON

Giustra, Sabrina Ramona, 2006, CCNM, ON

Gladstone, J. B. , 1962, ASN, MB

Gladstone, Sam A. , 1962, ASN, MB

Glasgow, Marina, 2006, CCNM

Glazer, Jennifer R., 2005, CCNM, ON

Glazer, Josie, 2000, CCNM, ON

Gleisberg, Peter, 1977, HSS Germany, SK

Gleixner, Martin, 2008, BINM, NB

Glew, Thomas J., 1982, NCNM, BC

Gluvic, Brian, 2000, Bastyr, BC

Gobindpuri, Rupinder (Rupi) see Mitha

Godfrey, Anthony J., 1990, OCNM, ON

Goehner, Jane A., 2001, CCNM, ON

Gokavi, Tanya Nandini, 2003, CCNM, SK

Gold, Leon Mann, c1927, Ohio, BC

Goldring, Julie Ann, 1996, CCNM, ON

Golikova, Olga see Cristal, Aloel

Golledge, Deborah Ellen, c1977, ON

Gonen, Julia Francine, 2006, CCNM, Israel

Gonzales, Carolyn, 2004, CCNM, ON

Good, Lisa, nee MacIntyre, 2008, BINM, BC

Goodwin, Mark C., c1953, ON

Gordon, Ashely J., 2003, CCNM, BC

Gordon, Christina, 2008, CCNM, ON

Gordon, Edward M., c1953, ON

Gordon, Shalima S., 2000, Bastyr, US

Goreshnik, Zilia, 1989, OCNM, ON

Gorrell, Darren, 2005, BINM, BC

Gould, Tutti Timmins nee Putnam, 1986, OCNM, QC

Govindji, Emynaaz S. (Emy), 2001, CCNM, BC

Gowan, Matthew J.E., 2003, CCNM, ON

Gowland, Jonathan Earle, c1953, ON

Grabreck, Reiner, 1990, OCNM, ON

Graham, George A., c1953, ON

Graham, Kathy Ann, 1993, CCNM, BC

Graham, Margaret Joy, see Banga

Graham, Russell W.W., 1997, CCNM, BC

Graham, Wm. L., c1953, ON

Grant, Christopher C., c1953, ON

Grant, Laura Kristin, 2004, CCNM, ON

Grant, Murie M., c1976, 1981, OCNM, ON

Grant, Ronald M., 1940, WSC, BC

Granzotto, Jason G., 2007, CCNM, ON

Gratton, Adam, 2008, CCNM, ON

Gray, James T., c1926, BC

Gray, Linden,

Gray, Megan, 2007, CCNM, ON

Gray, Samantha, 2001, NCNM, BC

Gray, William, c1926, BC

Green, Jennifer, 2000, CCNM, MI

Greenall, Jese, see Wiens

Greenhorn, Larry, 1978, NCNM, AB

Greggain, Carl N., 1990, OCNM, ON

Greib, Lowell Christopher, 2003, CCNM, ON

Grewal, Sonya, 2007, BINM, BC

Grey, Laurence A. K. (Larry), 1974, CMCC*, 1981, OCNM, ON

Griffith, Candice C., 2002, CCNM, BC

Griffith, Charles A., c1953, ON

Grime, Tammy C., 2006, CCNM, ON

Grinevitch, Lara, 1997, CCNM, AB, Australia

Grittani, Norman F., 1953, CMCC*, ON

Grizzle, Norman W., c1953, ON

Grobys, Sigrid nee Witek, 2007, CCNM, ON, Singapore

Grochocinski, Jennifer Ann, 2006, CCNM, ON

Grodski, Tom, 2006, CCNM, BC

Grossman, Barbara, c1981, ON

Grube, Lambert Kenneth (Bert), 1949, National, SK, MB, AB

Gu, Lei, 2007, CCNM, ON

Gucciardi-Mercurio, Giacomina, 1997, CCNM, ON

Guilmain, Luce, c1983, QC

Gullekson, B. L., c1959, AB

Gunther, Gustau, c1955, ON

Gurm, Sharon, 2005, CCNM, BC

Guruswami, Maya, 2004, CCNM, QC

Gustin, Darlene Carolyn, 1991, OCNM, ON

Guthrie, Amanda Rhiannon, 2006, CCNM, ON

Gutteridge, Susan E. see Joyce

Guy, Vivienne Therese, 2004, CCNM, ON

Gyuro, Maria, 1999, CCNM, ON

Habert, Emily, 2008, BINM, BC

Habib, Rahim B., 2000, CCNM, ON

Hack, Karen, 2001, CCNM, ON

Haessler, Jennifer Anne, 2003, CCNM, ON

Hafiz, Hasan, 1997, CCNM, AB

Hagarty, Corlyss Ellyn, 2001, CCNM, ON

Hainey, Brenda S. see Main

Hall, Catherine, 2003, CCNM, NY

Hall, Henry, MB

Hall, J. Alexander, 2000, CCNM, ON

Hallett, Harace C., c1953, ON

Hallsor, Ellis, 1937, NCNM, BC

Halm, Harry O., c1955, ON

Halonen, Joseph D., c1953, ON

Hamidani, Naureen, 2008, CCNM, ON

Hamilton, L.E., c1926, SK

Hamilton, Robert D., c1953, IN

Hamilton, Susan, 1991, Bastyr, BC, AB

Hammond, D. L. , c1960, BC

Hammond, John D., 1950, CMCC*, ON, AK

Han, Soo-Jung, 2006, CCNM, ON

Han, Wei-Wei, 2000, CCNM, ON

Hand, Darrow, 2000, CCNM, HI

Handford, Rebecca, 2007, BINM, BC

Handorf, Ernest W., c1953, ON

Hanlon, Angela, 2008, CCNM, ON

Hanlon, G. F., ON

Hann, David Charles, 1971, CMCC*, ON

Hannaford-Sterchi, Carolyn Jane, 2005, CCNM, NS

Hannaford, Sharon Elizabeth, 2006, CCNM, ON

Hannigan, Kelly Ann, 1997, CCNM, AZ

Hans, Karm, 2008, CCNM, ON

Hansen, Bernard Rudolph, 1949, NCDP, SK

Harb, Lindy, 2006, CCNM, ON

Hardman, Leonard A., 1967, CMCC*, ON

Hardy, Gary, 1986, OCNM, ON

Hardy, Randall (Randy), c1977, BC

Hardy, Sarah A., 2005, CCNM, Ont., NS

Hardychuck, Don, c1981, ON

Hare, Lois M., 1987, OCNM, NS

Harela, Eric Alan, 1981, OCNM, ON

Harknett, Kerry Ann, 2005, CCNM, ON

Harman, Marie Colette, 1990, OCNM, ON

Harney, Tracey Lynne, 2001, CCNM, Bermuda

Harper, Robert W., 1950, CMCC*, ON

Harris, H.M., c1926, NS
Harris, John F., c1926, AB
Harris-Janz, Ivan Nicholas, 2004, CCNM, MB
Harrison, Ellen E., c1953, ON
Harrison, J. R., c1953, ON
Hart, Jason William, 2005, CCNM, ON
Hartnett, Lydia see Starkovski
Harvey-Smith, Caroline J., 2001, CCNM, ON
Haskell, Alexander, 1986, NCNM, QC, Utah
Haskins, Douglas V., c1953, ON
Hassard, Mary Lynn, 1984, OCNM, ON
Hastings, Edward G., c1953, ON
Hauck, Sharon E., 2007, CCNM, ON
Haugh, I. Currie, c1953, ON
Haugh, I. R., c1953, ON
Hauk, Alfred, 1990, OCNM, ON
Haute, J. Oswaed (Haule), c1953, ON
Hauze, Judith, c1981, ON
Hauze, Robert, c1981, ON
Hawco, Sharleen, 2008, CCNM, ON
Hawley, Peter G., c1981, ON
Hawrylak, John Wayne, 1972, CMCC*, 1986, OCNM, NS
Hawthorne, Kathryn Louise, 2001, CCNM, ON
Hayes, Michael L., 1994, NCNM, OR
Hayhoe, Bruce A., 1969, NCNM, NB
Hayman, E. Kitchener, c1981, ON
Hayman, Rosalyn Joanne, 2005, CCNM, NS
Haynes, Anuj Gloria, c1995, ON
Hayte, Leroy, c1977, ON
Hazlitt, Katharine J. (Kate), 2006, CCNM, ON
He, Sen, 2004, CCNM, BC
Heald, Debra Gillott, 2008, BINM, AB
Healy, J. J., c1953, ON
Heard, Nettie, c1926, BC
Heath, Gayle, 2006, CCNM, AB
Heffernan, Susan Marie, 2003, CCNM
Heinen, Shirley J., 1992, OCNM, ON
Heins, Kristin Dagnia, 2006, CCNM, ON
Hellenbrand, Maria, 2008, CCNM, ON
Hembroff, Mary Anne, 2003, CCNM, MB
Henderson, Grant A., c1953, ON
Henderson, John A., 1911, RCC, ON

Henry, Nicole, 2008, CCNM, ON
Hepburn, James Hitchcock, 1928, PCC
Herington, Heather, 1987, Bastyr, BC, CA
Herod, Maria A. see Cronyn
Herrington, Craig, 2005, BINM, AB
Hershoff, Gregory Asa, 1974, CMCC*, 1981, OCNM, ON, CA
Herwig, Monika, 1999, CCNM, AB
Herzan, Martin George, 1997, CCNM, ON
Heskins, G. A., c1965, ON
Hess, Carrie M., c1953, ON
Hess, Rollo C., 1933, PCN, AB
Hetherington, John A., c1953, ON
Heuper, Herman, c1938, BC
Hibbs, Janet C., 2001, CCNM, ON
Hicks, Laurence V., 1990, OCNM, ID
Hiebert, Amy, 2006, CCNM, AB
Hill, Herbert A., c1953, ON
Hill, Thomas Ralph, 1976, CMCC*, ON
Hillemann, H. H.
Hiller, G., c1983, ON
Hillier, Jennifer Christina Ruth, 2003, CCNM, BC, ON
Hilton, Arthur Lyon Jr., c1940, BC
Hilton, Arthur Sr., 1936, WSC, BC
Hinze, Jack, 1986, OCNM, BC
Hippmann, Yvonne see Stiles
Hirji, Rahima, 2002, CCNM, ON
Hirst, Amber J. see Vance
Hlywka, Deanna, 2002, CCNM, ON
Hnatiuk, Rosemary, 2008, CCNM, ON
Hnatko, Cynthia, 2006, CCNM, AB
Hnatov, Vasilij, 2002, CCNM, ON
Ho, Cecilia C.Y., 2005, CCNM, ON
Hoang, Lily, 2008, CCNM, ON
Hoeffer, Maria, 2006, CCNM, OH
Hoffman, Edward R., c1953, ON
Hoffman, Trevor, 1997, SCNM, AB
Hoffmann, Michael, 2005, CCNM, AB
Hofner, Grazyna Wanda, 1988, OCNM, NS
Hogg, Joan Dorothy, c1977, ON
Holdaway, Janet I., c1953, ON
Holdaway, Lawrence J. R., c1953, ON

Holden, Ron, c1950, BC

Holder, Lee, c1920, BC

Holemar, Liliane, 1983, Bastyr, BC

Holenski, Erika, 2005, CCNM, BC

Holland, Margret Ann, 2004, CCNM, BC

Hollis, Michael J., 1997, CCNM, CA

Holloway, Amanda, 2002, CCNM, AB

Holm, Harry O., 1955, CMCC*, Sweden, ON

Holmes, William, c1953, ON

Holtum, Frederick Burt, 1938, ANA, BC

Holtum, Ronald Arthur, 1939, WSC, BC

Home, Jayda, 2003, CCNM

Homewood, A. Earl , 1956, PCN, ON, FL

Ho-Miecznikowski, Suzanne L., 2000, CCNM, ON

Hong, Jennifer, 2003, CCNM, SK

Hoo, Aaron Christopher, 2001, CCNM, BC

Hooper, Grant L., 1940, WSC, BC

Hopkinson, James, c1926, MB

Horne-Paul, Maureen C., 1995, CCNM, ON

Hornyak-Stewart, Andrea Ann, 2005, CCNM, ON

Horovitz, Robert, 2008, CCNM, ON

Hoskins, Douglas Pernon, c1926, ON

Hossard, Mary, c1981, ON

Hough, Eliot, c1959, MB

Hough, Ivan Currie, 1950, CMCC*, ON

Hough, Ivan Reginald, c1935, ON

Houle, J. Oswald, c1944, QC

Howe, Melissa McAthey, 1999, CCNM, ON

Howe, Roy M., 1951, CMCC*, ON

Howey, Martha, c1926, BC

Hoye, Ronald R. Sr., c1976, ON

Hoye, Ronald Raymond, c1978, ON

Hsu, Steven, 2007, BINM, BC

Huang, Beverly Patricia, 2004, CCNM, AB

Hudson, Henry, 1962, ASN, MB

Huepper, Herman, 1969, NCNM, AB

Huff, Harold (Hal), 1998, CCNM, ON

Huggins, Ernest C., 1950, CMCC*, ON

Hughes, Erika Michiko nee Shoyama, 2000, CCNM, ON

Hughes, Jason, 2003, CCNM, BC

Hui, Tom, 2002, CCNM, ON

Hunt, Barry R., 1952, CMCC*, ON

Hunt, J. Harold, c1953, ON

Hunt, Jeffrey James, 1992, OCNM, BC

Hunt, Stanley M., 1950, CMCC*, ON

Hunt, Verna, 1982, OCNM, ON

Hurd, Rebecca, 2006, BINM, BC

Hurtado, Alexandra, 2008, CCNM, ON

Huska, Colin J. L., 2005, CCNM, ON, NS

Hutchinson, Ted, 2000, CCNM, ON or BC

Hutchison, E. Pamela, 2000, CCNM, BC

Huynh, Thuong (Tina), 1988, OCNM, ON

Hyndman, Bryn, 2005, BINM, BC

Iarhox, Sidney B, c1953, ON

Ignatavicius, Alena, 2008, CCNM, ON

Ihara, Bruce T., 1984, NCNM, BC

Imola, Laura, 2003, CCNM, ON

Ingard, Ronald Anton, 1981, OCNM, ON

Ingoldsby, Philip

Ingram, Krista E., 2006, CCNM, BC

Ipsen, Leigh A., 2000, OCNM, NS

Ireland, Charles S., c1953, ON

Irving, I.S., c1926, AB

Irwin, Ernest W., c1953, ON

Irwin, Lindsay, 2005, CCNM, AB

Isaacs Langdon, Renee Lalitha, 2003, CCNM, ON

Isbister, Robert W., 1950, CMCC*, ON

Isles, Cynthia (Cindy), 1990, OCNM, BC

Ito, Akemi, 2002, CCNM, ON

Ivanovics, Suzanna, 2006, CCNM, ON

Jacks, Brenna, 2003, CCNM, BC

Jackson, J. W., AB

Jackson, Julia

Jackson, Kevin D., 1996, CCNM, BC

Jackson, Robert W., c1953, ON

Jacobs, Stephen M., c1962, CA, AB

Jacobson, Melanie S., 2005, CCNM, ON

Jain, Angelee, 2003, CCNM, ON

Jaklin, Teri A., 2002, CCNM, ON

James, Brandy, 2005, CCNM, AB

James, Earl Anglin, c1944, AB

James, Emile J., c2001

Jamieson, Douglas H. Neil, c1938, BC

Janczak, Bernadette, 2000, CCNM, ON

Janel, Kathleen, 1998, Bastyr, WA
Janssens, Susan, 2000, SCNM, AB
Janzen, Lori Mae, 2007, CCNM, MB
Jarvis, Keith I., c1953, ON
Jasarevic, Emina, 2008, Bastyr, WA, BC
Jasper, Deirdre nee Wiebe, 2003, CCNM, MB
Javanmardi, Mitra, 1985, NCNM, QC
Jebreen, Peter Joseph, 2005, CCNM, ON
Jenab, Arvin, 2000, CCNM, ON
Jenkyns, Eleanor Claire (Elly), 2002, CCNM, ON
Jennings, Stephanie Ann, 2003, CCNM, ON
Jensen, C.A., c1926, AB
Jensen, Jorgen E., c1953, ON
Jensen, Karen G., 1988, OCNM, AB, BC
Jensen, Nicholas, 2007, BINM, BC
Jheeta, Rajeshwar S. (Raj), 1987, NCNM, BC
Jiwa, Mubina, 2004, CCNM, ON
Jiwani, Nyla, 2003, CCNM, ON
Jiwani, Tahira, 1997, CCNM, BC
Jo, Debra E., nee Tol, 2004, CCNM, ON
Jobanputra, Maya, 2005, CCNM, ON
Jobin, Marika, 2006, CCNM
Johnson, Marguerite, 1986, NCNM, BC
Johnson, Mary, BC
Johnson, Melissa, 1999, CCNM, ON
Johnson, Shane, 2007, Bastyr, AZ
Johnson, William Roderick, 1989, OCNM, ON
Johnston, Bradley C., 2002, CCNM, AB
Johnston, Frank E., c1953, ON
Johnston, Lyman C., c1953, ON
Jones, Aranka, 2008, CCNM, ON
Jones, Stephen Frederick, 2001, CCNM, ON
Jones, Steven, 1999, CCNM, BC
Joshi, Kanu Priya, 2000, CCNM, ON, NS
Joslyn, Ethel V. Francis, 1935, WSC, BC
Jovin, Shantell M., 2004, CCNM, FL
Joyce, Susan E. nee Gutteridge, 2005, CCNM, ON
Jui, Danny Te-Yu, 2004, CCNM, BC
Juliao, Marita S., 2002, CCNM, ON
Jung, Georgina, 2008, CCNM, ON
Jurgens, Daphne L.R., 2003, CCNM, ON
Kabani, Aliya, 2006, CCNM, BC

Kablitsky, Irina, 1988, OCNM, NY
Kaganovsky, Alexey M., 1988, OCNM, ON
Kaganovsky, Carolyn Elizabeth nee Brunton, 1993, CCNM, ON
Kahrobaei, Sedige Jilla, 2003, CCNM, BC
Kalinowski, Edward, 1998, CCNM, ON
Kaloe, Sharon see Kang
Kang, Sharon nee Kaloe, 2005, CCNM, ON
Kantor, Laura M. see Bodner
Kanwal, Seema, 2006, CCNM, BC
Kao, Chih-Hsien (Bruce), 2007, CCNM, BC
Karain, Julie Ann nee Pegg, 1996, CCNM, ON
Karas, Josef, 1989, OCNM, Czecheslovakia
Karatzas, Irene, 2005, CCNM, BC
Karim, Rabia see Meghji
Karim, Shairoz (Shyrose), 2000, SCNM, BC
Karim, Zahra, 2001, CCNM, FL
Kassam, Neemez A., 2002, CCNM, ON
Kassam, Rehana nee Budhwani, 1997, CCNM, BC
Kassam, Tasleem, 1999, CCNM, AB
Kaster, Jennifer Lynne, 2007, CCNM, ON
Kaufman, Lauren A. see Linkner
Kaupp, Shannon Margret, 2003, CCNM, ON
Kaur, Sat Dharam, 1989, OCNM, ON
Kawai, Aki, 2007, CCNM, AB
Kawasaki, Misa, 2001, CCNM, Ont.
Kawecki, Henry S., 1962, MB
Kayoumedjian, Joseph, 1989, OCNM, ON
Keith, Karen see Parmar
Keller, R. August, c1953, ON
Kellerstein, Joseph, c1981, 1984, OCNM, ON
Kellerstein, Rebecca S., 2000, CCNM, ON
Kelly, Estella Maude, 1913, DCN, BC
Kelly, Mary-Ellen, 1996, CCNM, ON
Kelly, Sharon, 2005, CCNM, ON
Kelner, Jill D., 2000, CCNM, ON
Keltermann, Theodore, c1981, ON
Kemp Studer, Lesley Elaena, 2003, CCNM, BC
Kempling, Philip see Rayne, Braven
Kendall-Reed, Penelope A., 1997, CCNM, ON
Kende, Zsuzsanna Ilona, 1981, CMCC*, ON
Kennedy, Deborah A., 2006, CCNM, ON

Kennett, Jolene, 2006, CCNM, BC

Kenny, Andrea Bernadette see Beaubrun

Kerk-Hecker, Frederick, c1925, BC

Kerr, Denise, 2008, CCNM, ON

Kerr, Maxwell, c1953, ON

Kerr, Sherrie

Kerwin, Claire, 2002, CCNM, ON

Keserovic, Olga, 1999, CCNM, ON

Ketcheson, Melvin S., c1953, ON

Ketcheson, Orval J., c1953, ON

Keyes, Mary Katherine, 2006, CCNM, AB

Keyzer, Jacob, 1988, Bastyr, BC

Khalili, Afsoun, 2003, CCNM, ON

Khbeis, Jilan see Koch

Khoshkhosal, Nooshin nee Darvish, 1995, Bastyr, WA

Kian, Lena, 2004, Bastyr, CA

Kiani-Yazdi, Payam, 2005, CCNM, ON

Kiazyk, Catherine Maria, 2004, CCNM, MB

Kies, Roger F., 2002, CCNM, TX

Kieswetter, Anita R. nee Mirabelli, 2004, CCNM, ON

Kiklitsky, Irena, c1988, ON

Kim, Albert M., 2004, BINM, BC

Kim, Florie, 2000, CCNM, BC

Kim, Julie, 1996, CCNM, ON

Kim, Leena, 2003, CCNM, ON

Kim, Lena, 2003, CCNM, AB

Kimberley, Megan nee Mackenzie, 2000, CCNM, BC

Kind, Christoph, 1986, NCNM, BC

Kindopp, Lindsay see Martens

Kindy, Alden G, c1953, ON

King, Alison, 1999, Bastyr, BC

King, Wilbur F., c1959 AB

Kinnon, Sara Leslie, 2006, Bastyr, BC

Kinsman, Robert E., 1953, CMCC*, ON

Kipfer, Jacob, 2007, CCNM

Kirchner, Lessa A., 2003, CCNM, ON

Kirk, Angela S., 2002, CCNM, AB

Kirkbride, Douglas J., 1949, NCDP, BC

Kirsh, Shaila Alison see Schwartz

Kissun, Pushpa see Chandra

Kistler, James Edwin, c1962, Ohio, AB

Kitchen-Price, Melissa Erin, 2001, CCNM, ON

Klassen, Joseph, 2005, Bastyr, AB

Klassen, Peter Gerhard, 1997, CCNM, ON

Kleiker, Margot, 1994, Netherlands, NS

Kleiman, Asia, 1989, OCNM, ON

Klein, Elie E., 2003, CCNM, ON

Klein, Ronit, 2006, CCNM, NY

Kliber, Kazimiera Tanine, 1989, OCNM, ON

Klubal, Andrea, see Cleaver

Knappett, Bryan, 2006, CCNM, ON

Knetsch, Christie, 1993, CCNM, ON

Know, Lee Doug-June, 2003, CCNM, ON

Knudsen, Mary Louise, 2004, CCNM, AB

Ko, Daniel, 2004, CCNM, ON

Kober, Frank J. H., c1971, ON

Koch, Helmut G., 1989, OCNM, AB, YT

Koch, Jilan nee Khbeis, 2005, CCNM, AB

Koch-Kattenstroth, Sandra, 2000, CCNM, ON

Kodet, Antonin, 1998, NCNM, AB

Kodnar, Linda A., 1995, CCNM, AB

Koegler, Arno Rudolph, c1926, ON

Kolowicz, Katherine R., 2005, CCNM, ON

Komonski, Anita, 2008, CCNM, BC

Kong, Silvia, 2007, CCNM

Konstantinou, Fotini Tina, 2003, CCNM, ON

Koo Tze Mew, Ian, 2007, CCNM, ON

Koo, Linda, 1996, CCNM, ON

Kopp, Lisa, 2005, NCNM, AB

Korah, Dileep Varkey, 2003, CCNM, ON

Korsunsky, Sara, 2006, CCNM, AB, MB

Kozak, Loren T., 1984, NCNM, BC

Kozelka, Wendy M., 2000, CCNM, MI

Krasnov, Elena, 1990, OCNM, ON

Krebs, Albert Edward, 1932, NCNM, BC

Kresz, Eva, 2005, CCNM

Kristensen, Oscar Edward, c1926, ON, SK

Kroeker, George J., c1959, MB

Kroeker, J. A., c1959, MB

Kroeker, John G., c1959, MB

Kroeker, Melanie see MacIver

Kronhaus, Michael A., c1959, BC

Kropp, Gabrielle, 1994, ZFN Germany, NS

Krueger, Ardis M.C., 2002, CCNM, BC

Kruzel, Thomas A., 1987, NCNM, AB, AZ

Kuindersma, Cathy Mary Ann, 1993, CCNM, ON

Kuipers, Ralph P., c1959, AB

Kuker, Jaclyn Elizabeth (Jacie), 2007, CCNM, ON

Kulchyk, Joseph, 1988, OCNM, ON

Kulkarni, Preeti, 2007, CCNM, CA

Kullar, Sandeep, 2002, CCNM

Kuprowsky, Stefan, 1985, NCNM, BC

Kura, Martin, c1977, 1982, OCNM, ON

Kuramoto, Douglas, 1986, Bastyr, BC

Kurman, I.

Kush, Charlene T., 2003, CCNM, ON

Kushniryk, Nicole Paula, 2001, CCNM, AB

Kussmann-Armstrong, Heidi M., 2002, CCNM, ON

Kutlesa, Stjepan, 1996, CCNM, PA

Kutter, John, c1953, ON

Kuzmiski, Andrea Justine, 2004, CCNM, ON

Kuzniar, Leat Galimidi, 2004, CCNM, US

Kwok, Martin H.T., 1996, Bastyr, BC

Kwok, Moira Ye-On, 2007, CCNM, ON

Kyba, Georgia, 2005, NCNM, BC

La, Chi-Hung, 2006, CCNM, AB

La, Du H., 2002, CCNM, ON

LaBelle, Melanie A., 2004, CCNM, ON

Labriola, Daniel J., 1985, Bastyr, US

Lachance, c1944, QC

Lachowich, Leo Steve, c1981, ON

Lad, Ajay K., 2000, CCNM, ON

Lafond, Marie Martine Michèle, 1993, CCNM, ON

LaForge, Jonas, 2004, BINM, BC

Lafreniere, Justin, 2007, BINM, BC

Lagore, Susann, AB

Lai, Edmond M. L., 2001, CCNM, ON

Laic, Carol see Zoretich

Lainson, R.D., c1926, BC

Lalani, Noreen, 1999, CCNM, BC

Lam Man Yiu, David, c1973, ON

Lambert, Leslie Christopher, 1939, NCNM, BC

L'Ami, D.C., c1926, SK

Lander, Daniel, 2006, CCNM, OK

Landes, Wm. J., c1953, ON

Lane, J., c1954, AB

Langdon, Elizabeth, 1992, OCNM

Lange, Nina V.F., 2002, CCNM, BC

Langford, James A., c1961, ON

Langlais, L., 2000, CCNM

Langlois, M. Chantal, 2006, CCNM, ON

LaPlante, John Gerald, c1953, 1981, OCNM, ON

LaPointe, Kerri - Lynn, 2004, CCNM, ON

Lara, Ana Gabriela, 2004, CCNM, ON

Larouche, Bernard, 1991, NCNM, ON

Larry, Jodi Michelle, 2006, CCNM, ON

Lau, Lisa Cristine, 2001, CCNM

Lauermeier, Jane Lynn, 1992, OCNM, ON

Laugford, James A., c1953, ON

Lavallee, Michael A., 2001, CCNM, MB

Lavender, Julie M., 2005, CCNM, ON

Lavoie, Lisa A., 2003, CCNM, NS

Lawrence, Ann, 1999, CCNM, ON

Lawrence, Charles M., c1953, ON

Lawrence, H.C., c1926, SK

Lawrence, Herbert K., c1961, ON

Laxton, Glenda, 1998, NCNM, BC

Leah, Kathryn, 2008, CCNM, BC

Ledenac, Marianna, 2000, CCNM, ON

Lederman, Michael David, 1999, Bastyr, BC

Lee, Cynthia Joyce, 2007, CCNM, ON

Lee, Herbert K., 1941, NCC, ON

Lee, Jane I., 2001, CCNM, ON

Lee, Jason Chung-Ming, 2003, CCNM, ON

Lee, Jeffrey, 2005, Bastyr, BC

Lee, Joel see Villeneuve

Lee, Lexa W., 1982, NCNM, ID

Lee, Philip Khong Lip, 2007, CCNM, ON

Lee, Sooin, 2008, BINM, BC

Lee, Sung - Mee, 2003, CCNM, ON

Lee, Vanessa Z., 2004, CCNM, ON

Lefebvre, Giselle Lily, 2003, CCNM, ON, BC

Lefebvre, J. Edgar, c1953, ON

Lefebvre, Kadeja A., 2001, CCNM, QC

Legate, Oscar W., c1953, ON

Lemay, Pierre, 1989, OCNM, ON

Lemieux, QC

Lemmo, Walter U., 1999, Bastyr, BC

Lendvai, Raymond Perry (Ray), 1991, OCNM, MB, BC

Lensgraf, George H., c1926, AB

Leo, Colleen Marie, 2001, CCNM, ON

LePage, Anouk, 2005, CCNM, QC. ON

Leppelmann, Melaine, 2006, CCNM, MB

Lerman, Dana B., 2000, CCNM, ON

Lescanec, Heidi, 2002, NCNM, BC

Lescheid, David W., 2002, CCNM, ON

Lessard-Pereira, Brenda, 1999, CCNM, ON

Leung, Brenda, 1998, CCNM, BC, AB

Leung, Joanne, 2000, CCNM, YT

Leung, Kin Yan, 2008, CCNM, ON

Leung, Yu-Nan, 1972, CMCC*, ON

Levay, Ronald A., 1986, OCNM, ON

Levendusky, Paul, 1987, Bastyr, BC

Levesque, Donna, 1998, CCNM, BC

Levett, Suzie, Overseas

Levin, P., c1954, BC

Levine, Hollie, 1996, Bastyr, WA

Levine, Howard, 1986, OCNM, ON

Levine, Leonard, c 1981, ON

Levins, Todd Napier, 2004, CCNM, BC

Levitt, John, c1953, ON

Levy, Benjamin R., c1953, MI

Levytam, Shimon, 1998, CCNM, ON

Lewer, James, 1986, OCNM, NE

Lewis, E.H., c1926, ON

Lewis, Frederick F., c1953, ON

Lewis, Kenneth S., c1953, ON

Lewis, Kristy M., 2006, CCNM, ON

Lewis, Norman F., 1989, OCNM, ON

Lewis, T.A., c1926, BC

Lewis, Walter E., c1953, ON

Liang, Angela Fung-Ling, 1996, CCNM, ON

Liebscher, Michael Stephen, 1991, OCNM, ON, Taiwan

Lightstone, Deborah L., 2004, CCNM, IN

Lilly, Jennifer Lynn, 2005, CCNM, NS

Lim-Trotter, Aileen, 2006, CCNM, ON

Lin, Carol Yin-Hsiu, 2004, Bastyr, BC

Lin, Tobi Chong - Bi, 2004, CCNM, BC

Linehan, Shelly Lynn, 2003, CCNM, ON

Ling, EeVon, 2003, CCNM, ON

Linkner-Kaufman, Lauren Amy, 2004, CCNM, ON

Little, Robert, 1968, CMCC*, ON

Liu, Jessica Charmaine, 2006, CCNM, ON

Livdahl, Chad, 2001, CCNM, FL

Lloyd, Iva Rae, 2002, CCNM, ON

Lo, Muy-Ky, 2006, CCNM

Lo, Simon K., 1990, OCNM, ON

Lo, Theodora, 2001, NCNM, AB

Lobay, Douglas, 1991, Bastyr, BC

Lochowich, Leo, c1981, ON

Lock, Kandis, 2008, CCNM, ON

Loewen, Heidi Katherine see McGill

Loewen, William S., 1952, CMCC*, ON

Loffler, Fred William, 1943, WSC, BC

Lofting, Bruce, 1995, CCNM, AB

Logan, Alan C., 2001, CCNM, NY

Loken, Jason Allan, 2002, CCNM, ON

Long, Mary-Elizabeth see Welch

Long, Patricia see Rennie

Longaphee, Merlin, 1988, CHN in Utah, PEI

Lopez, Ana, 2007, BINM, BC

Loughead, Krista L. nee Wolfe, 2000, CCNM, ON

Louie, Laura A., 1994, Bastyr, BC

Love, Daria P., 1981, OCNM, ON

Lowes, Albert J. W., c1953, ON

Lubczynski-Mehta, Celina, 1989, OCNM, ON

Lubina, Jacqueline S., 2001, CCNM, ON

Luby, Kenneth P., 1990, OCNM, ON

Luck, Jennifer Danielle, 2006, CCNM, ON

Luhar, Faryal, 2003, CCNM, ON

Lukacena, Monika Maria, 2007, CCNM, ON

Lumley, Leonard S., c1953, MI

Lun, Bena Louise, 2007, CCNM, MB

Lunde, Charles, c1953, ON

Lurie, Vince, 2000, CCNM, BC

Lusis, Jonah, 2003, CCNM, ON

Lutchmansingh, Nadine A., 2001, CCNM, Trinidad

Lutes, Terri Lynn, 2002, CCNM, ON

Lycette, Cheryl A., 1993, CCNM, NS

Lynn, Joseph L., c1953, ON

Lyons, Robert J. W., c1959, MB

Lysander, Nesamoni, c1983, Calcutta, ON

Lytle, Millennia R., 2002, CCNM, ON
Ma, Carole H., 1998, CCNM, ON
Macart, Tara nee Whitford, 2000, CCNM, BC
MacDonald, Cathleen nee Coleman, 2000, CCNM, NB
MacDonald, Crista, 2006, CCNM, ON
MacDonald, Deidre, 1996, NCNM, BC
MacDonald, Lynne, c1994, NCNM, BC
MacDonald, Mary A., 2006, CCNM, ON
MacGilliaray, Charles Gordon, c1923, ON
MacInnis, Edna see Bailey
MacIntosh, John C., 2003, CCNM, ON
MacIntosh, Terrance I. (Terry), 1987, OCNM, ON
MacIntyre, Lisa see Good
MacIver, Melanie nee Kroeker, 2005, BINM, BC
Mack, Effrem L. M., c1953, ON
Mackay, J.S., 1926, AB
Mackenzie, D. Wayne, 1972, CMCC*, ON
Mackenzie, Megan see Kimberley
MacKimmie, Erin, 2008, CCNM, ON
MacKinlay, Tracey nee Simmons, 1995, Bastyr, BC
MacLachlan, Douglas James, 1987, OCNM, ON
MacLean, Gretchen E., 2002, CCNM, PE
MacLean, Theresa, 1997, SCNM, NS
MacLeod, Jade Lynn, 2007, CCNM, ON
MacMullin, Cara Leigh, 2006, CCNM, ON
MacNeil, Angela D., 2005, CCNM, ON
MacPherson, William H., c1926, NS
MacQuill, F., c1959, ON, NS
Mahadevan, Nirogini, 2004, CCNM, ON
Mahan, Edward, 1989, OCNM, SK
Maherali, Asifa, 1998, NCNM, BC
Main, Brenda S. nee Hainey, 2000, CCNM, ON
Maksimowich, Marika Ann see Berni
Maleki-Yazdi, Ellie, 2007, CCNM, ON
Malik, Tabish, 2007, CCNM, ON
Mallory, E.C., c1926, SK
Malone, Tracy Lynn, 2005, CCNM, ON
Maltais, Marie Lise, 1992, OCNM, BC, QC
Maltais, Stephen A., 2005, CCNM, ON
Manchester, Donald, 1988, NCNM, BC, OK
Mandel, Tanya K., 2001, CCNM, ON
Manji, Aisha, 2008, CCNM, ON

Mann, David, 1981, OCNM, ON
Mann, G. Edwin, 1951, CMCC*, ON
Mann, Kealy, 2008, CCNM, ON
Mann, Wm. John c1954, ON
Mannen, Eva, 1982, OCNM
Manning, David, 2008, CCNM, ON
Mansfield, Ernest A. C., 1926, ON
Manson, Philip R., BC
Manuel, Liona Siao-Ya, 2006, CCNM, ON
Marasco, Sylvia, 2008, CCNM, ON
Marcers, Morris, c1953, ON
Marchildon, Danielle, 2008, CCNM, ON
Mardian, Julie Elizabeth nee Trznadel, 2000, CCNM, ON
Margaritis, Ioannis, c2004, ON
Margaritis, John, 2002, CCNM, ON
Margaritis, Laura Kathleen nee Buckle, 2003, CCNM, ON
Marier, Denis T., 2000, CCNM, ON
Marinaccio, Heather J., 1979, NCNM, BC
Marino, Maria Pia, 2000, CCNM, ON
Marinzel, Helga, c1981, 1984, OCNM, ON
Markou, Elias, 2003, CCNM, ON
Markovitch, Elaine Beverly, 1981, OCNM, ON
Marquette, Mark R., c1986, BC
Marquis, George D., c1953, ON
Marquis, Jayne, 2008, CCNM, ON
Marr, Jason, 2007, CCNM, ON
Marrow, Cora I., c1953, ON
Marsden, Eric D., 2002, CCNM, ON
Marsden, Steven, 1999, NCNM, AB
Marsden-Gagne, Nathan, 2003, CCNM, BC
Marsh, Glenn E., c1959, AB
Marsh, Margaret H., c1959, AB
Marshall, c1920, BC
Marshall, H.C., c1926, ON
Marshall, Norina Rogue Estrellado (Rina), 2004, CCNM, ON
Martalog, Anca I., 1995, CCNM, ON
Martens, Lindsay nee Kindopp, 2005, CCNM, ON
Martin, Brian, 1995, NCNM, BC
Martin, Katrine C., nee Floegel, 2003, CCNM, ON
Martin, Philip Harold, 1966, CMCC*, ON

Martin, Virginia, 1998, CCNM, ON
Martindale, Thomas W., c1926, BC
Martindale, W.M., c1926, BC
Martin-Mueller, Christine C., 2007, NCNM, NB
Marx, Melanie, 2008, BINM, BC
Mason, Alexandra Carla, 2003, CCNM, ON
Mason, Mary G., c1953, ON
Mason-Wood, Michael, 2003, CCNM, YT, AB
Mass, Louis, c1953, ON
Mass, Samuel, c1953, ON
Matheson, Marie, nee Zalatan, 2005, BINM, BC, ON
Matheson, Christine Aileen, 2001, CCNM, ON
Matsen, Jonn G., 1983, Bastyr, BC
Matthews, Jennifer, 2004, Bastyr, BC
Matthie, Merrell H., c1953, ON
Matusik, Agnieszka, 2006, CCNM, BC
Mauro, Karlo Jr., 2000, CCNM, ON
May, Marilyn A., 1985, NCNM, ON
Mayell, Bertram, 1926, ASN, BC
Mayen, Oscar L., 1981, NWS, ON
Mayer, Alexander O., c1953, ON
Mayfield, A., c1977, ON
Mazariegos, Claudia P., 2002, CCNM, ON
Mazurin, Alexander, 1989, OCNM, BC
Mazurin, Natalie, 2007, BINM, BC
Mazzuchin, Chris Jason, 2003, CCNM, ON
McAvoy, Elizabeth M., 2000, CCNM, ON
McCallum, Frank B., c1926, MB
McCarthy, Johanne E., 2005, CCNM, ON
McCarthy, Joseph L., c1953, ON
McCarthy, Lorraine Michelle, 2004, CCNM, QC
McConnell, Christopher Sean, 2006, CCNM, ON
McConnell, Evelyn Marie, 1942, WSC, BC
McCoy, John-Douglas, 2001, CCNM, ON, HI
McCrorie, Richard David, 1986, OCNM, ON
McCulloch, Fiona Dianne, 2001, CCNM, ON
McDonald, Berendina Christina (Tina), 1997, CCNM, ON
McDonald, Edna K., c1953, ON
McEachern, Devin, 2008, CCNM, ON
McEachern, Tamara Jane, 2003, CCNM, AB
McElrea, Frank B., c1926, SK

McEwen, BC
McFarlane, J. E., c1961, ON
McGee, Karen, 2006, BINM, BC
McGill, Heidi Katherine nee Loewen, 2004, CCNM, ON
McGill, Howard W., c1953
McGill, William H. (Bill), c1970, BC, SK.
McGillicuddy, Irene E., c1953, ON
McGrath, Alana, 2004, CCNM
McGuinness, Kerry, 1985, NCNM, BC
McHan, Roger J., c1962, AB
McInnes, Daniel H., c1953, ON
McIntyre, Cameron, 2004, BINM, BC
McIntyre, Henry M., c1953, ON
McKeen, Julie Lauren, 2004, CCNM, NB
McKenna, Mary-Ellen, 1994, CCNM, ON
McKenzie, Janet, 2007, CCNM, ON
McKenzie, Kim D., 1982, OCNM, ON
McKeown, Charles J. W., 1938, NCNM, BC, Ont.
McKinlay, Marian W., c1953, ON
McKinney, Neil Harvey, 1985, NCNM, BC
McKinney, Violet, c1953, ON
McKinney, William E., c1953, ON
McKinstry, Barbara Lynne, 1988, OCNM, ON
McLachlan, Bonnie J., 2002, CCNM, ON
McLachlan, David Thomas, 1977, CMCC*, ON
McLaren, Tannis M., 2001, OCNM, ON
McLaughlin, C., 1999, CCNM, ON
McLean, John F., c1953, 1981, OCNM, ON
McLellan, Alexander, 1998, CCNM, NS
McLeod, John Benjamin, c1937, BC
McLeod, Melanie, 2008, CCNM, CA
McMillan, Robert Johnston, 1926, LCNT, BC
McMurrer, Lana L., 2006, CCNM, PE
McNally, Lynne Frances, 2004, CCNM, ON
McNamara, James, c1977, 1982, OCNM, ON
McNeilly, Laura, 1999, CCNM, ON
McNeil-White, Sara-Jane see White
McNinch, Gail, 2000, CCNM, ON
McNiven, Lisa A., 2001, CCNM, NS
McPhie, Heli, 1999, CCNM, BC
McQuarrie, Colleen M., 2002, CCNM, ON
McQueen, Kimberly nee Calder, 2001, CCNM, BC

Meacher, Jodi, 2005, BINM, BC
Meade, Michael J., 2002, CCNM, ON
Meale, John H., c1961, ON
Medrek, Robert, 1991, OCNM, ON
Meffe, Cristina, 2007, CCNM, ON
Meghji, Rabia, nee Karim, 2005, CCNM, AB
Meier, Nicole A., 2002, CCNM, ON
Meissner, Julek, 1983, NCNM, ON
Mekdeci, Zerlene Anne, 1997, CCNM, ON
Melanson, Margaret, 2000, CCNM, NS
Melondrez, Maureen F., c1987, ON
Menard, Joanne, 2006, CCNM, BC
Mendroff, Euon, c1981, ON
Menen, Hanifa, 1998, CCNM, ON
Mercer, Carolyn Frances, 2006, CCNM, ON
Mercer, Kathleen M., 2000, CCNM, NF
Mergard, Tanja, 2000, CCNM, ON
Merluza Coloma, Cristina, 2000, CCNM, BC
Merritt, Henry M., c1959, MD, AB
Meserey, J. E., c1960, BC
Messenger, C.E., c1926, AB
Messenger, H.H.F., c1926, AB
Meszaros, Caroline Margaret, 2001, CCNM, ON
Metha, Alexina, nee Alexander, 2008, BINM, BC
Meyer, Caroline F., 2005, CCNM, ON
Meyer, M. Michelle, 1997, CCNM, ON
Meyer, Thekla, NCNM, c1991, BC
Meyer, Ursula, 1994, NCNM, BC
Meyers, Helen, see Chang
Miaritis, Amalia, 2003, CCNM, Russia
Middleton, Christine, 2008, CCNM, ON
Middleton, F. David, c1953, ON
Mikhailova, Elena V., 2005, CCNM, ON
Milanovich, David, 2003, CCNM, BC
Milinkovic, Dragana, 1999, CCNM
Millar, Sarah, 2006, CCNM, ON
Miller, George E., c1953, ON
Miller, James Stanley, 1932, CCC, BC
Miller, John D., 1988, OCNM, ON
Miller, John Douglas, 1992, NCNM, AB, BC
Miller, Michael V., 1987, OCNM
Miller, R., c1926, ON

Miller, W. Murray, 1951, CMCC*, ON
Millington, Janice, 2000, CCNM, YT
Mills, Carla Danielle see Cameron
Milne, George W., 1976, CMCC*, 1987, OCNM, ON
Milroy, Pamela Ann, 1990, OCNM, ON
Minty, H.E., c1926, MB
Mirabelli, Anita R. see Kieswetter
Miranda, Sandra Janet, 2000, CCNM, ON
Mirza, Roxanna, 2002, CCNM, ON
Mirzaagha, Farahnaz, 2002, CCNM, ON
Mitchell, Chantelle, 2005, BINM, BC
Mitchell, Ernest Langworthy, BC
Mitchell, Tonia, 2007, CCNM, BC
Mitha, Rupinder (Rupi) nee Gobindpuri, 1999, CCNM, ON
Mithani, Sheheen, 2001, CCNM, BC
Mitrea, Lilieana nee Stadler, 2002, CCNM, ON
Mohan Ram, Sanjay, 2004, BINM, BC
Mokhtari, Tannaz, 2003, CCNM, ON
Mollier, Merri C., c1953, ON
Mollohan, Leah see Oster
Monforton-Everest, Michelle M., see Everst
Montgomery, Laurence, 2008, CCNM, ON
Montgomery, Sonya Leigh, 2001, CCNM, ON
Monto, James I., c1953, ON
Montroy, Natasha Tarja Talvikki, 2004, CCNM, BC
Moore, Angela M., 1989, OCNM, ON
Moore, Female, c1920, BC
Moore, Julie Ann, 2003, CCNM, BC
Moore, Male, c1920, BC
Morden, Dara, 2007, CCNM, MB
Mordy, Elliott, 2008, BINM, BC
Morello, Gaetano A., 1991, Bastyr, BC
Morley, Carol nee Zawada, 2003, CCNM, ON
Morphy, B. Herbert, c1953, ON
Morphy, Donna, c1981, 1986, OCNM, ON
Morris, Glenna Denise, 2001, CCNM, NS
Morris, William Walter (Bill), c1953, 1981, OCNM, ON
Morrison, Heather Rose, 2001, CCNM, ON
Morrison, Kathryn Anne (Kate), 2005, CCNM, ON
Morrison, Kyle, 2006, CCNM, BC
Morrison, Linda, 2007, CCNM, NS

Morrison, William, c1962, Ohio, AB

Morrow, Cora I., c1953, ON

Morton, Kathleen, 1994, CCNM, ON

Moscote, Nadia G., 2003, CCNM

Moshtagh, Rozita, 2006, BINM, BC

Moss, Jennifer, 2005, BINM, BC

Moss, L., c1962, PA

Moss, S., c1962, PA

Moulton, Rochelle, see Fenner

Moyer, Lindsay, 2008, CCNM, ON

Mrazek, Timothy R., 2000, CCNM, SK

Mudge,Charles R., c1926, ON

Mueller, Arthur Ernest, 2001, CCNM, ON

Mueller, Eva, c1981, ON

Mueller, Rudoph O., c1953, ON

Mullaly, Percy F., 1950, CMCC*, AB

Munkley, Alyson Kristen, 2004, CCNM, ON

Munkley, Shannon Elizabeth, 2007, CCNM, ON

Munro, Donald Stuart, 1975, CMCC*, ON

Murphy, Derek Christopher, 1998, CCNM, ON

Murphy, Amy, 2008, CCNM, ON

Murphy, Arthur Sterling, c1939, BC

Murphy, Jillian, 2006, CCNM, ON

Murphy, Sandra E., 2005, CCNM, NS

Murray, Lisa Marie see Doran

Mushtagh, Saeid, 2006, CCNM, NT

Muttart, Rebecca, 2001, CCNM, BC

Myers, c1954, AB

Naderiani, Nastia, 2008, CCNM, ON

Naesgaard, Heathir, 1993, Bastyr, BC

Naim, Judith, MB

Nakai, Ted, 1989, OCNM, AB

Nakajima, Ann Y., 2002, CCNM, ON

Naraynsingh, Chandra A., 1990, OCNM, Trinidad

Nardella, Jennifer, 1997, NCNM, AB

Nardini, Patrizio M., 2001, CCNM, ON

Neale, John H., c1953, ON

Neale, Peter Herbert, c1977, ON

Neilson, Stacey N., 2002, CCNM, BC

Neimor, Christopher J., 2002, CCNM, NF

Nelson, Brian Joseph, 1986, OCNM, ON

Nelson, Urban Albert Hans Edelmalm, 1990, OCNM

Ncmeth, Brenda Dawn, 2004, CCNM, AB

Nesbitt, Jessica, 2008, CCNM, ON, India

Newman, Maurice, 1967, NCNM, BC

Newton, E. Hazel Elliott, c1926, MB

Newton, J., c1926, MB

Ng, Caleb, 2001, CCNM, BC

Nghiem - Phu, Camille P., 2003, CCNM, ON

Nguyen, Christine, 2008, CCNM, ON

Nguyen, Mylinh, 2001, CCNM, ON

Nguyen, Nhi (Karen), 2007, CCNM, BC

Nguyen, Phuong-Thao, 1999, Bastyr, BC

Nicholl, Daniel Marcel, 1996, CCNM, ON

Nicholson, Andrew Dee, c1953, ON

Nicholson, William Reg, 1970, CMCC*, ON

Nicholson-Baker, Dannielle R., 2005, CCNM, ON

Nielsen, Albert M., c1953, ON

Nigh, Carol A., 2000, CCNM, ON

Nirdosh Taylor, Aparna, 2007, CCNM, ON

Niro, Maria Antonietta, 2007, CCNM, ON

Nobbe, Sonya Gabrielle, 2007, CCNM, ON

Noble, John Wesley, 1937, WSC, US

Nobrega, Kathryn, 2008, CCNM, ON

Noh, Elisa, 2005, CCNM

Nolan, Kevin R., 1989, OCNM, BC

Nomm, Inga, 1976, LMU, Germany, NS

Nonis, Stella, 2003, CCNM, ON

Nordin, Anna R., 1987, OCNM, TX

Norman, Simone, 2002, CCNM

Norman, Vernon Beverly, 1946, National, SK

Nortman, David, 2004, CCNM, ON

Nosworthy, Evelyn R., c1953, ON

Novak, Gabriela, 1989, OCNM, ON

Novakov, Slavica, 1988, OCNM

Nowazek, Michael G., 1997, CCNM, AB

Nowell, Herbert, 1924, ASN, BC

Nozari, Anahita (Ana), 2000, CCNM, ON

Nuraddin, Shiraz, 2002, CCNM, ON

Nurmi, Maria L., 1988, OCNM, BC

Oakes, Timothy Paul, c1981, ON

O'Brien, Tanya, 2008, CCNM, ON

O'Brien-Moran, Alison C.M., 2002, CCNM, ON

O'Connor, Danielle I. nee Rideout, 2003, CCNM, ON

O'Farrell, Erin S., 2002, CCNM, ON
Ogilvie, George E., c1953, ON
O'Grady, Michael J., 1990, OCNM, BC
Ogura, Stephanie C., 2001, CCNM, QC
Oh, Hong Keun David, 1991, OCNM, Korea
O'Hara, Dennis Patrick, 1986, OCNM, ON
Okabe, Dale, 1984, OCNM, ON
O'Leary, Sherisse, 2008, CCNM, NS
Olivastri, Angelo, 1995, CCNM, ON
Oliver, Peter Lawton, 1950, CMCC*, ON
Oliver, Hallie, 2007, CCNM
Olsen, Steven, 1987, Bastyr, BC, WA
Olson, Scott, c1953, AB, BC
O'Malley, Jane Alison nee Buckler, 2000, CCNM, ON
Omar, Fareed E., 1990, OCNM, ON
O'Neill, Deirdre, 2003, Bastyr, BC
O'Neill, James Christopher (Jim), 1982, OCNM, ON
O'Neill, Michelle L., 2002, CCNM, ON
Orbay, Mark C., 2003, NCNM, ON
Ordanis, Christine Elizabeth, 2006, CCNM, ON
O'Reilly, Mary Catherine, 1993, CCNM, ON
O'Reilly, Vincent P., 1989, OCNM
Orman, Marian, c1989, ON
Ormerod, Lucy C., 2003, CCNM, SK
Osborn, Russell E., c1953, ON
Osman, Diaa Seif Al - Nasr, 2003, CCNM, Minnesota
Ostafichuk, Katrina M.M., 2004, CCNM, ON
Oster, David Karl, 2004, CCNM, ON
Oster, Leah nee Mollohan, 2006, CCNM, ON
Oughtred, Ryan, 2006, BINM, BC
Ouley, Pearl R., c1953, ON
Ovens, Leslie Helena, 1992, OCNM, ON
Owens, Howard H., 2002, CCNM, ON
Owens, Rhiannon Alexandra, 2004, CCNM, AB
Owens, Wm. C., c1953, ON
Owens-Todd, Jamila, 2007, CCNM, MO
Oxbro, Kimberly Dianne, 2008, CCNM, ON
Packham, Lottie I., c1953, ON
Palmer, Craig, 1994, CCNM, ON
Palmer, Douglas, 1995, CCNM, ON
Palmer, Helen, Washington, 1979, NCNM, WA
Pan, Henry Sheng-Chieh, 2002, CCNM, ON

Pan, Tracy A., 2006, CCNM, ON
Panet, John, 1997, Bastyr, BC
Panych, Lynette Patricia, 2003, CCNM, AB
Papadogianis, Peter, 1996, CCNM, ON
Papaioannou-Bizios, Vivian, 2001, CCNM, ON
Papasodaro, Maria Melissa, 2007, CCNM, ON
Paquette, Karen Lee, 2005, CCNM, ON
Paradis, Renee, 2008, CCNM, ON
Parandian, Bijan, 1990, OCNM, ON
Parent, Gilles, QC
Parikh-Shah, Sejal, 1994, CCNM, ON
Park, Nari, 2003, Bastyr, BC
Park, Tracy Sung - Eun, 2003, CCNM, ON
Parks, Auromira A., 2003, CCNM, England
Parmar, Gurdev, 2000, CCNM, BC
Parmar, Karen nee Keith, 2000, CCNM, BC
Parmar, Perminder (Bobby), 2007, CCNM, BC
Paroo, Nina, 2001, Bastyr, WA
Parsons, D.C., c1926, ON
Parsons, Fred Edward, c1948, AB
Parsons, G.S., c1926, ON
Partlow, Roger K., c1953, ON
Paskins, William Arthur, 1935, WSC, BC
Past, Stanley J., c1953, ON
Pataracchia, Raymond John, 2001, CCNM, ON
Patel, Mukesh M., 1990, OCNM, ON
Patel, Poonam J., 2005, CCNM, ON
Patel, Rita J., 2004, CCNM, ON
Patton, Allison, 2001, CCNM, BC
Paul, Jeanne M. nee Albin, 1991, NCNM, BC
Pawlowska, Mariola, 1998, CCNM, ON
Pawlowska-Dobosz, Lidia, see Dobosz
Pawlowska-Wasiak, Maria T., see Wasiak
Payne, Maria see Boorman
Peacock, Jodie L., 2006, CCNM, ON
Pearman, Robert, 1985, NCNM, AB
Peddycoart, Nelson E., c1953, GA
Pegg, Julie Ann see Karain
Pelia, Rikninder Singh (Rick), 1992, OCNM, ON
Peltz, Stephanie, 2008, BINM, BC
Penner, Abram John, c1948, AB
Percival, Mark J., c1981, 1986, OCNM, ON

Peredery, Oksana P., 2001, CCNM, ON

Perkins, Carol, 2001, CCNM, IL

Perkins, Christine, 1997, CCNM, AB

Perley, Kirsten, 2007, CCNM, ON

Perrin, James Wordsworth, 1924, ASN, BC

Persaud, Reina M., 2001, CCNM, ON

Perser, C. M., c1961, ON

Peters, Caralei Elizabeth, 2004, CCNM, ON

Peters, Diane A., 2005, CCNM, ON

Peters, Michelle, 2005, CCNM, ON

Peterson, Clifford, c1954, AB

Petrykanyn, Walter J., 1953, CMCC*, ON

Pett, Edith (Edie), 1981, OCNM, ON

Pettit-Norfolk, Megan E., 2002, CCNM, ON

Pevac-Djukic, Marija, 2000, CCNM, ON

Phair, Deborah Anne, 1997, CCNM, BC

Pham, Jennifer To Trinh, 2004, CCNM, ON

Phibbs, M.B., c1926, SK

Phillips, Brett, 2007, BINM, BC

Phillips, Carl G., 1953, CMCC*, BC, AlB

Phillips, George A., c1953, NY

Phillips, Marian E., 2002, CCNM, ON

Phillips, Pascaline T., 2000, CCNM, ON

Pickrell, Christopher, 2008, CCNM, ON

Pidutti, John, 2004, Bastyr, BC

Pidutti, Nari, 2004, Bastyr, BC

Pierce, Jesse (Jessica), 2007, CCNM, ON

Piercell, Melissa, 2007, CCNM, ON

Piercey, Georgia A., c1926, N.S.

Pietrzak, Kimberlee (Kim) see Blyden-Taylor

Pikarchuk, Michael, 1952, CMCC*, ON

Pike, Tracey, 2003, CCNM, AB

Pikula, Ronald John, 1976, CMCC*, ON

Pincott, Ingrid, 1985, NCNM, BC

Pinter, Hajnalka, 2005, CCNM, AB

Pirie, John Scott, 1921, ANA, BC

Pitt, Gillian, 2006, CCNM

Plourde, Susan, 2002, SWCN, PE

Podwapinski, Michael, 1997, CCNM, Poland

Polewczak, Jolanta, 2002, CCNM, ON

Polinsky, Lisa, 1999, NCNM, BC

Pollard, Tracey Lynn, 2003, CCNM, PE

Pomeroy, Donald, c1962, OR, AB

Pontius, David Eugene, 1976, NCNM, BC

Poon, Karen K., 2001, CCNM, ON

Popal, Zarlashta, 2004, CCNM, ON

Pope, Nora Jane, 2002, CCNM, ON

Popov, Larissa Anne, 2006, CCNM, ON

Porter, Katelyn

Porter, Stephanie C.L., 2004, CCNM, ON

Posen, Eric, 1989, OCNM, BC

Posen, Robert Ian (Bob), 1988, OCNM, ON

Possamai, Mario R., 2005, CCNM

Potter, Janice, 1998, CCNM, ON, BC

Power, Kristina see Brooks

Pragnell, Norman Richard, c1976, 1981, OCNM, ON

Prange, Margaret A. nee Skazinska, 2002, CCNM, ON

Pratt, Lee C., c1953, ON

Prentice, Judith Anne (Jody), 2001, CCNM, ON

Presant-Jahn, Wendy M., 1995, CCNM, SK

Price, James A., c1941, ON

Price, Robert Allan, 2000, CCNM, ON

Pridham, Brandy Marie nee Rowley, 2004, CCNMM, ON

Prinsen, Adam Erris, nee Geerligs, 2003, CCNM, ON

Proctor, Cheryl Diane, 1988, OCNM, ON

Pronk, John C., 1999, CCNM, ON

Proulx, Andrea Renee, 2007, CCNM, ON

Prousky, Jonathan E., 1998, Bastyr, ON

Prtenjaca, Sandra, 2004, CCNM, ON

Prusin, William Slade, 1981, OCNM, ON

Prytula, Gregory W., 1997, CCNM, ON

Prytula, Michael A., 1988, OCNM, ON

Psota, Erin Gene, 2005, CCNM, ON

Pugliese, Connie A., 2002, CCNM, ON

Purcell, Pamela Gail, 2003, CCNM, NS

Putnam, Richard, 1984, OCNM, ON

Putnam, Tutti Timmins see Gould

Pyatt, Jennifer nee Clow, 2005, CCNM, AB

Pyatt, Matthew, 2005, CCNM, AB

Pycroft, C.A., c1926, SK

Pyne, Nora, 2006, CCNM, ON

Quach, Cindy, 2005, CCNM, BC

Quagliotti, W.R., c1926, BC

Quan, Eugene R., 2001, CCNM, AB

Quick, Donald Roy Morrell, 1977, CMCC*, ON

Race, Colin, 2006, CCNM, AB

Racioppo, Silvano

Rade, Bryan, 2008, CCNM, ON

Radhakrishnan, Vicky, 2006, BINM, BC

Radnor, Samuel, c1977, ON

Radosz, Caroline, 2008, CCNM, US

Radulovici, Cornelia, 2000, CCNM, ON

Rae, James McCheyne, 1951, CMCC*, ON

Ragbir, Rajesh, 2007, CCNM, ON

Rahman, Michael, 1996, CCNM, ON

Rahmaty, Oznoor, 2004, CCNM, ON

Raih, Harold N., c1953, ON

Raina, Rominder Singh (Romi), 2007, CCNM, ON

Rakhra, Raj-Inder, c1964, Punjab, AB

Rakic, Kristijana, 2005, CCNM, ON

Rampersad, Tanya, 2003, Bastyr, AB

Rampone, Tammy M., 2002, CCNM, ON

Ranch, Patrick, 1989, OCNM, ID, AB

Rappard, Daphne F., 1987, OCNM, ON

Rashvand, Parviz F., 2002, CCNM, United Arab Emirate

Raskin, Gannady, 1999, CCNM, Bastyr, US

Ratansi, Zayd P., 1998, Bastyr, BC

Rau, Kelly , 2005, CCNM, ON

Rawling, Nancy, 1997, CCNM, ON

Rawluk-Gendron, Tanya Krista, 2006, CCNM, ON

Rayat, Surender Singh, 1990, OCNM

Rayne, Braven nee Kempling, Philip, 1979, NCNM, BC

Rebellato, Nancy, 1998, CCNM, ON

Reeves, Joseph, c1928, BC

Reichert, Ronald, 1989, Bastyr, BC

Reid, Darlene Morgan, 2001, CCNM

Reid, Donna, 1993, CCNM, ON

Reid, Kathleen J., 2001, CCNM, ON

Reid, Michael David, 2007, CCNM, ON

Reid, Susanna, 1997, NCNM, HI

Reid, Toni, 2007, CCNM, AB

Reierson, Michael, 1997, NCNM, BC

Reilly, Harold J., c1953, NY

Reimer, William G., c1962, ID, AB

Reingold, Howard, c1983, ON

Reisinger-Oake, Frances, 2002, CCNM, NF

Rellis, J., c1953, ON

Rencher, Wm. D., c1953, ON

Rennicks, Robert A., 1952, CMCC*, ON

Rennie, Patricia nee Long, 1992, OCNM, ON

Resendes, Victoria, 2006, CCNM, ON

Resh, George F., c1953, ON

Reside, Jane, 2000, CCNM, BC

Reyn, Elina, 2003, CCNM, ON

Rezvani, Rashin, 2001, CCNM

Rezvani, Zahra Nooshin, 2000, CCNM, England

Rheaume, Kathryn E. (Kate), 2002, CCNM, ON

Riar, Lavleen, 2005, CCNM, India

Richards, Stacey Madrgiques, 2004, CCNM, ON

Richardson, Donald W., 1953, CMCC*, ON

Richardson, Sheryl Elizabeth Rose nee Cybulski, 2004, CCNM, ON

Richea, Michelle, 2006, CCNM, ON

Richmond, David Fuller, 2001, CCNM, AB

Rickford, Aubrey C., 1998, CCNM, ON

Riddell, R. Lyle, c1947, ON, MI

Riddle, Shaun Kevin, 2003, Bastyr, AB

Rideout, Danielle I. see O'Connor

Riedel, Rogers, c1953, ON

Ringdahl, Sally, 1992, Bastyr, BC

Rink, Ursula Meyer, c1993, ON

Ripley, Fred, c1946, MN

Riseing, Erin M., 2007, CCNM, ON

Ristimaki, Samantha Senja, 2005, CCNM, ON

Ristok, Erika, 1998, CCNM, ON

Ritcey, Susan J., 1996, CCNM, NS

Ritchie, Wm. A., c1953, ON

Rivard, Darcelle L., 1990, OCNM, ON

Rivers, Kaiten, 1990, Bastyr, WA

Rivet, Quinn, 1994, CCNM, BC

Riviere, Stacy Elizabeth see Foley

Rizothanassis, Vassiliki, 2008, CCNM, ON

Robert, Francois de Sales, 1968, LCNPS, QC

Roberts, Frederick E., c1953, ON

Roberts, H., c1926, ON

Roberts, Kenneth Gordon, 1960, CMCC*, ON

Roberts, Melina Ann, 2004, CCNM, AB

Robertson (Davies), Jordan, 2008, CCNM, ON

Robinson, Nicole, 2006, BINM, BC

Rochon, Denise, 1992, OCNM, BC

Rock, Doris

Rodak, Taras, 1992, OCNM, ON

Rode, Albert, 1988, NCNM, BC

Rodriguez, Christine

Rodriguez, Jorge Jacinto, c1981, ON

Rodriguez, Melissa, 2005, CCNM, ON

Rodriguez, Melodie Anne, 2003, CCNM, Barbados

Rody Parr, Kiersten J., 2004, CCNM, ON

Rogers, Everly Eldon, c1942, BC

Rogers, Martha L., 2004, CCNM, ON

Rogers, Thomas, 2000, Bastyr, WA

Rohn-Szabo, Suzanne, 1981, OCNM, ON

Rohon O'Halloran, Jane, 1987, NCNM, BC

Rohon, Juan F., 1986, NCNM, BC

Roke, Dorothy, 1994, CCNM, ON

Rolston, Christopher, 2000, NCNM, AB

Romanowski, Sarah J., 2003, CCNM, ON

Rongits, Carrie Ellen, 1999, CCNM, AB, ON

Rootes, Heidi, 2006, BINM, BC

Rooyakkers, Peter George, 1989, OCNM

Roscoe, Paulette, 1989, Bastyr, BC

Rose, Olivia Tamara, 2006, CCNM, ON

Rose, Ronald Edward, 1989, OCNM, BC

Rose, Zorana Mary, 2001, CCNM, ON

Ross, Marni Rebecca, 2004, CCNM, ON

Ross-O'Toole, Julie Anne, 2002, CCNM, ON

Roth, Amanda J. nee Ferris, 2004, CCNM, ON

Roth, George B., 1982, OCNM, ON

Roth, Harold W., 1950, CMCC, ON

Roth, Patricia, 1987, OCNM, ON

Rouchotas, Philip, 2004, CCNM, ON

Rowe, Robert William (Bob), 1975, CMCC*, BC

Rowles, Ida M., c1953, ON

Rowley, Brandy Marie see Pridham

Roy, Leo, c1971, 1981, OCNM, ON

Roy-Poulsen, Jytte, 1989, OCNM, AB

Rozbicka, Danuta Barbara, 1988, OCNM, ON

Rubino, Stephanie, 2002, CCNM, ON

Rudy, Andrea, 2008, CCNM, ON

Rushbrook, J. Ernest, c1953, ON

Russell, Albert Lysle, 1946, NCNM, BC

Russell, c1954, AB

Russell, Liz

Russell, Terrie

Russell, William (Bill), 1989, OCNM, BC

Russo, Petrina, c1953, NY

Ruth, Robert A., c1953, NY

Rutledge, Julie M. nee Zepp, 2004, CCNM, SK

Sabbagh-Ciraco, Olivia D., 2000, CCNM, ON

Sabourin, Donald, 1985, NCNM, BC

Sachdev, Amita A., 2002, CCNM, Ont.

Sackett, Ruth M., c1953, Ont.

Sadeh, Tali, 2003, CCNM, Ont.

Saeedi-Mepham, Parisa, 2003, Bastyr, WA, BC

Sagan, Rebecca Marie, 2003, CCNM, AB

Sahni, Ravinder Singh, 1975, NCNM, ON

Sainé, Andre G., 1982, NCNM, Ont, QC

Saini, Rena, 2008, CCNM, ON

Salaniuk, Andrzej (Andrew), 1992, OCNM, ON

Salewski, Alexandra Lydia, 1995, CCNM, Spain

Salib-Hubert, Jennifer Meghan, 2004, CCNM, NS

Salloum, Trevor K., 1986, NCNM, BC

Salsberg, Anne L., 2005, CCNM, ON

Samanta, Aaron, 2002, CCNM, ON

Samborski, Jeff, 2002, CCNM, ON

Samchuck, George Gerald, c1981, ON

Samet, Lisa, 1998, SWCN, QC.

Samieian, Shahab, 1992, Bastyr, BC. MT

Samuelson (Wittenberg), Lindsay, 2008, CCNM, England

Sanan, Rebecca Marie, c2003

Sanders, Albert, c1953, ON

Sandhu, Sam, 2004, BINM, BC

Sandhu, Sarge, 2005, BINM, BC

Sangra, Sandeep, 2002, CCNM, BC

Santimaw, Ricky, 2008, BINM, BC

Santos, Rodolfo Adrian (Rod), 2003, CCNM, BC

Sarchuk, Ed. H., 1973, NCNM, BC

Sarrasin, Shannon, 2007, CCNM, MB

Sauer, Gail, 2008, CCNM, ON

Sauls, James R. Jr., c1981, AL

Saunders, Albert, c1961, ON

Saunders, Paul Richard, 1990, OCNM, ON

Schad-Byers, Karen see Willow, Katherine
Schaeffer, Emil, 1950, WSCP, BC
Schafer, E. P., c1960, BC
Schafer, Garry Jerome, 1979, NCNM, BC, SK, AB
Schauch, Marita, 2005, CCNM, BC
Scheer, Jacob, 1987, OCNM, ON
Schemel, Gabriela B., 1999, Bastyr, BC
Schirmer, Jacob S., c1956, ON
Schlegel, Stefanie C.M., 2003, CCNM, BC
Schmidt, Anna I., c1956, ON
Schmidt, Hans, NS
Schmidt, Rachel, 2008, CCNM, ON
Schmidt, Stephanie Regina, 2006, CCNM, ON
Schmitt, R. H., c1954, PA
Schneider, Jason, 1999, NCNM, AB
Schneider, Martin John, c1953, ON
Schnell, Lawrence Franklin, c1954, AB, CA
Schnick, John Albert, 1923, NCC, ON
Schnurr, Kristin, 2005, CCNM, BC
Scholten, Andrea, 2008, CCNM, ON
Schrader, Dean, 1999, NCNM, MB
Schusky, Read, 1997, Bastyr, WA
Schwab, Felix J., c1953, ON
Schwartz, Owen, c1981, ON
Schwartz, Shaila Alison nee Kirsh, 2005, CCNM, CA
Schwartzman, Rachel, 2005, CCNM, ON
Sciortino, Nigma nee Talib, 2001, CCNM, BC
Scott, Jill, 2003, NCNM, BC
Scott, Leslie Evelyn, 1981, OCNM, ON
Scott, Michael, 1998, Bastyr, MD
Scott, R. D. Wayne, 1981, OCNM, ON
Scott, Susan Beverly, 1993, CCNM, AB
Scotten, David, 1993, Bastyr, BC
Scurtu, Simona, 2007, CCNM, ON
Sears, Glenna
Seeley, Mahlon R., c1954, ON
Seely, Dugald R., 2003, CCNM, ON
Segerstrom, Fredrik, 1930, NSP, BC
Segovia, Carlos A., 1993, CCNM, ON, St. Lucia
Segovia, Gayle Maria nee Devaux, 1995, CCNM, St. Lucia
Seifi, Mandana, 2006, CCNM, ON
Seim, George Martin, 1977, CMCC*, ON

Seligman, Trina, 1996, Bastyr, WA
Seliski, Lawrence J., 1990, OCNM, BC
Senaratne, Marlene S.R., 2003, CCNM, ON
Seth, Pankaj, 1992, OCNM, ON
Seth-Smith, Penelope (Penny), 1994, CCNM, BC
Seto, Stella, 2007, CCNM, BC
Shackleton, Robert Lorne, c1976, 1981, OCNM, ON
Shackleton, Sylvia Anne, c1976, 1981, OCNM, ON
Shah, Raza Ali, 2001, CCNM, ON
Shah, Sushma H., 2003, CCNM, ON
Shainhouse, Jill, 2004, CCNM, ON
Shalit, Jennifer, 2008, CCNM, ON
Shang, Yun - Jung Kitty, 2004, CCNM, ON
Sharma, Kavita, 2002, CCNM, ON
Sharpe, George T., c1953, ON
Sharpe, Harry W., c1963, ON
Sharpe, Lena T., c1953, ON
Shaw, Alana Kimberley, 2007, CCNM, ON
Shaw, George E., c1953, ON
Shaw, Louise, 2008, CCNM, ON
Sheehan, Edmond Man Lok, 2001, CCNM
Sheehan, Rachel, 2006, BINM, Japan
Sheehy, Chad T., 2003, CCNM, ON
Shen, Yendre W. 2001, CCNM, ON
Shibley, Stewart G., c1953, ON
Shih, David Chia-Hung, 2005, CCNM, ON
Shillington, Stacey Ly nn, 2006, CCNM, ON
Shin, Sindy, 2008, CCNM, ON
Shiroyeh, Haleh, 2006, CCNM, ON
Shortt, Nicole J., 2003, CCNM, BC
Shou, Jane, 2006, CCNM, ON
Shouldice, Janice, 1999, CCNM, ON
Shoyama, Erika Michiko see Hughes
Shrubb, Eric F., 1964, CMCC*, 1981, OCNM, ON
Shrubb, Frances Margaret see Eddleston
Shrubb, John Roy, c1953, ON
Shulman, Adrienne Rose, 2007, CCNM, ON
Shuster, Ruth, 2008, CCNM, ON
Sidhu, Harjot, 1991, OCNM, MN
Siebert, Horst, 1990, OCNM, ON
Silvea, Celest, NCNM, AB, BC
Simatovic, Karen Ann, 2006, CCNM, ON

Simbrow, Jordanna E., 2002, CCNM, ON

Simmauds, Wilfred E., c1953, ON

Simmonds, Kalmia (Kali), 1998, CCNM, PE

Simmons, Jill, 2000, CCNM, MB

Simmons, Tracey see MacKinlay

Simonson, Hilmer Steven, BC

Simpson, Jennifer Margaret, 2004, CCNM, ON

Simpson, Marguerite F., c1953, ON, CA

Sims, Gordon C., 1998, NCNM, MB

Sinclair, Danielle M. nee Soulliere, 2005, CCNM, ON

Singh, Onkar, 2001, CCNM, ON

Singh, Rana H., 2001, CCNM, ON

Singh, Rikninder, 1992, OCNM

Singh, Ujjagar, c1977, ON

Sirkis, Tama H., 2002, CCNM, ON

Sjoman, Eric W., c1953, ON

Sjovold, Sarah Louise, 2004, CCNM, BC

Skaken (Skakun, Dimitri M.) Colin, c1948, AB

Skaken, Luci, 1988, NCNM, AB

Skaken, Ross, 1947, SCCNP, AB, ON

Skaken, Sinnoi, 1988, NCNM, AB

Skazinska, Margaret A. see Prange

Skhirtladze, Olga, 2005, CCNM, ON

Slackhause, W. Lloyd, c1953, ON

Slanko, Edward, c1953, ON

Sleeth, Alex D., c1961, ON

Sleigh, Edward R. (Ted), 1982, Bastyr, BC

Sleith, Alexander D., c1953, ON

Slipacoff, Susan, 2005, CCNM, ON

Sloan, Tara Kathleen, 2006, CCNM, ON

Slonetsky, Christine T., c2002, ON

Smith, A.H., c1926, ON

Smith, Cheryl, 2000, Bastyr, US

Smith, Daniel Jeffrey, 1997, CCNM, ON

Smith, Ernest G., c1953, ON

Smith, Fraser A., 1997, CCNM, ON, IL

Smith, Gordon F., 1976, NCNM, YT

Smith, Hannah R., c1926, ON

Smith, Jaclyn, 2008, CCNM, ON

Smith, James P., c1962, CA, AB

Smith, Kayla, 1990, Bastyr, BC, CA

Smith, Kirsten, 2008, CCNM, ON

Smith, Michael John, 1995, CCNM, ON

Smith, Muriel W., c1953, ON

Smith, Salna Lee, 2005, CCNM, ON

Smith, Thomas M., c1953, ON

Smrz, Debbie A., 2007, CCNM, ON

Snider, Benjamin Robert, 2006, CCNM, ON

Snider, Pamela, 1982, Bastyr, ON

Snippe, Yasmin Danielle, 2005, CCNM, ON

Sockett, Ruth Melissa, c1925, ON

Soh, Erica J., 2000, CCNM, ON

Solli, Karen, 2006, BINM

Solomonian, Leslie Anne, 2005, CCNM, ON

Soloy-Theil, Megan L., 2002, CCNM, ON

Sommical, Samuel F., 1911, RCI, ON

Sommical, W., 1949, PCN, ON

Souch, Gordon, c1926, AB

Soulliere, Danielle see Sinclair

South, Lianne, 1986, OCNM, BC

Southichack, Sengpheth, 2004, CCNM, AB

Sovran, Vivian, 2007, Bastyr, WA

Sowton, Christopher Guy (Chris), 1988, OCNM, ON

Sozio, Linda nee DeLisi, 2002, CCNM, ON

Sparrow, Joanna Lynne, 2004, CCNM, ON

Speare, Jennifer, see Charron

Spevack, Edra C., 2002, CCNM, ON

Spicer, Farah A., 2004, CCNM, ON

Spoke, Lena, 2003, CCNM, ON

Spooner, Christopher R., 1998, CCNM, BC

Spring, James William, 1986, OCNM, ON

Srajeldin, Ayman, 2008, CCNM, ON

Srajeldin, Mohamed Fateh, 1990, OCNM, ON

Sraw, Kulwinder Singh (Kully), 2003, CCNM, BC

Sroczynski, Halina Barbara, 1988, OCNM, ON

Stackhouse, W. Lloyd, 1953, CMCC*, ON

Stadler, Lileana see Mitrea

Stagg, Jennifer, 2003, Bastyr, CT, WA

Standish, C.S., c1926, QC

Stanko, Edward, c1942, NY

Stapleton, Michelle L., 2000, CCNM, ON

Starkovski, Lydia, nee Hartnett, 1992, OCNM, ON

Statham, John Frank, c1973, FL

Stauffert, Kurt H., 2000, CCNM, ON

Staute, Edward V., c1953, ON

Stechnowych, Ihor, 2001, CCNM

Steckley, Durwin E., c1961, ON

Stedmann, Neall, 1984, OCNM, ON

Steels, Brenna C. L., 2000, CCNM, ON

Steely, Nancy, 2000, Bastyr, NV

Stein, Adrienne Hinda, 2004, CCNM, ON

Steinkamp, Paula, 1992, NCNM, MB

Steinke, Wayne, 1995, CCNM, AB

Stencell, Dennis C., c1953, ON

Stengler, Mark, 1995, NCNM, AB

Stephens, Anita M., c1953, ON

Sterchi, Carolyn Jane see Hannaford

Stevenson, John A., c1954, PA, AB

Stevenson, Scott, c1983, ON

Stewart, Dora H. nee Fleming, c1953, ON

Stewart, Rachel Frances, 2004, CCNM, BC

Stewart. Mary Norah Aileen, 1954, CMCC*, ON

Stickley, Durwin E., c1954, ON

Stiles, Yvonne nee Hippmann, 2006, CCNM, ON

Stimson, Elizabeth T., 2001, CCNM, BC

Stinson, Wm. A., c1953, ON

Stoddard, Joetha G, 2003, CCNM, ON

Storch, Fran, 1996, NCNM, NFLD, NS, CT

Storjohann, K. Elizabeth nee Varga, 1996, CCNM, ON

Storm, Cory Faye nee Webb, 2004, CCNM, MB

Storsberg, Susann , AB

Strang, Lynette M., 2002, CCNM, ON

Strasser, Trudy, 1997, SCNM, AB

Strattan, Bert W., c1953, MI

Strelec, Brandy K., 2002, CCNM, ON

Strong, Jennifer R., 2005, CCNM, ON

Stroud, Elaine Kujoko Sano, 1998, CCNM, ON

Strukoff, Teresa, 2000, CCNM, BC

Strzelec, Jolanta, 2005, CCNM, ON

Stuetzer, Paul, c1981, ON

Sturdy, Walter T., 1919, PCC, BC

Stuyt, Lorraine, 2005, CCNM, ON

Such, Herbert B., c1953, ON

Sud, Ruchira, 2004, CCNM, ON

Sullivan, Clare, 2008, CCNM, ON

Sullivan, Gene, 2003, CCNM, ON

Summerfield, Charlene Lillian, 1992, OCNM, ON

Sumner, Gordon Arthur, 1942, NCDP, BC

Sun, Sandy Yu-J, 2004, Bastyr, BC

Sunderji, Narmeena, 2002, Bastyr, BC

Suneja, Ashima, 2004, CCNM, ON

Sung, Ji-Hyun Julia, 2006, CCNM, AB

Susil, Monica H., 2002, CCNM, ON

Sussman, Avram H. (Avi), 1987, OCNM, ON

Sussman, Marda, 2004, CCNM, NY

Sutradhar, Priyanka, 2002, CCNM, ON

Swetlikoff, Garrett G., 1988, Bastyr, BC

Swetlikoff, Lorne G., 1994, Bastyr, BC

Swolfs, Lysianne, 1994, NCNM, BC

Sykes, Erika Dawn, 2004, CCNM, ON

Sykes, William, c1976, 1981, OCNM, ON

Szczurko, Orest M., 2003, CCNM, ON

Szymanski, Zbysek Geoffrey, 1988, OCNM, ON, BC

Ta, Kiet, 2000, CCNM

Taams, Pieter, 1986, OCNM, BC

Taddayoni, Dor, 2001, CCNM, CA

Tahiliani, Sasha A., 2004, OCNM, ON

Talib, Nigma see Sciortino

Talosi, Julie A. see Thurston

Tam, Jaty, 2008, CCNM, ON

Tamburic, Sanja, 2005, BINM, BC

Taneda-Brown, Timothy M., 1986, OCNM, BC

Tanner, J.H., c1926, ON

Tanner, Jennifer Elizabeth, 2005, CCNM, ON

Tanner, Sarah-Ann G., 2006, CCNM, NS

Tarasuk, Denise, 1999, SCNM, NS

Tardik, George, 2008, CCNM, ON

Targett, Matthew, 2000, CCNM, NS

Tasaka, Aloysius G., c1947, NV, AB

Tashakor, Taraneh see Ballew

Tavakoli, Kathrine, 2007, BINM, BC

Taylor, Lloyd W., 1953, CMCC*, ON

Taylor, Patricia E., 1999, CCNM, ON

Taylor, Shannon M., 2003, CCNM, ON

Tebruegge, Peter Joseph, 2006, CCNM, ON

Tellier Johnson, Joyce A.J., 2002, CCNM, ON

Tessis, Regan Ilana, 2005, CCNM, ON

Tessler, Neil, 1983, Bastyr, BC

Tettamanti-Ratvay, Lisa D., 2001, CCNM, BC

Thammasouk, Somphorn, 2005, CCNM, ON

Thempson, B., c1926, ON

Theriault, Serge A., c1973, ON

Thibodeau, Margaret, 2006, CCNM, NC

Thiessen, Joanna Marjorie, 2006, CCNM, ON

Thistle, Diane Elizabeth, 1998, CCNM, ON

Thompson, Caryn A., 2003, CCNM, ON

Thompson, Emma Victoria nee Caird, 1925, USC, BC

Thompson, Gerald B., c1953, ON

Thompson, Jennifer, 2008, CCNM, ON

Thomson, Keith, 1982, OCNM, ON

Thonne, J. B., c1959, MB

Thornton-Pow, Pamela Jane, 1998, CCNM, ON

Thorpe, Heather Stephanie, 2003, CCNM, AB

Thorpe, Julie Carmel, 2003, CCNM, ON

Thuna, Jacob R. (Jack), c1959, QC

Thurlow, Charles K., c1962, NS

Thurston, Julie A. nee Talosi, 2002, CCNM, ON

Thut, Albert J., 1930, National, ON

Tibelius, Carolyn, 2000, CCNM, MB

Timothy, Bryan, 1989, OCNM, ON

Ting, Katharine, 2005, Bastyr, US

Tintinalli, Lynn J., 2001, CCNM, ON

Toale, A. Clarkson, c1953, ON

Tocher, Rebecca Laurel, 2001, CCNM, AB

Tokiwa, Jonathan Jason, 2005, CCNM, ON

Tol, Debra E., see Jo

Tolzmann, Louise, 1997, Bastyr, OR

Tom, Winston C., 2001, CCNM, ON

Tomlin, Victor K. E., c1953, ON

Tonskamper, Gudrun, 1983, NCNM, BC

Toplak, Anthony R., 1987, OCNM, ON

Torrance, Patricia, 1988, Bastyr, BC

Torreiter, Michael Anton, 2005, CCNM, ON

Tournianski, Anna, 1997, CCNM, ON

Townsend, Kimberley Anne, 1998, CCNM, ON

Trabert, Jennifer, 2006, CCNM, ON

Tran, Neil, 2006, CCNM, BC

Trenciansky, Stephanie N., 1997, Bastyr, BC

Trethewey, R.A., c1926, BC

Trevorrow, Marianne, 2006, Bastyr, BC

Trick, Julia see Fountain

Tripodi, Robert, 1982, OCNM, ON

Tripodi, Stephen J., 2000, CCNM, ON

Trotter, Makoto O., 2004, CCNM, ON

Truelane, Paul, c1981, ON

Truong, Diana, 2002, CCNM, ON

Truscott-Brock, Erin C., 2000, CCNM, ON

Trznadel, Julie Elizabeth see Mardian

Tsui, Teresa C. O., 2005, CCNM, ON

Tuck, Percy E., c1953, ON

Tucker, Lealand A., c1953, ON

Tucker, Ralph H., c1953, ON

Tucker, Terry, c1981, ON

Tung, Amy Jennifer, 2004, CCNM, ON

Tunstall, Richard D., 1987, OCNM, ON

Tupper, James F., 1932, LACC, BC

Turcasso, Aura-Taina Eerika, 2005, Bastyr, BC

Turcinskas, Danute Novogrodskaite, 1989, OCNM

Turcotte, Alison, 2000, CCNM, ON

Turgeon, Madeliene, c1982, QC

Turk, Frances W., 2006, CCNM, ON

Turner, Christopher, 1986, NCNM, MB

Turner, Natasha, 1999, CCNM, ON

Turpin, Tricia, 2005, CCNM, ON

Turska, William, c1962, ID, AB

Tutt, Frances O., 2000, CCNM, ON

Tweedle, Amy Beth, 2005, CCNM, ON

Tyler, A. Scott, 1986, NCNM, BC

Tyler, Allen N., 1949, PCN, Ont, BC, WA, BC

Tymoshenko, Nadia, 1996, CCNM, ON

Um, Michael, 2002, CCNM, ON

Upcott, Kelly Lee, 2003, CCNM, ON

Uraz, Zeynep, 2006, CCNM, ON

Ure, Audrey Shanley, 1988, NCNM, BC

Ure, Sherry, 1990, NCNM, BC

Vacirca, Amy, 2008, CCNM, ON

Valchar, Jan Scott, 1981, OCNM, ON

Valiquette, V., c1959, QC

Vallee, Brian L., 1981, NCNM, BC

Vallieres, Lucien, c1970, QC

van Alstyne, Terrie D., 2001, CCNM, BC

van Gaver, Aaron Lewis, 2003, CCNM, BC

van Hoogenhuize, William, c1981, ON
van Horlick, Robert H., 1988, NCNM, BC
van Lierde, Kathleen, 2005, CCNM, ON
van Loon, Isis Marianne, 1995, Bastyr, BC
Vance, Amber J. nee Hirst, 2001, CCNM, ON
Vandekerkhove, Alison, 2004, BINM, BC
VandenBerg, Rachel, 2005, CCNM, ON
Vanderheyden, Terry Anthony, 1994, CCNM, ON
Vanderhym, Jeff, c1981, ON
Vanderlinden, Kim, 1991, Bastyr, BC
Vanzhov, Filip, 1987, NCNM, BC
VanZilurden, J., c1991, ON
Varadi, Lisa, 2005, CCNM, ON
Varga, K. Elizabeth see Storjohann
Vecchi, Lisa Marie, 2005, CCNM, ON
Veeravagu, Arjuna, 2002, NCNM, BC
Veitch, Wm., c1954, ON
Verge, Alexandra M. E., 2001, CCNM, ON
Verslycken, Matthew, 2007, CCNM
Vetiska, Jana, 1990, OCNM, ON
Vetter, Krista Dawn, 2004, CCNM, ON
Vigliotti, Julian Chris, 1991, Bastyr, BC
Villazan, Orna F., 2005, CCNM, QC
Villegas, Pilar Elizabeth, 2007, CCNM, ON
Villeneuve, Joel nee Lee, 1991, OCNM, ON
Vinge, Robin, 1998, Bastyr, AB
Vinnen, Herman, c1953, ON
Vitsas, Zafiria Roula. 2000, CCNM, ON
Vivian, Kimberly Jo (Kim), 2003, CCNM, ON
Vlahopoulos, Christina, 2004, CCNM, ON
Vo, Lan, 1998, CCNM, ON
Vo, Mylinh, 1997, Bastyr, WA
Voitenko, Zoya, 2006, CCNM, ON
Vojtisek, David, 2007, CCNM, AB
Vok, Jitka, 1997, CCNM, ON
Vollmer, Amanda, 2008, CCNM, ON
von Glatz, Ilse, 1997, CCNM, ON
VonWagoner, Mark, c1981, ON
Voortman, Lynn, 1998, CCNM, ON
Vosloo, Werner, 2006, NCNM, OR
Voss, c1926, BC
Vowles, c1926, QC

Vu, Alan Lam-Huan, 2006, CCNM, ON
Wachtler, Marnie, 2006, BINM, AB
Waddington, Philip, 1996, CCNM, ON
Wadland, William H., c1923, ON
Waechter, Fernando, c1962, ON
Wagstaff, S.Craig, 1982, NCNM, BC
Walden, Watson, 1937, National, ON
Waldron, Gemma, 2008, CCNM, QC, ON
Wales, Patricia J., 1981, OCNM, Ont, AB
Walji, Rishma, 2002, CCNM, ON
Walker, Jennifer, 2000, CCNM, Hong Kong
Walker, Lindsey Dawn, 2005, CCNM, ON
Walker, Meghan, 2007, CCNM, ON
Walker, Susan Anita, 2004, CCNM, ON
Wall, Claude C., c1926, ON
Wallace, Christy Leigh Kerr, 2005, CCNM, ON
Wallace, Kelly Beth, 2004, CCNM, ON
Wallace, Norman George, 1989, OCNM, SK
Wallace, Thomas Frederick, c1953, ON
Waller, Natalie Bianca, 2004, CCNM, AB
Walls, Colin Bell, c1940, PA
Walsh, Harvey E., c1953, ON
Walsh, Robin Lynn, 2003, CCNM, ON
Walters Saddler, Cassandra D., 2002, CCNM, ON
Wang, David, 1990, OCNM, BC
Wang, George Nelson, c1953, ON
Wang, Richard P., 2005, CCNM, China
Wang, Rida, 2005, Bastyr, US, BC
Warchter, Fernando, c1953, ON
Ward, John, c1953, ON
Ward, Tawnya Frances, 2004, CCNM, BC
Warden, Douglas, c1953, ON
Warren, Donald G., 1984, NCNM, ON
Warren, Susan Elaine, 2001, CCNM, NB
Warshavsky, Olga, 2001, CCNM, ON
Wasiak, Maria T. nee Pawlowska, 1989, OCNM, Poland
Wasylynko, David E., 1989, OCNM, BC
Watkins, Carrie R., 2007, CCNM, ON
Watson, Lisa, 2007, CCNM
Watters, Daniel Jin, 2005, CCNM, ON
Watts, Colin B., c1953, ON
Waunch, Paul, 1984, OCNM, ON

Weaver, Charles A., c1953, ON

Webb, Cory Faye see Storm

Websterm, c1926, SK

Weeks, Lisa Margaret, 2007, CCNM, ON

Weene, Samuel M., c1958, OR, BC

Weidenfeld, Hana, 1999, CCNM, ON

Weiler, Victoria Lynn, 2008, CCNM, ON

Weinberg, Jyll, 2002, CCNM, ON

Weir-Teal, Joan, 1988, OCNM, ON

Weisenburger, Jennie, 2006, BINM, BC

Weiss, Barbara Lynn, 2006, CCNM, ON

Weiss, Sid, 1980, NCNM, BC

Weissberg, Wm., c1953, NY

Welch, Mary-Elizabeth nee Long, 1999, CCNM, ON

Wells, Elizabeth Amy, 2003, CCNM, BC

Welton, Stacey, 2007, CCNM, ON

Wendler, Carly Roxanne, 2006, CCNM, ON

Wesenberg, W., c1926, ON

West, Samuel H., c1953, ON

Wharton, Katherine S. (Kate), 2003, CCNM, ON

Whatmough, Howard B., 1950, CMCC*, ON

Wheeler, Jennifer (Jen), 2008, CCNM, ON

Whitaker, Kim L., 2004, CCNM, ON

Whitby Lipson, Stephanie A., 2002, CCNM, ON

White, John Vernon, 1953, CMCC*, ON

White, Jack, 1949, PCN, BC

White, John W., 1958, CMCC*, ON

White, Sara-Jane nee McNeil, 2003, CCNM, ON

White, Tanja, 2006, BINM, BC

Whitfield, Laurence O., c1953, ON

Whitford, Tara see Macart

Whitmore, Joseph D., c1953, ON

Whitney, Lyle, 1989, OCNM, AB

Wichels, Herbert J., c1953, ON

Wickland, Karina, 2006, BINM, BC

Wiebe, Deirdre see Jasper

Wieder, William, c1953, NY

Wiens, Jese Anne, nee Greenall, 2007, BINM, BC

Wikenheiser, David, 1995, NCNM, BC

Wiley, Erin Elizabeth, 2007, CCNM, ON

Wilkinson, Selene, 2007, CCNM, ON

Wilkes, Leonard H., c1926, ON

Wilks, Penelope nee Brand, 1999, CCNM, ON

Willems, Jacinta P., 1995, Bastyr, ON

Williams, A., c1926, ON

Williams, John A., c1953, ON

Williams, Maureen, 1995, Bastyr, BC.

Willis, Michelle, 2006, BINM, BC

Willms, Heidi Marie, 2003, CCNM, ON

Willoughby, William Bryce, c1953, ON

Willow, Katherine nee Schad-Byers, Karen, 1983, NCNM, ON

Wilson, Danielle nee Comeau, 1998, CCNM, ON

Wilson, Frederick Charles, c1981, 1984, OCNM, ON, US

Wilson, James Leslie, c1977, 1981, OCNM, AZ

Wilson, L.C., c1926, SK

Winter, Kathy, 1998, CCNM, ON

Winters, John, c1991, MB, US

Winton, Morgan, 2003, CCNM, ON

Witek-Grobys, Sigrid see Grobys

Wolf, John Brian, 1990, OCNM, ON

Wolf, Natasha, 2002, Bastyr, US

Wolfe, Heather Jerrine, 2001, CCNM, ON

Wolfe, Krista L. see Loughead

Wolfe, Patricia Cecelia, 1987, OCNM, BC

Wolter, Audrey, 2005, CCNM, BC

Wong, Alfonso W. H., 1988, OCNM, China

Wong, Catherine, 2002, CCNM, ON

Wong, G. N., c1962, PA

Wong, Ina, 1998, CCNM, BC

Wong, Jasmine, 2006, CCNM, BC

Woo, Maylynn, 1995, Bastyr, BC

Wood, Alexander Allan (Sandy), 1977, CMCC*, 1982, OCNM, ON

Wood, Eric, 2008, CCNM, US

Woodman, Cheryl A., 2001, CCNM, ON

Woodworth, Scott, 2000, CCNM, NS

Word, Rebecca Rodgers, 2007, CCNM, ON

Worts, Shelby A., 2004, BINM, ON

Wrenshall, Natasha Dawn, 2003, CCNM, Ireland

Wright, Joseph c1936, BC

Wright, Masina A., 2000, CCNM, ON

Wright, Robert D'Arcy, 1935, WSC, BC

Wright, W. G., c1985, ON
Wyatt, Julie, 1999, CCNM, ON
Wyatt, Robert A., c1953, ON
Wyer, Sarah S., 2004, CCNM, ON
Wylde, Tanya R. S., 2005, CCNM, ON
Wynn, Richard S., c1953, ON
Wyse, Tiffany D., 2007, CCNM, ON
Xin, Rong, 2005, CCNM, ON
Yakimovich, Shawn Robert, 2006, CCNM, ON
Yam, Peter Chun-Ting, 1989, OCNM, BC
Yang, Hannah, 2007, CCNM, England
Yang, Jenny, 2004, CCNM, BC
Yap-Yu, Marilyn J., 1989, OCNM, PE
Yaremovitch, A., c1946, MB
Yarish, Michael, 2007, CCNM, ON
Yarnell, Eric, BC
Yates, Harry A., c1954, ON
Yates, Seth, 2008, CCNM, ON
Yau, Alice, 2001, CCNM
Yawrenko, David, 1989, OCNM, AB
Yee, Jennifer Pui Ling, 2006, CCNM, ON
Yehia, Houyda, 2002, CCNM
Yeong, Siu-Hong Adrian, 2008, BINM, BC
Yeung, Man-Yee, 2005, CCNM, AB
Yhap, Kelly V., 2004, CCNM, BC
Yik, Ardyce, 2005, CCNM, ON, Hong Kong
Yik, Patricia, 2006, CCNM, AB
Yik, Stephanie C., 2001, CCNM
Yim, John, 1994, Bastyr, BC
Yores, Anthony James, 2003, CCNM, ON
Younano, Melissa, 2008, CCNM, ON
Young, Karrin Anne see Fairman
Young, Lorraine, 2000, CCNM, NS
Young, Robert Goddard (Bob), 1950, CMCC*, ON
Young, Whitney, 2008, CCNM, ON
Youngs, Gilbert H., c1953, NY
Yu, David, 1984, OCNM, ON
Yuan, Alexander, 1986, OCNM, China
Yun, Jennifer, 2008, CCNM, ON
Yurko, Jackie, 2000, CCNM, AB
Zabol, Shirley, 1994, CCNM, ON
Zaidi, Syed Rehan Ali, 2004, CCNM, ON

Zaidman-Averbuck, Shelly, 1995, CCNM, ON
Zajmalowski, Natasha, 2002, CCNM, ON
Zalatan, Marie see Matheson
Zambri, Saveria Andrea (Rena), 1991, OCNM, ON
Zamojski, Donuta Mary, c1979, ON
Zamost, Israil, c1953, PA
Zarei, Mona, 2008, CCNM, ON
Zarzeczny, Dominika, 2008, CCNM, ON
Zawada, Carol see Morley
Zeifman, Mitchell Bram, 2003, CCNM, ON
Zelina, Fedor, 1984, OCNM, BC
Zeoli, David, 1999, NCNM, BC
Zepp, Julie M. see Rutledge
Zettel, Paulina nee DeLaCampa, 2002, CCNM, ON
Zhang, Zhe Thomas, 1997, CCNM, ON
Zickler, Nicole, 2003, Bastyr, BC
Zimmermann, Rachel Anke, 1991, OCNM, ON, BC
Zoretich, Carol nee Laic, 1998, CCNM, ON
Zytaruk, Emily, 2008, CCNM, AU

Information Guide

Information is reported as last name, first name, year of graduation, naturopathic school, location of practice
Incomplete records indicate that information was unavailable at the time or printing
'c' prior to the date refers to the date that the name first appeared in correspondence. This is used when no record was found that confirmed year of graduation
Underlined words refer to the name that the person goes by.
'( ) are used to denote the short-form of a name that is used
'see' followed by a name is used when a person's name has changed, such as with marriage
'nee' followed by a name is used to denote a maiden name.
CMCC* - prior to 1978 graduates of CMCC were able to take additional courses and then write an exam in order to achieve their Drugless Therapy (DT) license. Naturopathic Doctors in Ontario were initially regulated under the term of Drugless Therapy.

HISTORY OF
NATUROPATHIC TERMINOLOGY

THE DEFINING OF NATUROPATHIC MEDICINE has been an ongoing process since it was first established. Not because the founders and doctors of naturopathic medicine have been unclear, but because the profession is based on specific philosophies and principles, yet over the years, due to regulatory and governmental requirements, the definitions have needed to become more structured with the profession defined by its scope and treatments versus by its underlying philosophies. There has always been the challenge of maintaining terminology that serves both purposes.

Throughout the years there have been many meetings and discussion within the profession with aim of agreeing on naturopathic terminology. The following takes a look at the terminology that has been used over time.

1902 – "Naturopathy" as defined by Benedict Lust

The term naturopathy 'stood for the reconciling, harmonizing and unifying of nature, humanity and God.' Lust went on to explain that the term 'Naturopathy' is a hybrid word and 'it is purposely so. No single tongue could distinguish a system whose origin, scope and purpose is universal – broad as the world, deep as love, and high as heaven. Fundamentally therapeutic because men need healing; elementally

educational because men need teaching; ultimately inspirational because men need empowering, it encompasses the realm of human progress and destiny. Dietetics, physical culture, and hydrotherapy are the measures upon which Naturopathy is to build; mental culture is the means, and soul-selfhood is the motive.

. . . The scope of naturopathy is from the first kiss of the new-found lovers to the burying of the centenarian whose birth was the symbol of their perfected oneness. It includes ideally every life-phase of the id, the embryo, the foetus, the birth, the babe, the child, the youth, the man, the lover, the husband, the father, the patriarch, the soul.'"

1918 - Universal Naturopathic Directory

"The natural system for curing disease is based on a return to nature in regulating the diet, breathing, exercising, bathing and the employment of various forces to eliminate the poisonous products in the system, and so raise the vitality of the patient to a proper standard of health.

Official medicine has in all ages simply attacked the symptoms of disease without paying any attention to the causes thereof, but natural healing is concerned far more with removing the causes of disease, than merely curing its symptoms. This is the

glory of this new school of medicine that it cures by removing the causes of the ailment, and is only rational method of practicing medicine. It begins its cures by avoiding the uses of drugs and hence is styled the system of drugless healing. . . .
The prime object of natural healing is to give the principle of life the line of least resistance, that it many enable man to possess the most abundant health. . . .

Naturopathy, on the other hand, so far as it has been developed, and so far as official medicine will allow it to act, leaves no such trail of disease, disaster, and death behind it. Natural healing is emancipation from medical superstition, ignorance and tyranny. It is the true Elixir of Life.
. . . For thousands of years medical doctors have been educating the public into the false belief that poisonous drugs can give health. This belief has become in the public mind such a deep-seated superstition, that those of us who know better and who would like to adopt more sensible, natural methods of cure, can do so only at the peril of losing practice and reputation. The program of Naturopathic Cure includes:

Elimination of Evil Habits – e.g., overeating, alcoholic drinks, drugs, the use of tea, coffee and cocoa that contain poisons, meat eating, improper hours of living, waste of vital forces, lowered vitality, sexual and social aberrations, worry, etc.
Corrective Habits – correct breathing, correct exercise, right mental attitude, moderation in the pursuit of health and wealth.
New Principles of Living – proper fasting, selection of food, hydrotherapy, light and air baths, mud baths, osteopathy, chiropractic and other forms of mechano-therapy, mineral salts obtained in organic form, electropathy, heliopathy, steam or Turkish baths, sitz baths, etc.

Natural healing is the most desirable factor in the regeneration of the race. It is a return to nature in methods of living and treatment. It makes use of the elementary forces of nature, of chemical selection of foods that will constitute a correct medical dietary. . . . There is really but one healing force in existence and that is nature herself, which means the inherent restorative power of the organism to overcome disease. . . . The practical application of these natural agencies, duly suited to the individual case, and true signs that that art of healing has been elaborated by the aid of absolutely harmless, congenial treatments, under whose ministration the death rate is but five percent of persons treated as compared with fifty percent under the present allopathic methods."

Early 1900s – What is Naturopathy, Ludwig Staden ND

". . . Let us now recapitulate in brief the essence of Naturopathy.
It is the method of healing all diseases without medicines, drugs, poisons, and almost without any operations.
It is based on the highest scientific principles: (a) on the harmony of our perceptive faculties with the physiological and psychological laws of nature; it stands on reason, conscience and experience. (b) The change of matter functioning normal or abnormal is the standard of physical health or disease. All physical life is based upon the change of matter of the cell or upon the vibration within the cell. The vibrative process in the cell being disturbed more or

less must be the physical cause of all disease and this is the problems which has to be solved in healing disease.

The power of healing is within us; Nature only, Nature alone, solves the problem, man presses the button, nature does the rest.

Naturopathy knows that there is but one disturbance which manifests itself in different forms, symptoms and names.

Being but one disturbance or disease, there can be but one original cause; this is divided into a psychical and a physical one; the first is the impure thought; the second the disturbed vibrative process in the cell, as mentioned above. The occasional causes are infinite just as the symptoms and forms are.

The most important differences of form and symptoms in disease that Naturopathy recognizes are acute and chronic disease.

Naturopathy's material medica consists of the principal elements which are derived from nature: light, air, water, heat and clay, beside non-stimulating diet, exercise and rest, electricity, magnetism and massage, calisthenics, physical culture, mental culture, etc., etc.

Naturopathy attacks always the original cause of every disease. The human body being an organism containing thousands of nerves, blood vessels, etc., which are all most intimately connected, Naturopathy consequently is always treating the entire body.

It looks upon the fever as the greatest natural healing process, which should never be suppressed by poisons like quinine, antipyrin, etc., but should be guarded like a wild fire. No healing method has ever had such an immense success in treating fever diseases as Naturopathy. Suppressed fever diseases cause chronic diseases. Chronic diseases therefore are developed if there is insufficient vitality in the system; if nature is healing a chronic disease it always produces a crisis of a more or less acute form, which may be repeated several times and finally finishes up with a fever. The fever is the sick man's greatest friend.

In the action and reaction of extreme heat and cold Naturopathy finds the greatest physical power to correct the inharmonious change of matter.

The food question is divided into a raw food diet consisting of fruits, berries and nuts of all kinds, besides such vegetables and cereals that can be eaten raw, and in a cooked food diet, based on the saline vegetarian theory of Dr. H. Lahmann, Dresden.

Stimulating and nerve-irritating food of any kind is entirely eschewed by strict Naturopathy, especially alcohol, in any form, coffee and tea, meat, beef juice, beef extract, vinegar, spices, etc."

1939 – Association of Naturopathic Practitioners of British Columbia (ANPBC)

"A Naturopathic Physician, by philosophy and by law, practises those fields of preventive and therapeutic healing which are "natural". Natural fields of healing utilize those substances which are found and developed by nature and those forces which produce normal physiological responses within the body. These fields include the use of the following:

Plant life –both in the field of nutrition and herbology.

Body mechanics, which includes remedial exercises, posture, manipulations, and prosthetics.

Physical agents such as water, light, air, sound, and electricity.

Remedial psychology such as psychosomatics and counselling.

Natural therapeutics are particularly suited for the management and correction of many human ailments and injuries and can accomplish much towards the improvement of health standards in the community. These fields, used singly or in combination as required, fill a place in the healing arts which the Naturopathic Physician feels should be more adequately stressed.

The Naturopathic Physician is not adverse to, nor does he condemn the methods of treatment of the other healing arts; rather he recognizes there is a place for each of the healing professions and his frequent referrals testify to his evaluation of them. The Naturopathic Physician believes that public should not be restricted exclusively to any one branch of the healing arts.

Naturopathy, as an exact science, takes its place with the other healing arts in properly accepting its responsibility in the treatment of disease."

1941 – The New Gould Medical Dictionary, first edition

"Naturopathy is a therapeutic system embracing a complete physianthropy employing nature's agencies, forces, processes, and products, except major surgery."

1946 – Manitoba Naturopathy Act

"Naturopathy is the science of Physiological Medicine in which its methods employ only those forces and remedies which are inherently natural to the human organism.

We believe that sickness is a deviation from health due to disturbances of a hereditary or environmental nature or from poor living habits. We approach the problem of ill health with the firm conviction that true healing can only be produced from within the body and that Nature herself can and will perform the necessary adjustments if the antagonistic influences are removed, and that the best results are obtained in treating the sick by the use of proper nutrition.

We believe the best method of treating altered vital function (disease) to be by creating better living habits of nutrition, body mechanics, remedial psychology and by the judicious utilization of such natural forces as heat, light, air, electricity, water, etc. The relief of symptoms, which are really Nature's warnings, is considered secondarily because when the cause of ill health has been located and removed, the symptoms automatically disappear.

We believe that there are no superfluous parts in the body and that surgery should only be used when absolutely essential and not until the body has conclusively demonstrated its inability to heal the diseased part."

1948 – 'What is Naturopathy', Dr. Lambert ND

"Naturopathy is the science of Physiological Medicine in which its methods employ only those forces and remedies which are inherently natural to the human organism.

We believe that sickness is a deviation from health due to disturbances of a hereditary or environmental nature or from poor living habits. We approach the problem of ill health with the firm conviction that true healing can only be produced from within the body and that Nature herself can and will perform the necessary adjustments if the antagonistic influences are removed, and that the best results are obtained in treating the sick by the use of proper nutrition.

We believe the best method of treating altered vital function (disease) to be by creating better living habits of nutrition, body mechanics, remedial psychology and by the judicious utilization of such natural forces as heat, light, air, electricity, water, etc. The relief of symptoms, which are really Nature's warnings, is considered secondarily because when the cause of ill health has been located and removed, the symptoms automatically disappear.

We believe that there are no superfluous parts in the body and that surgery should only be used when absolutely essential and not until the body has conclusively demonstrated its inability to heal the diseased part."

1951 – Summit Meeting at Deep Cover Vancouver Island on August 19th

"Definition of Naturopathy: Naturopathy is the application of the laws of biology to the maintenance of health and the treatment of disease.

Definition of Disease: Disease is a process manifested as altered vital function and this alteration is produced by failure to maintain the coordination of the physiological and psychological processes of the body.

Definition of Health: The vital function of the body which makes health possible, can only be maintained by the proper coordination of all the physiological and psychological processes of the body. These processes are biochemical in their nature."

1955 – CNA Incorporation Document

"Naturopathy is the prevention, diagnosis, and treatment of human injuries, ailments, diseases and deformities by means of any one of more of the psychological, physical, mechanical, chemical or material forces or agencies of nature."

1955 – United States Department of Labor, "Dictionary of Occupational Titles," 2nd edition

"Doctor, Naturopathic, Naturopathic Physician: A healer; diagnoses, treats and cares for patients, using a system of practice that bases its treatment of all physiological functions and abnormal conditions on natural laws governing the body; utilizing physiological, psychological, and mechanical methods, such as air, water, light, heat, earth, phytotherapy, food, and herb therapy, psychotherapy, electrotherapy, physiotherapy, minor and orifacial surgery, mechanotherapy, naturopathic corrections and manipulations, and all natural methods or modalities, together with natural medicines, natural processed foods, and herbs and nature's remedies. Naturopathy excludes use of major surgery, X-ray and radium for therapeutic purposes, and drugs."

1955 – Naturopathy Act of Alberta

"'Naturopathy' means a system of therapy that treats human injuries, ailments or diseases by methods of nature including any agency of nature, and employs as auxiliaries for such purposes, the use of electrotherapy, hydrotherapy, body manipulations and dietetics.

The immense scope of this science is perhaps more readily understood when "Natural Methods" are recognized as all the constructive therapeutic fields which produce natural physiological reactions within the human body. The science embraces not only the physical fields of physiotherapy and its closely related branches of electrotherapy, hydrotherapy, and mechanotherapy, but also the equally important therapies affecting the chemical (nutritive) welfare of the human body, as well as the psychosomatic relations.

In the correction and maintenance of human health, these therapies must be applied, not as isolated units to treat the separate organs or parts, but as a unified group to both the symptomatic and causative factors.

This is particularly necessary in treatment by physical therapeutics. The combination of the natural healing forces of physiotherapy, (electrotherapy, hydrotherapy, and mechanotherapy) with the specialized branches of body mechanics (manipulative techniques, posture, corrective exercises), produce quicker and more permanent correction of the body tissues."

1962 – ANPBC official definition

"Naturopathic medicine is a therapeutic and diagnostic art and science which is concerned with the application of the biological and physiological principles of the human body for the restoration and preservation of health; these inherent processes of the body are assisted through the use of nature's agents, forces, and products.

Scope: "Nature's agents and forces embrace the therapeutics of light, air, water, electricity, vibration, sound, temperature and life; the physical mechanics of the body (manipulations); nature's products – the therapeutics of food, food supplements and concentrates, of plant and mineral substances, of animal substances which form components of the body; and nature's processes include the therapeutics of the emotions, of conscious and sub-conscious mind and the physio-chemical processes of the body. These fields of practice constitute "natural therapeutics". Naturopathic principles and practice do not employ the therapeutics of radium, x-ray, and major surgery."

1965 – CNA official definition

"Naturopathic Medicine is the philosophy, science and art of healing with assists the self-recuperative processes of the body, by the use of natural, physical, biochemical and psychological forces, in an integrated system of optimum physiological effect, through the application of the natural laws of life to the whole man for the restoration and maintenance of health and prevention and treatment of disease."

1966 – 'The Nature of A Naturopath', a CNA document

"Naturopathic Medicine is
- A philosophy, science, art and practice
- Based on the natural laws of life and living and nature
- Integrated into a system of diagnosis of causes of disease, of the underlying and/or predisposing factors/circumstances in disorders of the health, vitality and healing ability of all organs of the body and of factors which may impede healing
- A comprehensive compendium of natural, health restoring therapies, consisting

of biochemical, psychological, physical, body immunity, life force restoration and ecological methods and procedure

• Essential to the comprehensive treatment of the total person, his/her lifeforce, lifestyle, emotions, environment, physical, biochemical and structural nature

• Oriented to the patient's self-recuperative processes, to the restoration and maintenance of optimum health, to the treatment of disease, and to the prevention of future illness

• With emphasis on educating patients to clear understandings of the causes and nature of their health problems so that they are able to assume and do assume responsibility in regaining and maintaining their own health."

1960s brochure – Alberta Association of Naturopathic Practitioners

"Naturopathic Medicine is essentially an in depth study of the scientific and philosophical principles taught in accredited Naturopathic Colleges.

Naturopathy, as a profession and science, uses wisdom from the past and from modern science. Most of its concepts of physiological therapy are based on modern research – on the vast libraries of newly discovered information by medical researchers delving into the secrets of the world of the living cell.

Naturopathy does not discard methods because they are old. Nor does it endorse and arbitrarily embrace ideas, techniques and remedies because they are new. Only concepts, methods, techniques and therapies, rigidly tested upon the anvil of time and experience are accepted and used.

Naturopathic medicine favors modern, scientific advancement and techniques which extend the life and health of the human body, providing such approaches do not violate natural or biological laws.

A great deal of what has been Naturopathy for a long time, is being accepted and incorporated into practices of a considerable number of more eclectic, broad scope thinking and somewhat maverick doctors of Chiropractic, Osteopathy, and of Medicine. Many of these go under the name of "Holistic Medicine": and of "Preventative Medicine" doctors.

Prejudices, still prevalent against the minority healing professions by the firmly ensconced establishment, are not reciprocated. Naturopathic physicians openly, and with pleasure, co-operate with any licensed doctor in the other healing professions when such co-operation is in the best interests of the patient(s)."

1971 – 'Naturopathic Medicine – A Separate and Distinct Healing Profession', a CNA document

"There are certain distinct features, unique to the profession of Naturopathic Medicine which readily differentiate it from other healing professions such as medicine or surgery, osteopathy, chiropractic and podiatry. These are as follows:

• The Naturopathic Physician is concerned with the whole man rather than a specific anatomical area, in his diagnostic and therapeutic efforts.

• While Naturopathic Physicians are concerned with the immediate causative factors of an illness, equal consideration or treatment is given to the basic, underlying causal factors or circumstances so frequent in many disorders. Particular emphasis is place on the maintenance of health (or prevention of disease) through health education in nutrition, mental hygiene, physical fitness and other aspects of bodily care.

• Naturopathic Physicians are true "doctors" (latin root - 'docere'; meaning 'to teach') and true physicians ("one who heals" – Oxford dictionary 4th edition) in that patients, in conjunction with the therapeutic efforts of the Naturopathic Physician, are frequently instructed on what THEY must do to regain and maintain their health.

• Naturopathic Medicine includes a complete physianthropy with the emphasis on natural methods with evoke a biological response – therapeutic in nature.

• Naturopathic treatment is "physiological" in nature. i.e. Treatment assists the inherent physiological processes as they relate to healing and biochemistry. Any method or form of treatment that violates natural or physiological law is considered unnatural especially if such "treatment" causes a new or different illness (iatrogenic disease) or complicates the existent disease process.

• Naturopathic Physicians rarely employ a singular method or purely symptomatic approach to bodily disorders but combine in one well-ordered system of therapeutics the best of all forms of natural healing, by a combination of multiple methods or approaches best suited for the particular illness being treated.

• Naturopathic therapeutics involves a multi-disciplinary approach to most chronic health problems; i.e. a botanical or herbal medicine may be used in conjunction with – a nutritional or metabolic supplement, diet, ultrasound and spinal manipulation in the treatment of an arthritic patient.

• Naturopathic therapeutics include treatment directed to the neurological, biochemical and endocrine systems of the body, in contradistinction to chiropractic, which involves a singular neurological approach, or medicine which involves a chemological approach, or surgery which involves the repair or removal of tissue.

• Naturopathic Physicians treat any and all conditions that come within the realm of general practice. (Cardiovascular problems; neurological, musculoskeletal, and orthopedic diseases; gastro-intestinal, genitor-urinary, respiratory and dermatological problems are treated frequently as are pediatric or geriatric illnesses.) Naturopathic physicians co-operate freely with any licensed doctor in the healing profession, when such co-operation is in the best interests of the patient. Problem cases are frequently referred for specialty care.

• Naturopathic services should not be considered ancillary or paramedical in relation to the medical profession.

• Naturopathic Physicians have met a standard of qualifications that compares favourably with medical graduates of medical schools and they are equally scientifically oriented to perform and interpret diagnostic procedures.

The name "Naturopathy" is of comparatively recent date, but its philosophy and practices can be traced to antiquity. It does not discard a method because it is old, neither does it embrace a technique because it is new. Its methods and techniques have been tested upon the anvil of time and experience and proven effective.

In consideration of the above, it must be emphasized that Naturopathic medicine is very much in favour of all modern, scientific advancement and techniques, (many of which have verified naturopathic concepts and principles) which extend the life and health of the human body, providing such scientific endeavours do not violate natural or biological law.

New concepts of micro-biology, neurophysiology, physio-therapeutics and psycho-therapeutics have been incorporated into daily practice. Indeed there is a tendency for many doctors of other healing professions to employ various aspects of contemporary Naturopathic Medicine."

1984 – A Brief Presented to the Caucus of the Government of BC

"Naturopathic medicine is a health care system based upon the irrefutable principle that human beings like other organisms, possess intrinsic mechanisms for health maintenance and spontaneous repair. This perspective has ancient roots and has until recently formed the backbone of the art and science of medicine. In their practice naturopathic physicians strive to assist these inherent curative forces by the use of agents and therapies which support the organism in its efforts. This is in direct contrast to the use of many allopathic drugs, which by definition are antagonistic to natural processes and therefore often cause unnecessary and undesirable side effects.

From the perspective of naturopathic medicine, the ideal of health is a person who is a complete and integrated whole, with physical, mental and emotional dimensions all in a positive state of balance. Health problems arise when a given state of balance is upset for any period of time. An imbalance may at first appear on only one of these levels, but if uncorrected will eventually have effects on all the others. Therefore, rational therapy should seek to

recognize and correct imbalances as early as possible, and at as many levels of organization as possible. This requires taking the health problems of an individual in the total context of his or her life – environmental, familial, social, and so on. The attempt to understand disease from a lifestyle point of view is central to the renewed concept of holistic medicine, and naturopathic physicians are, by conviction and training, in a unique position to practise in this way."

1989 – American Association of Naturopathic Doctors definition, adopted by the CNA

"Naturopathic medicine is a distinct method of primary health care - an art, science, philosophy and practice of diagnosis, treatment and prevention of illness. Naturopathic physicians seek to restore and maintain optimum health in their patients by emphasizing nature's inherent self healing process, the vis medicatrix naturae. This is accomplished through education and the rational use of therapeutics."

1994 – Board of Directors of Drugless Therapy – Naturopathy

"Naturopathic medicine is the promotion of health, the assessment of the physical and mental condition of an individual and the diagnosis, prevention and treatment of diseases, disorders and dysfunctions, through education and by assisting, supporting and stimulating the individual's inherent self-healing processes."

2000 – CNA Summit

"Naturopathic Medicine is a unique profession of primary healthcare that emphasizes disease prevention and the promotion of optimal health through natural therapeutics. Naturopathic medicine is an art, science, philosophy and practice of diagnosis, treatment and prevention of illness. Naturopathic medicine is distinguished by the principles which underlie and determine its practice. These principles are based upon the objective observation of the nature of health and disease, and are continually reexamined in the light of scientific advances. Methods used are consistent with these principles and are chosen upon the basis of patient individuality. Naturopathic doctors are primary healthcare practitioners, whose diverse techniques include modern and traditional, scientific and empirical methods.

Naturopathic medicine encourages the self-healing process and blends centuries-old knowledge of natural therapies with current advances in the understanding of health and human systems. Its scope of practice includes all aspects of family and primary care, from pediatrics to geriatrics, and all natural medicine modalities.

Naturopathic doctors (N.D.'s) are the most extensively trained practitioners in the broadest scope of naturopathic medical modalities. In addition to the basic medical sciences and conventional diagnostics, naturopathic education includes: therapeutic nutrition, botanical medicine, homeopathy, natural childbirth, classical Chinese medicine, hydrotherapy, naturopathic manipulative therapy, pharmacology and minor office procedures. Naturopathic doctors tailor care to the individual patient, emphasizing prevention and self-care."

2008 – CAND Documents

"Naturopathic Medicine is a distinct primary health care system that blends modern scientific knowledge with traditional and natural forms of medicine. Naturopathic medicine is the art and science of disease diagnosis, treatment and prevention using natural therapies including botanical medicine, clinical nutrition, hydrotherapy, homeopathy, naturopathic manipulation, traditional Chinese medicine / acupuncture, and lifestyle counseling."

History of

Naturopathic Curriculum

Naturopathic medicine was founded in Europe based on the therapies of hydrotherapy and hygiene. Many of the practitioners that embraced natural therapies and that were influential in the early years were trained in conventional medicine and were looking for alternative ways of healing. Naturopathic medicine was established at the same time that chiropractic, osteopathic, physical medicine and forms of energetic healing. Many of the early practitioners were trained in multiple systems of medicine, hence the practice of naturopathic medicine has always been eclectic and diverse in the methods of treatments practiced.

The following is a historic look at the therapies that were a part of naturopathic medicine. Much of the language that was used has been retained to capture the essence of that time period.

1940's – ANPBC document

The natural methods employed for the naturopathic purposes are: manipulations, body mechanics, hydrotherapy, light therapy, nutrition, herbology, electrotherapy, and remedial psychology. The following is how each aspect was defined:

Manipulation

By manipulating the different body segments of the spinal column to restore them to their normal relative positions and thus to insure a free and unhampered movement of the joints, the functions of the nervous system can be directly affected. The nerves passing through the intervertebral foramina can be stimulated or inhibited generally or locally to produce the desired reaction in the affected organs of the body.

Recently the art of manipulation has been applied to the soft tissue of the body reportably with a considerable degree of success. This phase of the subject has become known as "bloodless surgery", because of the fact that it has saved many people the agonies and expense of medical surgery. Its purpose is the replacing of the organs to their proper positions and so promoting a better circulation of blood and lymph to and from the cells, establishing an unhampered nerve supply, and preventing and "breaking down" fibrous adhesions.

Body Mechanics

This method is defined as "the mechanical correlation of the various systems of the body with special reference to the skeletal, muscular, and visceral systems and their neurological associations. Normal body mechanics may be said to be obtained when this mechanical correlation is most favourable to the functions of these systems." The essence of this method is the formation and development of good postural habits; and so increase the vitality and resistance of the body to disease. It includes the use of braces and other mechanical aids; remedial muscle and breathing exercises; active and passive massage; and the proper methods of carrying the body in the standing, sitting, and resting positions. Its application to the body in conjunction with Manipulations is particularly valuable. The proper relationship of the different organs and tissues to one another is first accomplished by the manipulations and this is followed by such measures as exercises and rest etc, as will strengthen the body and prevent re-occurrences of the condition.

Hydrotherapy

This is defined as the "science that treats disease with water as a therapeutic agent." Water is recognized as a universal solvent and its presence is essential to all cell life. Taken internally in large quantities it acts as the eliminative processes. Applied externally in the forms of baths, douches, packs, compresses, and enemas, it produces its effect on both the nervous and circulatory systems. It might be well to quote at this time Baruch's Law – 'The effect of any hydrotherapy procedure is in direct proportion to the difference between the temperature the water is above or below that of the skin, the effect is stimulating; when the two temperatures are the same the effect is sedative.' Besides this effect of the nervous system, it is one of the most reliable measures in the regulation of the volume of the blood in different organs.

Light Therapy

The beneficial properties of sunlight used therapeutically has been recognised for ages past. It is now know that these light vibrations are of varying wavelengths and that set groups of these wavelengths produce definite physiological responses in the body. At one extreme there is the infra red rays, at the other the ultraviolet rays, while between the two are the rays which form the visible spectrum. Science today has discovered the way to produce each of these three groups through artificial means, and though the effect will never equal that from the natural source, there are definite advantages in its use. The infra red rays focused on the sin cause heating of the superficial tissues and stimulation of the specialized nerve endings in the skin. The visible light rays, used in Deep Therapy equipment, are more sedative to the nervous system and far more penetrating than the longer infra red. The shorter ultra violet rays are bactericidal in action and produce chemical changes in the bloodstream.

The visible spectrum is a composite mixture of all the colors; each color having a different rate of vibration. Each color also exerts a characteristic reaction in the body. For example, red is warming, blue is cooling, and green is soothing. The therapeutic use of colors, called, "Chrometherapy", is advantageous in the treatment of certain cases.

Nutrition

The nutritive elements of the environment, food and air, are carried by the bloodstream to all the cells of the body.

The ultimate source of all food is plant life. Plants have the capacity to change the mineral elements of the earth and combine this chemistry with the energy of the sun into organic compounds which the animal cells can assimilate, digest, and metabolize. A secondary source is animal life and its products. Since inorganic minerals cannot be utilized by the body cells, their presence in the bloodstream is toxic and destructive, and care must be exercised in the formulating of diets, to prevent or eliminate them from it.

From a chemical standpoint food is divided into five distinct classes – carbohydrates, fats, proteins, organic minerals, and vitamins. Each of these groups must be chemically complete; and available to the cells in a sufficient quantities to sustain life and health. There therapeutically, these groups given in definite proportions and combinations in the dietary of ailing patients, are of tremendous value. Their use can re-vitalize the body as whole and in turn promote the healing of local conditions.

Beside supplying all the essential needs of the body chemically, the diet must also be aesthetic to the patient. The failure to allow for this factor in the diet of each individual has been the cause of many disappointments in the application of this measure. Then too, the time consumed at each meal, and the state of the individual's emotions during the meal, are other important factors which must be considered, if the full benefit of the diet is to be expected.

In addition to the nutritive value of plants, it has been found that certain of these contain active chemical substances which have a marked healing effect on various body structures in disease. The art of administering these plants as infusions decoctions, poultices, for the treating of sickness has created the science of "herbology"

Air is a nutritive factor, necessary to cell life because of its oxygen content. An abundance of fresh air is advocated in all feverish conditions, in anemias, in resuscitation and so forth. Adequate ventilation of all public and private buildings is now provided to ensure that presence of this vital environmental force for the maintenance of health. "Air – conditioning" is the latest innovation in this regard.

Electro-Therapy

Though an enormous amount of research has been conducted on the therapeutic effect of the electric current, the manner in which these various currents exert their effect in the body is still largely a theoretical problem. It is the writer's contention that each cell in the body is a potential source of electro-chemical energy. Every cell can be compared to a battery; the protoplasm contains carbon and electrolyte acid in reaction, the surrounding lymph fluid also is an electrolyte alkaline in nature. Each cell then can accumulate and generate electrical energy, which can be converted into the other forms when needed.

In the employment of those electrical currents which have become standardized, for example diathermy, galvanism, sinusoidal, the physiological effects are produced not only through the customary channels, the blood and the nervous systems, but also directly on the body tissues. Consequently besides the action of stimulating or inhibiting the nerves to the part, and promoting changes in the composition and circulation of the bloodstream, which in turn will affect the individual cells, the current can directly produce changes beneficial or destructive in the protoplasm of the cells. The strength, duration, and extent of application as well as the type of current employed will determine the local or general sedative, stimulative, or destructive effects.

Notwithstanding the little knowledge that there is at present on the basic principles of electricity applied to the body, Electrotherapy is already one of the outstandingly successful methods within the scope of Naturopathy. And with the further development of the newer currents such as shortwave and electronics, and with a better understanding of the effects they produce in the body, this branch of the drugless arts will fill an even more prominent place in the treatment of human diseases.

Remedial Psychology

In the development of the nervous system in man, the anterior section of the neural canal becomes enlarged and specialized to form the brain. The segmental arrangement which existed previously becomes over-shadowed somewhat by the control which the brain exerts over all the rest of the body.

In childhood the sum of environmental influences impress themselves upon this specialized region to form the mind. And as previously mentioned this specialized part of the nervous system has the ability to discharge these impression (impulses) at some future time. So it may happen that relatively slight changes in the environment may affect the mind in such a way as to produce excessive reactions in different parts of the body.

This disturbance can only be corrected by applying a knowledge of Remedial Psychology to the individual in such a man-

ner that he himself can regain control of this vital center. This is often a long and tedious task, but persistence in teaching the individual the "art of living" eventually has its reward, and the results can be astonishing.

As a therapeutic measure, Remedial Psychology is becoming a necessary part of the armamentarium of every Naturopathic physician.

Naturopathy therefore embraces all these methods in the treatment of disease. Each has its place in treatment, and is most suitable for certain types of conditions. To attempt to treat all the body ailments with one method to the exclusion of all the rest is a common error made today by many physicians and one which should be corrected. Again in every case to use all the above therapeutic agents is considered extremely unscientific and unnecessary. These methods must be used intelligently and in the combinations that are indicated by the condition of the individual. Only then may one expect uniform successful results in the majority of cases.

1956 – Naturopathic Therapies

The studies of Naturopathic Therapies consideration must be given to the methods of application, indications for usage and the contra-indications of all methods of naturopathic armamentaria. The subject matter may be grouped, for convenience, into: (1) Physical and Mechanical and Manipulative Therapies; (2) biochemical Therapies; (3) Psychotherapies.

Physical and Mechanical Manipulative Therapies:

• Irradiation therapy (helio, light, ultraviolet, infra-red, chrome, etc.)

- Electrotherapy (galvanic, faradic, sinusoidal, diathermic devices, etc.)
- Thermotherapy (the use of heat in artificial fevers and sweatbaths, packs, etc.)
- Vibrotherapy (the use of oscillations, concussion, vibration and spondylotherapy)
- Remedial Exercises (kinesiotherapy, medical gymnastics, body mechanics, active and passive exercise)
- Manipulations (osseous and soft tissue manipulations, mobilization and immobilization techniques, spinal therapy, manipulative and orificial surgery, and minor surgery)
- Vasomotor Control (control of circulation from the vaso-motor area of the spine)
- Hydrotherapy
- Mechanical Therapy (the use of supporters, prosthetics, belts, casts, pneumatotherapy, zone therapy, orthopaedic devices, etc.
Crymotherapy (the use of cold as a therapeutic agency)

Biochemical Therapies:

- Nutritional Therapy (the employing of hygienic and corrective nutrition in diseases, and the correction of nutritional deficiencies.)
- Phytotherapy (the use of all naturopathic botanicals, herbal and vegetable materials listed in the Naturae Medicina)
- Biochemic Therapy (the use of all tissue minerals, and cell salts-Schuessler-; vitamins; endocrines, etc.
- Vapotherapy (vapors and gases for therapeutic prouposes)
- Colon Therapy (should include, no only the use of colonic irrigatins, but also the use of natural botanic and other products in the treatment pathoses of this region.)
- Autotherapies

- Climatiotherapy
- Antiseptics, germicides, local anesthetics, etc.

Psychotherapies:

Applied psychology
Suggestotherapy and auto-suggestion
Therapeutic hypnotism
Occupational therapeutics
Psychosomatic therapy
Psychiatry

1966 – The Nature of a Naturopath, CNA

Biochemical Therapies:

Botanical and Herbal Therapies, unguents, salves, balms and counter irritants. (ref. Naturopathic Materia Medica)
Homeopathic Remedies: Hahnemann modalities, Bach Flower Remedies
Corrective Nutrition: dietetics, physiological, cell and tissue concentrations, biological normalizers
Metabolic, biochemical, glandular balancing and restoration

Detoxification Methods

Fasting therapy
Using enemas, colonics, laxatives
Restoring and intensifying the functioning of the multiple organs of detoxification and of elimination

Therapy of Body Mechanics and Structure

Body mechanics: anatomical and orthopaedic adjustments, manipulations of solid organs and of soft tissues. Balancing and manipulating of bones and body structures – This includes: rehabilitation devices: torque resistance units, shoulder wheels, exercise pulley, hydraulic exercise units, training walkers. Prosthetic devices: lumbosacral belts supports and splints. Decongestive therapy; vaso-pneumatic devices

Physiotherapies and Physical Medicine

The application of energy forces, short-wave diathermy, ultra-sound, various frequency vibrations, balancing body energies, etc.
Active and Passive Exercises
Electrotherapy: galvanic currents, sinusoidal, faradic and pulsating currents, and other life force normalizers.
Light and Color Therapy: The use of ultra-violet, infra-red and thermal radiation lamps and chrome therapy.
Hydrotherapy, Kneipp therapy, sprays and douches
Acupuncture, acupressure, Needles, helium and neon lasers, TENS (transdermal electro neuro stimulators)

Psychological Therapies

Naturopathic Medicine recognizes the relationship between the mind and the body in the development of disease. The employment of the principles of psychology, in private practice, has become increasingly valuable in diagnosis and as a treatment. Psychology therapies include:
Patient counselling; remedial psychology; suggestion and/or hypnotherapy; restoring of self awareness, moral, and self image. Gestalt, Reality, Psychoanalysis; Scream Therapy and others.
In illnesses where psychogenic causes

are specific, the Naturopathic Physician seeks to adjust or to adapt the individual to the circumstances of "stress" – or to aid in the removal of the stress excesses, wherever possible.

Restoration of Life Forces, Energy Reserves, Healing Ability

Neuro biochemical restoration and revitalisation
Relaxation therapy, Polarity therapy
Electro-pulsating magnetic force fields

Clinical Ecology

2008 – CAND documents

The therapies taught and used by naturopathic doctors include:

Clinical Nutrition

Nutrition and the therapeutic use of foods have always been a cornerstone of naturopathic medicine. A growing body of scientific knowledge in this area is reflected in nutrition and dietary sciences, validating the naturopathic approach to diet and nutrition. Many medical conditions can be treated as effectively with foods and nutritional supplements as they can by any other means, but with fewer complications and adverse effects.

History and Symptomatology: The collecting of all data relating to the specific nature of disease and body disability – its causes and influence – through the use of organized questionnaires and systematized methods of correlating all information and findings. To the Naturopathic Physician, comprehension of a complete and accurate history is essential to determine the pre-disposing and etiological factors of disease. These underlying causes of the ailment are give special attention in formulating treatment, especially on a systemic level.

Comprehensive Physical Examinations

To be complete, the physical examination requires a thorough use of auscultation, palpation, percussion, the "reading" of body shapes and appearance and the inspection and visualisation of as many as possible of the different organs and tissues of the body. The use of sphygmomanometer, stethoscope, laryngoscope, nasocope, otoscope, oesophagoscope, gasgtroscope, sigmoidoscope, protoscope, rectal and vaginal speculae, cystoscope, other orifice examining speculae, dilators and catheters thermometer, tape measures, are standard procedures. Iridology, visualizing the iris of the eye through a magnifying glass or microscope can provide valuable information concerning the stages f tissue and organ changes and breakdown, even long periods of time prior to recognizable symptoms or physical changes.

Physiological Tests

Most physical examinations of the past included an evaluation of the structures of the body, only. Early stages of disease and degeneration frequently manifest, first through changes in the functions of the different organs. Special emphasis is placed upon the assessment of the functional and neurological activities of the organs and tissues. The physiology and early changes can be recognized through such instruments as the Endo(phono) cardiograph, heartometer, and/or Doppler.

Circulation physiology is readily evaluated through the use of an oscilloscope – and by visualizing the fundus of the eye by means of an opthalmoscope or a retinoscope.

Neurological examinations are valuable and possible by use of simple instruments such as the reflex hammer, tuning fork, brush and needle.

Total body organs are evaluated through instruments such as the Voll Diagnostic instrument.

The Bioscript readily determines and pinpoints vitality, degeneration, nerve and organ irritation and inflammation in various segments of the body.

A respirometer and other vital capacity measuring devices can be evaluations essential to a complete diagnosis.

Other valuable testes: Photometric diagnostic apparatuses, electromyographs, photomographs, thyroid testing devices.

Accepted Laboratory Procedures: blood, urine, feces, and hair analysis procedures. Simple laboratory tests to evaluate haemoglobin, urine and feces are easily performed in office practices. These can include: blood sugars, blood proteins, blood sedimentation rates, hematocrits, urine calcium, urine potassium, etc. Blood coagulation cross matching testes set ups are available for determining many fo the common allergies. Other tests involving more complicated or more expensive laboratory equipment are readily available for doing different blood tests. Serological and bacteriological and more complex tests are best referred to competent laboratories.

Nutritional Surveys: Many Naturopathic Physicians include this as a part of the routine health evaluation procedure. Some use computerized forms of nutritional evaluation to determine specific deficiencies and body needs.

X-Ray Diagnosis: Whenever required, radiology is used in establishing a diagnosis. Many naturopathic physicians provide X-ray facilities in their offices.

Interpretations and evaluations of all clinical findings: Including diagnostic summaries, computer correlation and interpretations, and the use of various charts and manuals.

2008 – CAND documents

The therapies taught and used by naturopathic doctors include: ***Clinical Nutrition***
Nutrition and the therapeutic use of foods have always been a cornerstone of naturopathic medicine. A growing body of scientific knowledge in this area is reflected in nutrition and dietary sciences, validating the naturopathic approach to diet and nutrition. Many medical conditions can be treated as effectively with foods and nutritional supplements as they can by any other means, but with fewer complications and adverse effects.

Botanical Medicine

Many plant substances are powerful medicines, with advantages over conventional drugs. They are effective and safe, when used properly, in the right dose and in the proper combinations with other herbs or treatments. Herbs can be prepared in many forms – teas, tinctures or capsules. Naturopathic physicians are trained in both the art and the science of botanical medicine.

Homeopathic Medicine

This powerful system of medicine is more than 200 years old, and is widely accepted in other countries. Homeopathic remedies are made from specific dilutions of plant, animal, and mineral substances. When carefully matched to the patient they are able to affect the body's "vital force" and to stimulate the body's innate healing forces on the structural, functional, and psychological level, with few adverse effects. Some conditions that conventional medicine has no effective treatment for respond well to homeopathic medicine.

Oriental Medicine / Acupuncture

The key principle that defines and connects all of Chinese medicine is that of Chi, or vital energy. The chi of all organs must be in balance, neither too active nor too dormant, for a person to be healthy. The chi of the body's organs and systems are all connected in meridians or channels that lie just under the skin. A Naturopathic Doctor will use Eastern herbs and acupuncture to assist the body in regulating the Chi and achieving balance. Acupuncture is the use of very thin needles which are inserted into specific meridian points. The practice of acupuncture has been around for over two thousand years and has proven to be very effective especially for pain relief and chronic illness.

Physical Medicine

In the last 100 years, various methods of applying treatments through the manipulation of the muscles, bones and spine have been developed. Naturopathic medicine has its own techniques, collectively known as naturopathic manipulative therapy. Physical medicine also includes, but is not limited to, physical therapy using heat and cold, electrical pulses, ultrasound, diathermy, hydrotherapy, and exercise therapy.

Lifestyle and Stress Management Counselling

Mental attitudes and emotional states can be important elements in healing and disease. Addressing all aspects of a person's life, identifying and addressing the impact that stress and life events have a person's health are an important aspect of naturopathic treatment. Naturopathic doctors are trained to counsel on diet, lifestyle, specific stressors, exercise and occupational or environmental hazards as an integral part of the naturopathic treatment program.

Other Natural Therapies

The naturopathic therapies used varies by practitioner and by province. Some Naturopathic Doctors have additional training in other naturopathic therapies such as :
- IV therapies
- Chelation therapy
- Minor Surgery
- Colon Therapy
- Acupuncture
- Vibrational medicine – including sound therapy, light therapy, and other new technologies.

TIMELINE

Early BC: The concepts of vitalism and holism are the basis of health and disease
             The use of botanicals and herbal medicine
             The use of acupuncture
             Food, exercise, hot baths and following the laws of nature were used to heal the sick

460-377 BC   Hippocrates: father of conventional and naturopathic medicine
             Hippocrates: embraces the concepts of vitalism and holism

469–399 BC   Socrates: one of the founders of Western philosophy, defines vitalism

428-348 BC   Plato: one of the founders of Western philosophy

384-322 BC   Aristotle: one of the founders of Western philosophy, defines vitalism

129-200 BC   Galen: vital processes in an organism must be interpreted in relation to its environment

1004   Quarantine concept introduced as a way of limiting spread of infectious diseases such as tuberculosis

1135 – 1204 Moses Maimonides: emphasized diet, exercise, and positive mental outlook

1223   The term 'physician' is coined

1300 – 1650 Renaissance period: body is starting to be understood on the basis of chemistry and physics

1348   Venice establishes 1st institutionalized system of quarantine

1439   Johannes Gutenberg: invents the mechanical printing press

1493 – 1541 Paracelsus: disease due to toxins in food and drink
             Paracelsus: advocates talk therapy
             Paracelsus: explains disease as chemical process

1590   Zaccharias Janssen and his son Hans: two Dutch spectacle makers, invented the technology for the microscope

1596 – 1650 René Descartes: introduces dualism, the theory that mind and body are separate
             Descartes: introduces mechanistic concept of human beings

1623 – 1723 Anton van Leeuwenhoek: builds the first microscope in Holland

1624 – 1689 Thomas Sydenham: focuses on identifying the cause of disease - often lifestyle - and the natural healing ability of the body

1643 – 1727 Isaac Newton: provides theories of gravitation, the laws of motion, and the ground work for classical mechanics

1660 – 1734 George Ernst Stahl: reintroduces the concept of a soul or vital essence in humans

1693   The first mail delivery happened between Quebec City and Montreal

1712 – 1778 Jean Jacques Rousseau: fuels the nature cure movement

1755 – 1843 Samuel Hahnemann: founder of homeopathy

1762 – 1836 Christoph Wilhelm Hufeland: founder of holistic medicine, uses hydrotherapy, air and light therapies, vegetarian diets and herbal remedies

1774   Benjamin Jesty: a farmer in England, first recording of vaccinating humans –inoculated his wife and two sons with smallpox

1798   Edward Jenner: coined the term vaccination from the latin root for cow: 'vacca' from his use of preventing small pox infection by inoculation

1798 – 1856   Johann Schroth: student of Priessnitz, introduces moist heat therapy, recom mends fasting and dry food

1799 – 1851   Vincent Priessnitz: founder of hydrotherapy, uses cold water therapy

Late 1700s   Anatomy and physiology integral part of medicine

1765   The first US medical school is opened in Philadelphia, USA

1794 – 1851   Graham Sylvester: an American practitioner, one of the founders of the hygienic school of thought

1798 – 1859   William Alcott: an American practitioner, one of the founders of the hygienic school of thought. Prior to early 1800s medicine is done by layman and is domestically oriented

1805 – 1848   J.H. Rausse: first to lay down the scientific principles of water cure

1809 – 1882   Charles Darwin: separation of man from his environment, survival of the fittest

1812 – 1877   Russell Thacker Trall: promotes hydropathic and hygienic treatments and eclectic practice, a prolific author

1816   René Laënnec: a French physician who invents the stethoscope

1821 – 1894   Father Sebastian Kneipp: promotes hydrotherapy and holistic healthy lifestyle Kneipp: link between European nature cure and American naturopathy

1823 – 1906   Arnold Rikli: founder of light and air cures, introduces contrast water baths, and the use of steam

1824   The first Canadian medical school is opened in Montreal

1824 – 1883   Theodor Hahn: furthers hydrotherapy, vegetarianism and promotes self-responsibility

1825   Hans Burch Gram (1787-1840): brings homeopathy to America

1830s   Isaac Jennings, Sylvester Graham and William Alcott: fathers of hygiene movement

1831 – 1903   Dr. Emily Stowe, MD: One of the first Canadian woman physicians. Trained in the United States, as Canadian medical schools did not allow women in those days. Also trained as a homeopath. She practiced in Toronto and focused on women's health.

1833   Dr. Constantine Hering (1800-1880): immigrates to America and later became known as the father of American Homeopathy

1834   William Kelly: introduces idea of preventing the spread of disease via sanitation

1835 – 1907   Louis Kuhne: introduces concept of "unit of disease" and disease due to excess foreign matter or food in the body. A prolific author, advocates vegetarian diet and raw food

1839   College of Physicians and Surgeons is established (incorporated in 1869)

~1840   Chas. Lauterisser: opens 1st Kneipp sanatorium, in New Jersey

1843 - 1903   F.E. Blitz: popularizes water cure and coordinates many natural systems of healing, renames Schroth treatment to regenerative treatment, opened a Nature Cure sanitarium, prolific author including an encyclopaedia of Nature Cure

1844   The Canadian Medical Assocation (CMA) is started, an official association in

1867

1844   American Institute for Homeopathy is formed, the first national medical association in the United States.

1844	Russell Trall: opens the second water cure sanatorium in America
1846	American Medical Association (AMA) is founded
1850 – 1924	Ernst Schweninger: establishes first nature cure hospital, located in Berlin
1851	Hermann von Helmholtz from Germany: invents the ophthalmoscope
1852	Russell Trall: establishes the 1st school of natural healing arts, New York Hygieo-Therapeutic College that has a 4-year curriculum and which grants the degree of Medical Doctor upon graduation.
1852 – 1942	John Tilden: propounded theory of auto-intoxication or toxaemia, prolific author
1852 – 1943	John Harvey Kellogg: prolific author, patents first 'health food' cereal
1853:	Term psychotherapeutics is coined
1856 – 1926	Emanuel Felk: introduces clay poultices
1859 – 1939	Adolph Just: introduces concept of healing crisis, promotes self-care and responsibilities
1860 – 1905	Heinrich Lahmann: one of the first scientific nature doctors
1861 – 1865	American Civil War
1862 – 1924	Henry Lindlahr: founder of scientific naturopathy
1863	James Caleb Jackson: creates granola
1864	Louis Pasteur (1822 – 1895): a French microbiologist: furthers the understanding of the germ theory
1865 – 1885	Homeopathy flourishes in America
1865 – 1933	Franz Schönenberger: one of the first University professors for nature cure methods
1866	British Columbia becomes a Colony of the British Empire, and the regulation of medicine in B.C. comes under English common law. According to common law persons are free to practice any school of medicine – from homeopathy to surgery – as long as they do not misrepresent their credentials; the public are free to choose from the full range of medical practitioners, but are also respon sible for the consequences of their choice. Medicine at this time is pluralistic in its theories and divided among several.
1867	Dominion of Canada formed uniting Ontario, Quebec, New Brunswick and Nova Scotia
1867	The Governor and Legislative Council of the Colony of B.C. enacts The Medical Ordinance to enable persons to distinguish qualified from unqualified practitioners.
1868 – 1925	Louisa Lust: naturopathic doctor, wife of Benedict Lust, financially supports the early growth of naturopathic medicine
1868 - 1955	Bernarr Macfadden: leader of the physical culture movement
1870	Manitoba and Northwest Territories joined Canada
1870s	Medical schools start to introduce hands-on approach
1871	British Columbia added to the Dominion of Canada
1871	Harvard University creates the 1st four-year medical educational curriculum in America
1872 – 1945	Benedict Lust: father of American naturopathy
1873	Prince Edward Island (PEI) added to the Dominion of Canada
1873 – 1948	Fredrick W Collins: embraces the eclectic aspect of naturopathic medicine, establishes the first free naturopathic clinic
1874	Andrew Taylor Still (1828 – 1917): founds osteopathy
1876	Alexander Graham Bell: invents the telephone. First call occurred in Mount

	Pleasant, Ontario
1879 – 1962	Otis G. Carroll: introduces constitutional hydrotherapy and the concept of food sensitivities
1880s	Prior to this anyone could hang up a shingle, with no formal education, and call themselves a doctor
1885 – 1992	Niels Bohr: a Danish physicist who contributed to quantum mechanics and how received a Nobel prize in physics in 1922
1886	B.C. enacts The Medical Act to regulate the practice of medicine (including homeopathy) and surgery
1887 – 1961	Erwin Schrödinger: an Australian theoretical physicist who contributed to the discovers of quantum mechanics, especially the Schrödinger equation, for which he received the Nobel prize in 1933
1889 – 1946	Joe Shelby Riley: embraces eclectic aspect of naturopathic medicine, introduces acupuncture, reflexology and zone therapy into naturopathic medicine
1891	A. Reinhold: opens a Kneipp Sanitarium, located in New York
1891	John's Hopkin's University and other schools adopt a four-year medical program
1892	Andrew Steel, MD: founds the first school of Osteopathy, American School of Osteopathy in Missouri
1893 – 1966	George Ohsawa: a Japanese philosopher who founds the macrobiotic diet
1895	Daniel David Palmer: a Canadian born in Port Perry, Ontario establishes chiropractic
1895	Dr. John Scheel: a German homeopath who coins the term Naturopathy. The term was purchased by Benedict Lust in 1902.
1895	Wilhelm Konrad von Roentgen from Germany: invents the X-ray
1896	Benedict Lust: brings Nature Cure to America
1897	First school of chiropractic, Palmer School of Chiropractic, is established in Iowa
1897	James T. Kent: publishes his first homeopathic repertory
1897	Ernst Duchesne: describes the antibiotic properties of penicillium sp.
1898	Yukon added to Canada
1898 – 1964	Alfred Brauchle: cooperation between natural and allo pathic medicine: The great nature cure experiment in Dresden hospital
1898 – 1991	Arno R. Koegler: influential Canadian ND, teacher, involved in securing Ontario regulation, promoted the use of homeopathy and iridology.
1900	Benedict Lust: opens 1st naturopathic school, American School of Naturopathy in New York City
1900 – 1958	Wolfgang Pauli: an Australian theoretical physicist who was instrumental in the development of quantum mechanics
1901	American Osteopathic Association is founded
1901	*Journal of the American Medical Association* begins
1901	Robert Foster: establishes a naturopathic school in Idaho
1901	Kneipp convention which is held in New York marks the birth of Naturopathy in America
1901 – 1976	Werner Heisenberg: a German theoretical physicist who asserted the uncertainty principle of quantum theory
1901 – 1978	Margaret Mead: an American cultural anthropologist who contributed to the discovery of Systems Theory
1902	Benedict Lust: opens Yungborn Sanitarium in New Jersey
1902 – 1944	Linus Pauling: scientist who won two Nobel prizes, focused on the healing

	power of Vitamin C.
1904	AMA creates Council on Medical Education
1904 – 1980	Gregory Bateson: a British anthropologist who contributed to the discovery of Systems Theory
1905	Saskatchewan and Alberta added to Canada
1906	Lindlahr Sanitarium for Nature Cure and Osteopathy opens in Chicago
1909	Pacific College of Chiropractic opens
1909	State of California is the first State to acquire legislation for naturopathic medicine
1909	Paul Ehrlich: develops the narrow spectrum antibiotic salvarson which is used for syphilis. Early 1900s Government run hospitals are started
1910	The Carnegie Foundation issues the Flexner report sponsored by the AMA
~1910	Henry Lindlahr: founds the Lindlahr College of Nature Cure and Osteopathy, later renamed to the Lindlahr College of Natural Therapeutics, a leading naturopathic college of its day.
1912 - 1995	John Bastyr: father of modern day naturopathic medicine
1914	Benedict Lust: opens Yungborn Sanitarium in Florida
1915	Drugless Physicians Association is formed in Ontario, later dissolved in 1952
1916 – 1987	Joseph A. Boucher: an inspiring teacher and advocate of naturopathic medicine
1917 – 1937	Halcyon years for naturopathic medicine
1917 – 1992	David Joseph Bohm: an American-born quantum physicist who made significant contributions in the fields of theoretical physics, philosophy and neuropsychology
1918	First airmail delivery, occurred between Montreal and Toronto
1920	Over 20 naturopathic schools in the United States
~1920	Ragnar Berg (1873 – 1956): introduces acid/alkaline concept
1920	Allopathic physicians and surgeons are licensed in all jurisdictions in the United States
1920	British Columbia (BC) provincial association starts
1920	Connecticut licenses naturopathic doctors
1921	Amendment to the B.C. Medical Act allows the practice of naturopathy and chiropractic
1922	Fredrick Banting and J.J.R. Macleod, two Canadian scientists: discover insulin
1923	Northwest College of Naturopathy is founded
1923	British Columbia regulated under *The Medical Act*
1925	Ontario regulated under umbrella legislation *Drugless Practitioner's Act*
1927	Beginning of residency programs in hospitals
1927	2000 NDs in America, 10,000 practitioners at naturopathic conferences
1928	Alexander Fleming: discovers penicillin
1929 – 1939	Great Depression
1930	Many of the naturopathic schools had either closed or were hanging on by a thread
1930	Institute of Naturopathic Sanipractic Physicians is formed
1932	Pacific College of Chiropractic is reorganized and renamed Western States College
1936	British Columbia is regulated under *Naturopathic Physician's Act*
1936	Association of Naturopathic Physicians of British Columbia (ANPBC) is established as both the provincial association and the regulatory board
1937	Ontario's regulation is revised
1938	BC's regulation is revised

1939 – 1945	World War II
1940s	Hahnemann Medical School, last US medical school to teach homeopathy discontinues its program
1944	Naturopathic Association of Alberta is established
1944	Ontario's regulation is revised
1946	Manitoba regulated under *The Naturopathy Act*
1946	Manitoba Naturopathic Association (MNA) was incorporated as both the provincial association and the regulatory body
1948	Alberta regulated under *Drugless Practitioner's Act*
1948	BCs regulation is revised
1948	Alberta Association of Naturopathic Practitioners (AANP) is established as both the regulatory body and the provincial association
1949	Newfoundland joined Canada
1949	Canadian national association started under the name Canadian Association of Naturopathic Physicians (CANP), name is later changed to CNA when it is incorporated in 1955
1950	Ontario Naturopathic Association (ONA) is established
1950	Alberta's regulation is revised
1952	AANP is incorporated
1952	Alberta's regulation is revised, name changes to *The Naturopathic Act*
1952	Ontario's regulation is revised
1953	23 states have received government recognition or licensure
1954	National College in Chicago closes
1954	Saskatchewan is regulated under *The Naturopathy Act*
1954	Saskatchewan Association of Naturopathic Practitioners (SANP) was established as both the provincial association and the regulatory board
1955	Alberta's regulation is revised
1955	Canadian Naturopathic Association (CNA) is incorporated
1955	Western States Chiropractic College (the last in the US to have a ND program) discontinues its ND program
1956	Ontario's regulation is revised
1956	National College of Naturopathic Medicine (NCNM) is founded
1956	Inaugural convention for Northwest Naturopathic Physicians Convention
1956	Board of Directors of Drugless Therapy – Naturopathy (BDDT-N) is established
1957	Canadian government passes Hospital Insurance and Diagnostic Services Act (HIDS)
1958	NCNM moves to Seattle
1958	National Association of Naturopathic Physicians (NANP) is formed by merging The American Association of Naturopathic Physicians (different organization than present AANP) and the American Naturopathic Association
1958	BC's regulation is revised
1961	All provinces agree to start HIDS
1961 – 1965	Royal Commission on Health Services
1962	Saskatchewan's Medical Care Insurance Act – 1st Canadian comprehensive public health-care system
1963	Quebec Naturopathic Association of Physical Therapy (QNAPT)
1963	AMA refuses to continue to examine chiropractors for licensure
1963	Chiropractors establish their own examining boards

1963	AMA establishes the committee on quackery for the purpose of discrediting alternative practitioners
1963	Unity meeting between Canada and the US with respect to the definition of naturopathic medicine
1964	Ontario Chiropractic Association urges members not to renew their ND license
1965	ND services are covered partly under BC's medicare
1965	Saskatchewan's regulation is revised
1966	Malpractice insurance first instituted in Canada
1966	Amendment to the B.C. Medical Act which effectively eliminated the legal practice of homeopathy (by medical doctors). Naturopathic doctors were still allowed to practice homeopathy as it was part of their curriculum
1968	National medicare in Canada
1969	Osteopathic doctors are granted full active membership in the AMA
1970	Joint CNA and Northwest Naturopathic Convention
1971	The College of Emporia agrees to teach the 1st and 2nd years of NCNM
1972	CNA publishes booklet *Naturopathy*
1973	College of Emporia closes
1973	NCNM transfers first two years of program to Kansas Newman College
1974	Chiropractors licensed in all 50 States
1974	ONA requests that NCNM teach acupuncture
1975	Number of US states that have naturopathic regulation drops to seven
1976	NCNM moves back to Portland
1977	The AMA's Judicial Council adopts new opinions which permitted medical physicians to refer patients to chiropractors
1977	Canadian Memorial Chiropractic College (CMCC) ends it naturopathic program
1978	Ontario College of Naturopathic Medicine is founded
1978	John Bastyr College of Naturopathic Medicine (Bastyr) is founded
1978	Council of Naturopathic Medical Education (CNME), the Federation of Naturopathic Boards, and the Federation of Naturopathic Colleges are formed
1978	Saskatchewan's regulation is revised
1979	First medical residencies are offered by NCNM
1979	BC's regulation is revised, name changes to *The Naturopath's Act*
1980	Alberta's regulation is revised
1982	National Association of Naturopathic Physicians (NANP), the oldest professional naturopathic organization in the United States files for bankruptcy.
1983	Global AIDs concern
1983	Institute of Naturopathic Education and Research (INER) is established
1984	Canada Health Act – prohibits user fees and extra billing
1984	Saskatchewan's regulation is revised
1985	American Association of Naturopathic Physicians (AANP) is founded
1985	Textbook of Natural Medicine is published by Dr. Joe Pizzorno, the first new naturopathic textbook since mid 1940s
1986	Alberta is deregulated
1986	Naturopathic Physicians Licensing Exams (NPLEX) is founded
1986	BC's regulation is revised, name changes to *Naturopath's Act of British Columbia*
1987	CNME is formally recognized by the US Department of Education
1987	Nova Scotia Association of Naturopathic Doctors (NSAND) is established

1988	Internet begins and is opened for commercial interests
1988	Canadian Naturopathic Educational Research Society (CNERS) is established
1992	Southwest College of Naturopathic Medicine (SCNM) is founded
1992	OCNM name changes to Canadian College of Naturopathic Medicine (CCNM)
1993	British Columbia Naturopathic Association (BCNA) splits from ANPBC
1994	Nova Scotia Association of Naturopathic Doctors (NSAND) is formed
1995	Quebec Professional Association of Naturopathic Physicians (QPANP) / Association Professionelle Des Médicins Naturopathes Du Québec is formed
1997	ONA changes its name to Ontario Association of Naturopathic Doctors (OAND)
1997	Bridgeport University's naturopathic medical program is created
1997	CNERS changes it name to Canadian Naturopathic Foundation (CNF)
1997	ONA changes its name to OAND
1998	CNME approval is withdrawn by US Department of Education
1998	QPANP is renamed to Quebec Association of Naturopathic Medicine (QANM) / Association de Medicine Nauropathique Du Québec (ANMQ)
1999	Nunavut joins Canada
2000	CCNM receives full accreditation from CNME
2000	CNA Summit is held at CCNM
2000	ANPBC changes its name to College of Naturopathic Physicians of British Columbia (CNPBC)
2000	Phil Waddington ND is appointed Executive Director for the Office of Natural Products and in 2001 becomes the 1st Director General of the Natural Health Products Directorate (NHPD) in Ottawa
2000	North American Board of Naturopathic Examiners (NABNE) is established
2001	Boucher Institute of Naturopathic Medicine is founded
2001	New Brunswick Association of Naturopathic Doctors (NBAND) is formed
2001	American Association of Naturopathic Medical Colleges (AANMC) is formed
2003	CNME approval is reinstated by the US Department of Education
2001	Yukon Naturopathic Association (YNA) is founded
2004	CNA name changed to Canadian Association of Naturopathic Doctors (CAND)
2004	Prince Edward Island Association of Naturopathic Doctors (PEIAND) is formed
2006	Newfoundland Association of Naturopathic Doctors (NLAND) is formed
2007	CNF administration transferred to the CAND
2008	Alberta is re-regulated under the *Naturopathy Act*
2008	Ontario's regulation is revised and the name changes to the *Naturopathy Act*. Once it passes through the transition council, the regulation will fall under the Regulated Health Professions Act (RHPA) of Ontario
2008	Nova Scotia receives title protection under the *Naturopathic Doctors Act* 2008 BINM receives full accreditation from CNME

Canadian Association of Naturopathic Doctors (CAND)
www.cand.ca

Association History
1949   National association started under the name Canadian Association of Naturopathic Physicians (CANP).

1955   Canadian Naturopathic

1995   CNA headquarters moved from Calgary, Alberta to Toronto, Ontario.

2004   Name changed from CNA to Canadian Association of Naturopathic Doctors (CAND).

Founding Members
Dr. Fred Parsons ND
Dr. Ruth Else Budd ND
Dr. Ross Skaken ND
Dr. Lawrence Schnell ND
Dr. Verdean Fulton ND

Honourary Lifetime Members
Honourary Lifetime Members are members in good standing whose contribution to naturopathic medicine has been recognized by the CAND board of directors.
Dr. Gerald Farnsworth ND
Dr. Ross Skaken ND
Dr. Robert Fleming ND
Dr. Fred Loffler ND
Dr. Carl Phillips ND

Founders Club
Founder's Club members are active members in good standing who have supported the CAND through a one-time $5,000 contribution.

Dr. Fareed Omar ND
Dr. Wayne Steinke ND
Dr. Christopher Turner ND

Interim Chairperson of CANP
1949 - 1955   Dr. Fred Parson ND

Chairs of the CNA
1955 - 1957   Fred Parson ND
1957 - 1958   Albert Russell ND
1958 - 1960   Ross Skaken ND
1960 - 1965   Douglas Kirkbride ND
1965 - 1974   Lawrence Schnell ND

1978 - 1980   William Morris ND
1980 - 1985   Joseph Boucher ND
1985 - 1987   Roger McHan ND
1987 - 1989   John Cosgrove ND
1989 - 1991   Philip Kempling ND
1991 - 1994   Kelly Farnsworth ND
1994 - 1996   Donald Warren ND
1996 - 1999   Lois Hare ND
1999 - 2001   Robert vanHorlick ND
2001 - 2003   Wayne Steinke ND

Chairs of the CAND
2003 - 2004   Kevin Jackson ND
2004 - 2005   Walter Lemmo ND
2005 - 2008   Iva Lloyd ND
2008 -   Jason Boxtart ND

Membership
1960: 22
1964: 47 (~300 NDs in Canada)
1970: 80
1996: 110
2000: 313
2002: 448

2005: 862
2008: 1179

Canadian Naturopathic Foundation (CNF)
www.cand.ca

Association History
1988 Canadian Naturopathic Educational Research Society (CNERS) established as chartable society.

1997 Name changed to Canadian Naturopathic Foundation (CNF) and converted to a charitable foundation.

2007 Administration transferred to the CAND.

Founding Members
Dr. Robert Fleming ND
Ann Fleming

Chairs of the CNERS
1987 - 1990	Anthony J. Boucher
1990 - 1993	Scott Tyler ND
1993 - 1995	Robert Fleming ND
1995 - 1996	Edward Sleigh ND
1996 - 1997	Robert Fleming ND

Chairs of the CNF
1997 - 1999	Robert Fleming ND
1999 - 2000	Cindy Franklin
2000 - 2002	David Wang ND
2002 - 2003	Brian Martin ND
2003 - 2006	Walter Lemmo ND
2006 - 2008	Gerald Farnsworth ND
2008 -	John Cosgrove ND

Scholarships
Dr. Joseph Boucher Scholarship
Awarded to a third year student who demonstrates the highest overall level of achievement, both scholastically and clinically.

Mrs. Angeline Fleming Scholarship
Awarded to a second year student who has achieved sound academic standing, exhibited perseverance and dedication, and performed volunteer service of benefit to the school and the student body.

Dr. Wendy Bayley Scholarship
Awarded to a student who is of sound academic standing and has made exceptional contributions of time and energy to the advancement of naturopathic medicine.

CNF Scholarships
1989	Sheree Campbell	Bastyr
	Sherry Ure	NCNM
	Anke Zimmerman	OCNM
1990	Susan Hamilton	Bastyr
	Bernard Larouche	NCNM
	Saveria Zambri	OCNM
1991	John Miller	NCNM
	Jeffrey Hunt	OCNM
	Dorothea Durward	Bastyr
1992	Lawrence Brkich	NCNM
	Cameron Dodds	Bastyr
	Kathy Graham	OCNM
	Robert Ewing	Bastyr
	Ursula Meyer	NCNM
	Lysianne Swolfs	NCNM
1993	Todd Farnsworth	NCNM
	Ruth Anne Baron	OCNM
	Lorne Swetlikoff	Bastyr
1994	Suzanne Danner	NCNM
	Mark Stengler	NCNM
	Gayle Devaux	CCNM
	MayLynn Woo	Bastyr
1995	Laura Kantor	CCNM
1996	Zerlene Mekdeci	CCNM
1997	Elaine Stroud	CCNM
	Heli McPhie	CCNM
1998	Tanya Baldwin	CCNM
	Arvin Jenab	CCNM
1999	Molly Brass	CCNM
	Caleb Ng	CCNM
2000	Jennifer Forgeron	CCNM
	Howard Owens	CCNM
2001	David Lescheid	CCNM
2002	Shawna Darou	CCNM
2004	Caroline Meyer	CCNM
	Suzanna Ivanovics	CCNM

British Columbia Naturopathic Association (BCNA)

www.bcna.ca

Regulation History

Status: regulated
Initial Regulation: 1923 - The Medical Act
First ND Regulation: 1936 c204 - Naturopathic Physicians Act
Revised: 1938 - Naturopathic Physicians Act
Revised: 1948 c239 - Naturopathic Physicians Act
Revised: 1958 - Naturopathic Physicians Act
Revised: 1979 c 297 - Naturopaths Act
Revised: 1986 - Naturopaths Act of British Columbia

College of Naturopathic Physicians of British Columbia (CNPBC)

www.cnpbc.bc.ca

Association History

1936 Association of Naturopathic Physicians of British Columbia (ANPBC) - both the provincial association and the regulatory body.

1993 Split between Regulatory Board and Provincial Association. Provincial Association adopted the name British Columbia Naturopathic Association (BCNA).

2000 Name of Regulatory Board changed from ANPBC to College of Naturopathic Physicians of British Columbia (CNPBC).

Chairs of the ANPBC

1936 - 1939	W. Arthur Paskins ND
1939 - 1940	Joseph Wright ND
1940 - 1942	Arthur Hilton ND
1942 - 1946	W. Arthur Paskins ND
1946 - 1948	Frank Dorchester ND
1948 - 1959	Albert Russell ND
1959 - 1966	Ronald Holtum ND
1966 - 1977	Douglas Kirkbride ND
1977 - 1981	Allen Tyler MD ND
1981 - 1983	Joseph Boucher ND
1983 - 1987	Malcolm Cass ND
1987 - 1988	Brian Vallee ND
1988 - 1990	Kelly Farnsworth ND
1990 - 1992	Stefan Kuprowsky ND
1992 - 1993	Kerry McGuinness ND
1993 - 1995	Lisa Connoly ND
1995 - 1996	Heather Marinaccio ND
1996 - 1997	Kelly Farnsworth ND
1998 - 1999	Heathir Naesgaard ND

Chairs of the CNPBC

2000 - 2003	Brian Martin ND
2003 -	Lorne Swetlikoff ND

Chairs of the BCNA

1993 - 1998	Eugene Pontius ND
1998 - 2000	Braven Rayne ND
2000 - 2002	David Wang ND
2003 - 2007	Garrett Swetlikoff ND
2007 -	Christoph Kind ND

Membership

1989: 54
2000: 149
2008: 279

Points of Interest

1959 All members charged $5 per month to support a public relations program.

1965 September 1st, the British Columbia provincial health care plan was launched. The BC plan included naturopathic physicians at the rates of $6 for the first office visit; subsequent office visits at $5; house call - first visit was $8 and additional house calls were $6. There was also a limit of $50 per patient and a maximum of $100 in any one year per contract. Lab services and X-rays were not paid under the plan. In

1972 the fees were raised to $10 for an emergency, $9 for the first house call, $7 for subsequent house calls, $8 for the first office visit and $6 for subsequent consult.

1972 The ANPBC included a "school assessment" fee in the quarterly dues. Each member contributed $5 per month to support National College of Naturopathic Medicine.

1978 The ANPBC established a Minimum Fee Schedule for the first time.

1993 The BC regulatory and provincial associations split. The provincial association adopted the name BCNA, the regulatory board kept the name ANPBC.

Alberta Association of Naturopathic Practitioners (AANP)

www.naturopathic-alberta.com

Association History

1945 The Naturopathic Association of Alberta was incorporated under the Societies Act.

1948 Alberta Association of Naturopathic Practitioners (AANP) was incorporated as both the provincial association and the regulatory body.

Regulation History

Status: regulated
Initial Regulation: 1948 c84 - Drugless Practitioner's Act
Revised: 1950 c 21 - Drugless Practitioner's Act
Revised: 1952 c 61 - The Naturopathy Act
Revised: 1955 - The Naturopathy Act
Revised: 1980 - The Naturopathy Act
Revised: 1986 - deregulated, Naturopathy Act was repealed
Revised: 2008 - Naturopathy Act

Chairs of the AANP

1945 - 1947	Colin Skaken ND
1947 - 1948	Ross Skaken ND
1948 - 1952	Fred Parsons ND
1953 - 1954	Ross Skaken ND
1954 - 1959	Fred Parson ND
1959 - 1964	Clifford Peterson ND
1971 - 1984	Roger J. McHan ND
1984 - 1986	Ross Skaken ND
1986 - 1999	Roger McHan ND
1999 - 2000	Karen Jensen ND
2000 - 2001	Karen Jensen ND and Patricia Wales ND
2001 - 2007	Michael Nowazek ND
2007 -	Allissa Gaul ND

Membership

1963: 32
2000: 38
2008: 98

Points of Interest

1951 Naturopathic Drs. Fred Parson and Ruth Budd met with college officials from CMCC to propose the financial support of a department of naturopathic medicine at CMCC.

1959 All healing arts were placed under the jurisdiction of the Minister of Health.

1960 NDs lost the use of the government supported diagnostic laboratories.

1961 The Medical Act was amended to prevent anyone but a member of the College of Physicians and Surgeons from using the title or designation "physician".

1962 X-ray bill was introduced that would limit the access of naturopathic doctors. Due to vigilance and a fairly large expenditure of funds the association was included in the exemption section along with medicine, dentistry, chiropractor, etc.

1976 July 1st - The Alberta Health Plan program was inaugurated. At that time it covered naturopathic services, yet the coverage was on an optional basis and a double premium had to be paid. The initial payment schedule was $6 for the first visit and $4 for each additional office visit with a maximum of $100 per patient per year and a flat $10 rate for X-rays.

Saskatchewan Association of Naturopathic Practitioners (SANP)

www.sanp.ca

Association History

1954   Saskatchewan Association of Naturopathic Practitioners (SANP) was incorporated as both the provincial association and the regulatory body.

Regulation History

Status: regulated
Initial Regulation: 1954 c75 - The Naturopathy Act
Revised: 1965 c324 - The Naturopathy Act
Revised: 1978 n4 - The Naturopathy Act
Revised: 1984 c16 - The Naturopathy Act

Chairs of the SANP

1954 - 1970s	Bernard Hansen ND
1970s - 1989	William McGill DO
1989 - 1998	Edward Mahan ND
1999 - 2005	Douglas Amell ND
2005 -	Alana Barmby ND

Membership

1954: 3
1989: 4
2000: 5
2008: 17

Manitoba Naturopathic Association (MNA)

www.mbnd.ca

Association History

1946   Manitoba Naturopathic Association (MNA) was incorporated as both the provincial association and regulatory body.

Regulation History

Status: regulated
Initial Regulation: 1946 c106 - The Naturopathy Act

Chairs of the MNA

1946 - 1963	Fred Ripley ND
1963 - 1965	J. B. Gladstone ND
1965 - 1971	Frank Amsden ND
1985 - 1986	Royce Baker ND
1986 - 1987	Lambert Grube ND
1987 - 2004	Christopher Turner ND
2004 - 2005	Cameron Dodds ND
2005 - 2007	Christopher Turner ND
2007 - 2008	Gordon Sims ND
2008 -	Cory Storm ND

Membership

1961: 15
2000: 10
2008: 19

Ontario Association of Naturopathic Doctors (OAND)

www.oand.org

Association History

1950   Ontario Naturopathic Association (ONA) is incorporated.
1987   Name changed to the Ontario Association of Naturopathic Doctors.

Chairs of the ONA

1949 - 1952	James Price ND
1952 - 1958	Victor Tomlin ND
1958 - 1960	Albert Thut ND
1960 - 1961	Victor Tomlin ND
1961 - 1962	Robert Farquharson ND
1962 - 1963	Werner Arnet ND
1963 - 1971	Harold Drescher ND
1971 - 1974	Robert Farquharson ND
1974 - 1975	John LaPlante ND
1975 - 1977	William Morris ND
1977 - 1982	Eric Shrubb ND
1982 - 1983	John LaPlante ND
1983 - 1985	John Cosgrove ND

Chairs of the OAND

1985 - 1991	Patricia Wales ND
1991 - 1992	Alan Bell DC ND
1992 - 1995	Mark Percival ND
1995 - 1996	James Farquharson ND
1996 - 2002	Richard Dodd ND
2002 - 2007	Ruth Anne Baron ND
2007 -	Shelley Burns ND

Ontario Board of Directors, Drugless Therapy – Naturopathy (BDDT-N)
www.boardofnaturopathicmedicine.on.ca

Regulation History
Status: regulated
Umbrella Regulation: 1925 c149 - Drugless Practitioners Act
Revised: 1937 c229 - Drugless Practitioners Act
Revised: 1944 - Drugless Practitioner's Act
Revised: 1952 c25 - Drugless Practitioner's Act
1956   Board of Directors of Drugless Therapy – Naturopathy was formed.
Revised: 1956 - Drugless Practitioner's Act
New Regulation: 2008 - Naturopathy Act. Ontario regulation now under the RHPA

Chairs of the BDDT-N
1952 - 1956	Leonard Bailey ND
1956 - 1961	Eric Sjoman ND
1976 - 1981	John LaPlante ND
1981 - 1983	William. Morris ND
1983 - 1986	Eric Shrubb ND
1986 - 1993	James Spring ND
1993 - 2008	Angela Moore ND
2008 -	Patricia Rennie ND

Membership
1962: 125
1967: 79
2000: 360
2008: 917

Points of Interest
1952   Victor K.E. Tomlin DC ND – 1st to write NDs exam in Ontario.

1953	ONA starts offering monthly CE courses to registrants.
1959	BDDT-N attempted to change the name of the Act from Drugless Practitioner to Naturopath.
1974	ONA requests that NCNM add acupuncture to its curriculum.
1974	BDDT-N applied to the Ontario Government for regulation of acupuncture under the Drugless Therapy Act.
1975	ONA listed in the phone book for the first time.
1977	Radiology was no longer allowed.
1979	The ONA gave presentations to the World Symposium on Humanity.

Quebec Association of Naturopathic Medicine (QANM)/ Association de Medicine Naturopathique Du Québec (ANMQ)
www.qanm.org

Association History
1995	Quebec Professional Association of Naturopathic Physicians (QPANP) / Association Professionelle Des Médicins Naturopathes Du Québec (APMNQ).
1998	Name changed to Quebec Association of Naturopathic Medicine (QANM)/ Association de Medicine Nauropathique Du Québec (ANMQ).

Regulation Status: unregulated

Chairs of the QANM
1995 -   Andre Sainé ND

Membership
1995: 8
2008: 12

New Brunswick Association of Naturopathic Doctors (NBAND)

www.nband.ca

Association History

2001   New Brunswick Association of Naturopathic Doctors (NBAND) was formed.

Regulation Status: unregulated

Chairs of the NBAND

2001 - 2005   Cathleen Coleman ND
2005 -   Judah S. Bunin ND

Membership

2000: 2
2008: 12

Nova Scotia Association of Naturopathic Doctors (NSAND)

www.nsand.ca

Association History

1994   Nova Scotia Association of Naturopathic Doctors (NSAND) was formed.

Regulation History

Status: regulated
Title Protection: 2008 – The Naturopathic Doctor's Act

Chairs of the NSAND

1994 - 1997   Lois Hare ND
1997 - 2008   Margo Kleiker ND
1998 - 2001   Lois Hare ND and Margo Kleiker ND
2001 - 2008   Sarah Baillie ND and Jyl Bishop-Veale ND
2008 -   Rosalyn Hayman ND and Glenna Morris ND

Membership

2000: 13
2008: 36

Prince Edward Island Association of Naturopathic Doctors (PEIAND)

www.peiand.com

Association History

2004   Prince Edward Island Association of Naturopathic Doctors (PEIAND) was formed.

Regulation Status: unregulated

Chairs of the PEIAND

2004 - 2005   Kali Simmonds ND
2005 -   Gretchen MacLean ND

Membership

2000: 1
2008: 5

Newfoundland Labrador Association of Naturopathic Doctors (NLAND)

Association History

2006   Newfoundland Labrador Association of Naturopathic Doctors (NLAND) was formed.

Regulation Status: unregulated

Chairs of the NLAND

2006 - Kathleen Mercer

Membership

2008: 1

Yukon Naturopathic Association (YNA)

Association History

2001   Yukon Naturopathic Association (YNA) was formed.

Regulation Status: unregulated

Chairs of the YNA

2001 -   Joanne Leung ND

Membership

2001: 1
2008: 3

Northwest Territories

Association History: no association

Regulation Status: unregulated

Membership
2008: 1

Canadian College of Naturopathic Medicine (CCNM)
www.ccnm.edu

Association History
1978   Ontario College of Naturopathic Medicine (OCNM) is founded.
1981   Purchased K-W Art Gallery building located at 43 Benton Street, Kitchener.
1983   Formation of INER.
1984   Moved from Benton St. Kitchener to 1263 Bay Street, Toronto.
1986   Moved from Bay St. to 60 Berl Ave., Toronto.
1992   Name changed to The Canadian College of Naturopathic Medicine (CCNM).
1997   Moved from Berl Ave. to 2300 Yonge St., Toronto.
1999   Moved from Yonge St. to 1255 Sheppard Avenue East, Toronto
2000   Receives full accreditation from CNME.

Founding Members
Dr. Robert B. Farquharson DC ND
Dr. G. Asa Hershoff DC ND
Dr. John G. LaPlante DC ND
Dr. Eric F. Shrubb DC ND
Dr. Gordon Smith ND
Dr. William Morris DC ND

Presidents of OCNM / CCNM
1978 - 1989	Arno R. Koegler ND President Emeritus
1978 - 1981	Eric F. Shrubb ND
1982 - 1983	Robert Farquharson ND
1988 - 1990	Steve Hambly
1990 - 1991	Patricia Hutchinson
1991 - 1993	Kenneth Pownall DDS
1993 - 1996	Donald Warren ND
1996 - 2003	David Schleich PhD
2004 -	Bob Bernhardt

Chairs of the INER
1983 - 1984	John LaPlante ND
1984 - 1988	Alexander Wood ND
1988 - 1990	Robert Farquharson ND
1990 - 1990	Alan Nell ND
1990 - 1993	Donald Warren ND
1993 - 1997	Robert Schad
1997 - 2003	Jeremy Kendall
2003 - 2004	John Cosgrove ND
2004 - 2007	Susan Langley
2007 -	Kim Piller

Annual Tuition
1983: $5,000
1986: $7,000
1990: $7,900
1994: $8,900
1996: $12,000
2000: $14,000
2008: $21,455

Points of Interest
~1980 Dr. Gordon Smith ND purchased two bookcases of textbooks from Dr. Irlma Kennedy-Jackson's, MD estate auction for $1,000. Dr. Kennedy-Jackson was one of the first women to graduate from the University of Toronto Medical School; she practiced homeopathic psychiatry.
1991   CCNM students became eligible for OSAP and federal student loans.
1993   The first open house was held on November 28th 1993.
1993   Eight founding members of the CNA committed $1000 each from 1992 to 1995 to CCNM to support specific education projects. This was the start of the Mentor's Club.

Boucher Institute of Naturopathic Medicine (BINM)
www.binm.org

Association History
1999 West Coast Naturopathic Medical College was established.
2000 West Coast Naturopathic Medical Society was incorporated.
2001 Name of school is changed to BINM.
2008 Full accreditation from CNME is received.

Founding Members
Rowan Hamilton
Neil McKinney ND
Geri Martin
Kevin Nolan MD ND
Cidalia Paiva PhD
David Scotten ND
Isis van Loon ND
David Wang ND
Patricia Wolfe ND
Maylynn Woo ND
Eric Yarnell ND

Presidents of the BINM
2000 - 2007   David Scotten ND
2007 - 2009   Patricia Wolfe ND
2009 -   Alexander Cortina

Annual Tuition
2008: $17,200

National College of Natural Medicine (NCNM)
www.ncnm.edu
Note: although this College is in the United States it is included in this section due to the importance to Canadian naturopathic history and the involvement that Canadian NDs had in its formative years.

Founding Members
Dr. Charles R Stone ND
Dr. Martin Bleything ND
Dr. Frank G. Spaulding ND
Dr. Joseph Boucher ND
Elizabeth Murray
Dr. Gerald Farnsworth ND
Dr. Carl Kennedy Sr. ND
Dr. Dorothy Johnstone ND
Dr. Henry M Merritt ND

Annual NCNM Tuition
1956: $500
1965: $450
1972: $650
1974: $1500 for 3rd / 4th years at NCNM
$2090 for 1st / 2nd years at Kansas College
1978: $2,500

Points of Interest
1959   NCNM debuts the Naturopathic Missionary Medical Course intended to train Christian mis sionaries to serve overseas. Program discontinued in 1965.
1960s The salary for teaching, if you were paid at all, was in the range of six to eight dollars per contact hour.
1970   Dr. Bastyr paid for NCNM's x-ray machine out of his pocket at a cost of $5,000.
1972   ONA requests the NCNM include acupuncture in its pro gram.
1977 - An extension program was offered
1979   in Arizona for chiropractors and medical doctors which allowed them to be licensed as naturo pathic doctors after passing the course and exams.
1979   Medical residencies were started.
1990   As in all medical educational pro grams, the majority of students were male, but by 1990 females made up over seventy percent of each class, a trend that has con tinued at NCNM and in most naturopathic programs in Canada and the United States.

Naturopathic Physicians Licensing Examinations (NPLEX)

www.nabne.org

Chairs of the NPLEX

1986 - 1988	Ed Hoffmann-Smith ND
1988 - 1990	Robin Moore ND
1990 - 1995	Ed Hoffman-Smith ND
1995 - 2000	Christopher Turner ND
2000 -	Paul Saunders ND

North American Board of Naturopathic Examiners (NABNE)

www.nabne.org

Chairs of the NABNE

2000 - 2002	Michael Traub ND
2002 - 2005	Robin Moore ND
2005 -	James Spring ND

Council on Naturopathic Medical Education (CNME)

www.cnme.org

Presidents of the CNME

1978 -	M.W. Loftin ND
	Jeffery Bland PhD
1985 - 1987	Joe Pizzorno ND
1987 - 1989	Carlo Calabrese ND
1990 - 1991	Randall Bradley ND
1992 - 1993	William (Bill) Tribe
1994 - 1997	Randall Bradley ND
1997 - 1998	Eric Jones ND
1998 - 2001	G.S.S. Khalsa ND
2001 - 2005	Donald Warren ND
2005 - 2009	Marcia Prenguber ND
2009 -	Rita Bettenburg ND

Journals and Newsletters

Early Naturopathic Journals

1896 - 1901	Amerikanische Kneipp-Blätter in English as The Kneipp Water Cure Monthly
1902 - 1915	The Kneipp Water Cure Monthly renamed to The Naturopath and Herald of Health
1916 - 1922	renamed Herald of Health and Naturopath
1923 - 1927	Naturopath
1925 - 1953	Nature's Path
1934 - 1944	Naturopath and Herald of Health
1919	1st Universal Naturopathic Directory and Buyer's Guide

CNA / CAND – Brochures and Documents

1956	"CNA" State of the Profession
1960	Nature's Way to Health (shared with the American national association, AANP)
1962	A Brief Respecting National Health Services
1963	A Brief Respecting Hypnosis for Diagnostic and Therapeutic Purposes
1964	Naturopathic Medicine in Canada, CNA's first public relations booklet
1966	Statement on Naturopathy
1967	revised edition, Naturopathic Medicine in Canada
1971	revised edition, Naturopathic Medicine in Canada
1972	Naturopathy: A Separate and Distinct Healing Profession
1972	Naturae Medicina and Naturopathic Dispensatory, updated from the original by Kutz Cheraux
1972	A Comparison Between the Scope and Practice of the Naturopathic Practitioner and the Chiropractor, prepared by the CNA Committee on Education
1994	Clinical Nutrition Update
2001	Naturopathic Practice in Canada
2008	revised, Naturopathic Practice in Canada

CNA / CAND – Professional Journals

1955 - 1958	The Naturopathic Practitioner Journal (jointly with the AANP)
1964 - 1979	Canadian Journal of Naturopathic Medicine a bi-monthly journal, year ly subscription cost was $10
1983 - 1991	The Canadian Naturopathic Association / Association Canadienne de Naturopathie Newsletter
1991 - 1995	Naturopathic Newsletter
1995 -	Vital Link

CNA / CAND – Consumer Journals

1956 – 1959	Health for You (jointly with AANP)
1963 - ~1972	Reflections, a bimonthly magazine for the public.

BCNA – Professional Journals

1994 - present	BCNA Bulletin
1994 -	BCNA: Quarterly News and Views

BCNA – Public Journals

1995 -	Your Health

AANP – General Publication

1951	Theory of Nature Cure and Its Relation to Treatment
1960	Medicina Naturae and Naturopathic Dispensary
1960	Basic Naturopathy

AANP – Professional Journals

1953 - ~1955	Alberta Naturopathic Bulletin: quarterly issues
~1960 - ~1970	Newsletter of the Alberta Association of Naturopathic Practitioners

MNA – Public Journals

1935 - ~1960	Healthy Living Digest
1935 - ~1960	Handy Home Doctor

ONA / OAND – General Documents

~1964	Naturopathy, rehabilitation of the total person through natural therapies and ecology
1970	Reference File on the Naturopathic Profession
~1980	Introduction to Naturopathic Medicine – The Natural Choice for Health Care
1986	Overview of Naturopathy in Ontario

ONA / OAND – Professional Journals

1962 - ~1970	ONA News Bulletin
1974 - ~1984	Friends of Naturopathy Journal
1975 - ~1976	Natural Health World and Naturopath
1979 - ~1980	The Healing Crisis
1984 - 1987	ONA Newsletter
1987 - 1990	ND Reports – Publication of the ONA
1990 - 1992	Nature FAX
1995 - 1999	The ONA Pulse
1999 - 2002	OAND Journal
2002 -	OAND Pulse

ONA / OAND – Public Journals

1999 - 2006	Natural Path

Consumer brochures on a number of health concerns

OCNM / CCNM

1980 - 1983	OCNM Journal
1983 - 1992	OCNM Newsletter
1992 - ~1995	CNM Update
2000 - 2000	Naturopathic Connections
2000	Taxarcum, CCNM's first creative writing journal
2001 - 2006	Sage Source Newsletter
2006 - 2008	CCNM Quarterly Supplement
2008 -	Body, Mind, Spirit

CCNM NSA

2001 -	The Vine

ACRONYMS

AANMC – Association of Accredited Naturopathic Medical Colleges: www.aanmc.org

AANP – Alberta Association of Naturopathic Practitioners: www.naturopathic-alberta.com

AANP – American Association of Naturopathic Physicians: www.naturopathic.org

AMA – American Medical Association: www.ama-assn.org

ANA – American Naturopathic Association, see AANP

ANPBC – Association of Naturopathic Physicians of British Columbia, split and renamed to CNPBC and BCNA

ASN – American School of Naturopathy

Bastyr – see BU

BCNA – British Columbia Naturopathic Association: www.bcna.ca

BDDT-N – Board of Directors of Drugless Therapy – Naturopathy: www.boardofnaturopathicmedicine.on.ca

BINM – Boucher Institute of Naturopathic Medicine: www.binm.org

BNM – Board of Naturopathic Medicine: see BDDT-N

BNSA – Boucher Naturopathic Students' Association: www.binm.org

BU – Bastyr University: www.bastyr.edu

CAN – Citizen's Alliance for Naturopathy

CAND – Canadian Association of Naturopathic Doctors: www.cand.ca

CCA – Canadian Chiropractic Association: www.ccachiro.org

CCNM – Canadian College of Naturopathic Medicine: www.ccnm.edu

CEA – Conference Exchange Agreement

CHN – College of Health and Nutrition, University of Utah

CHPA – Canadian Health Protection Act (B.C.)

CJNM – Canadian Journal of Naturopathic Medicine

CMA – Canadian Medical Association: www.cma.ca

CMCC – Canadian Memorial Chiropractic College: www.cmcc.ca

CNA – Canadian Naturopathic Association, name changed to CAND

CNDA – College of Naturopathic Doctors of Alberta

CNERS – Canadian Naturopathic Education and Research Society, name changed to CNF

CNF - Canadian Naturopathic Foundation: www.cand.ca

CNME – Council of Naturopathic Medical Education: www.cnme.org

CNPBC – College of Naturopathic Physicians of British Columbia: www.cnpbc.bc.ca

DNM – Doctor of Naturopathic Medicine

DP – Drugless Practitioner

DPA – Drugless Practitioners Act (Ontario)

FNME – Federation of Naturopathic Medical Examiners, Inc.

HC – Health Canada: www.hc-sc.gc.ca

HIDS – Hospital Insurance and Diagnostic Services Act

HPA – Health Professions Act (British Columbia)

HPLRC – Health Professions Legislative Review Committee (Ontario)

HPRAC – Health Professions Regulatory Advisory Council (Ontario): www.hprac.org

ISNP - International Society of Naturopathic Physicians: www.isnp.net

LACC – Los Angeles City College

LCNPS – Lincoln College of Naturopathic Physicians and Surgeons Inc.

LMU – Ludwig Maximilian University of Munich, Germany

MNA – Manitoba Naturopathic Association: www.mbnd.ca

MOH – Ministry of Health

MRA – Mutual Recognition Agreement

NABNE – North American Board of Naturopathic Examiners: www.nabne.org

NANP - National Association of Naturopathic Physicians (NANP), formed in 1956 by merging American Naturopathic Association (ANA) and the American Association of Naturopathic Practitioners (AANP).

National – National College of Chiropractic Medicine

NBAND – New Brunswick Association of Naturopathic Doctors: www.nband.ca

NCC – Naturopathic Coordinating Council

NCDP – National College of Drugless Physicians

NCNM - National College of Naturopathic Medicine, name changed to National College of Natural Medicine: www.ncnm.edu

ND – Naturopathic Doctor

NDI – Natural Doctors International: www.ndimed.org

NHPs – Natural Health Products

NHPD – Natural Health Products Directorate: www.hc-sc.gc.ca/dph_mps/prodnatur/index_eng.

NLAND – Newfoundland & Labrador Association of Naturopathic Doctors

NMSA – Naturopathic Medical Student Association: www.naturopathicstudent.org

NPLEX – Naturopathic Physicians Licensing Examination Board: www.nabne.org

NSA – Naturopathic Students' Association (of CCNM): www.nsa-ccnm.com

NSAND – Nova Scotia Association of Naturopathic Doctors: www.nsand.ca

NWC – see NWCC

NWCC – Northwestern College of Chiropractic

NWNPC – North West Naturopathic Physicians Convention: www.nwnpc.com

OAND – Ontario Association of Naturopathic Doctors: www.oand.org

OCNM – Ontario College of Naturopathic Medicine, name changed to CCNM

ONA – Ontario Naturopathic Association, name changed to the OAND

ONHP – Office of Natural Health Products

PCN - Pacific College of Naturopathy

PCN – Philadelphia College of Naturopathy

PEIAND – Prince Edward Island Association of Naturopathic Doctors: www.peiand.com

QANM – Quebec Association of Naturopathic Medicine: www.qanm.org

RHPA – Regulated Health Professions Act (Ontario)

SANP – Saskatchewan Association of Naturopathic Physicians: www.sanp.ca

SCCNP – Southern California College of Naturopathic Physicians and Surgeons, Los Angeles

SCNM – Southwest College of Naturopathic Medicine and Health Sciences: www.scnm.edu

UBCNM – University of Bridgeport College of Naturopathic Medicine: www.bridgeport.edu/

WCB - Workers Compensation Board

WCNMC – West Coast Naturopathic Medical College, see BINM

WSC: Western States College

YNA - Yukon Naturopathic Association

BIBLIOGRAPHY

Alberta Association of Naturopathic Practitioners (AANP) 1940s – 2008. Documents, letters and journals

Abramson JH, Abramson ZH 2008 *Research Methods in Community Medicine, surveys, epidemiological research, programme evaluation, clinical trials.* John Wiley & Sons, England

American Chiropractic Association (ACA) 2007 http://www.amerchiro.org

American Medical Association (AMA) 2006 http://www.ama-asson.org

American Osteopathic Association (AOA) 2006 http://www.osteopathic.og

Arntz W, Chase B, Vicente M 2005 *What the Bleep Do We Know.* Health Communications, Florida

Baer HA 1992 *The potential rejuvenation of American naturopathy as a consequence of the holistic health movement.* Medical Anthropology, 13, pg. 369-383.

Bailey RD Kent and Gokavi Tanya 2001 *Naturopathic Practice in Canada.* Canadian Naturopathic Association

Barrett Stephen 2001 A Close Look at Naturopathy

British Columbia Naturopathic Association (BCNA) 1930s to 2008. Documents, letters and journals

Beinfield H and Korngold E 1991 *Between Heaven and Earth, a guide to Chinese Medicine.* Ballantine Wellspring, New York

Boon Heather 1996 The *Making of a Naturopathic Practitioner: The Education of "Alternative" Practitioners in Canada.* University of Toronto

Boon Heather 1996 *Canadian Naturopathic Practitioners: The Effects of Holistic and Scientific World Views on Their Socialization Experiences and Practice Patterns.* Thesis, University of Toronto

Boon Heather 1998 *Canadian Naturopathic Practitioners: Holistic and Scientific World Views.* Social Science Medicine Vol. 46 No9, pp 1213-1225

Canadian Association of Naturopathic Doctors (CAND) 1949 to 2008. Documents, letters and journals

Cant S.L. & Sharma U, 1996 *Professionalization of complementary medicine in the United Kingdom.* Complementary Therapies in Medicine. Vol4, pg157-162.

Carter JP 1992 *Racketeering in Medicine, the suppression of alternatives.* Hampton Roads, Norfolk, VA

Canadian College of Naturopathic Medicine (CCNM) 1977 to 2008. Documents, letters, journals and course calendars

Chaitow Leon 2008 *Naturopathic Physical Medicine, theory and practice for manual therapists and naturopaths.* Edinburgh, Elsevier

Canadian Naturopathic Association (CNA) 1971 *Naturopathic Medicine in Canada.* CNA

Canadian Naturopathic Association (CNA) 2001 *Naturopathic Medicine in Canada – A Strategic Template for the Growth and Development of the Naturopathic Profession.* CNA

Cody George 1985 History of naturopathic medicine. *History of Natural Medicine*, 1, 1-23 in A Textbook of Natural Medicine, JE Pizzorno and MT Murphy, eds. Seattle, WA: John Bastyr College Publications

Collins F.W. 1971 *The National University of Therapeutics*

Cooper Richard A and Stoflet Sandi J. 1996 *Trends in the Education and Practice of Alternative Medicine Clinicians*. Health Affairs, Vol15, No3 pg226 – 238.

Cottrell Katherine 1995 *The Age of Alternatives*, Chatelaine

CNME 1998 *Handbook of Accreditation for Naturopathic Medical Colleges and Programs*. Council on Naturopathic Medical Education

Cullin F.A. 1953 *A Thesis on the Therapeutic Sciences*. British Columbia

Duffin Jacalyn 2007 *History of Medicine, a scandalousy short introduction*. University of Toronto Press, Toronto

Eisenberg David M, Kessler Ronald C, Foster C, et al 1993 *Unconventional Medicine in the United States, prevalence, costs, and patterns of use*. The New England Journal of Medicine, Vol328, No4 pg246-252

Esmail Nadeem 2007 *Complementary and Alternative Medicine in Canada: Trends in Use and Public Attitudes, 1997 – 2006*. The Fraser Institute, British Columbia

Farnsworth Earl W. 1956 *A Thesis on Naturopathy To The Naturopathic Examining Board*. British Columbia

Farnsworth G.R. 1993 *The History of Naturopathic Medicine in British Columbia: 1886 – 1975*. BCNA

Finken Dee Anne 1886 *Naturopathy, America's homegrown alternative healing art*. Medical Self-Care, November-December.

Gershanek S 1926 *The Naturopathic and Chiropractic Directory*. New York

Glover 2004 A People Centered Model for Health: An Open Letter to the Ministries of Health

Gort Elaine 1986 *A Social History of Naturopathy in Ontario: The Formation of an Occupation Master's Dissertation*. Department of Behavioural Science / Community Health, University of Toronto, Toronto

Gort Elaine H and Coburn D 1988 *Naturopathy in Canada: Changing Relationships to Medicine, Chiropractic and the State*. Social Science Medicine Vol26, No10, pg1061-1072

Haller John S 1997 *Kindly Medicine, Physio-Medicalism in America 1836-1911*. Kent State University Press, Ohio

Hillemann, Howard H. 1960 *The Illusion of American Health and Longevity*. Lee Foundation for Nutritional Research

Holtum Ronald A 1937 *A Thesis on the Philosophy of Naturopathy*, British Columbia

Hough Holly J, Dower C, O'Neil Edward H 2001 *Profile of a Profession: Naturopathic Practice, Center for the Health Professions*. University of California, San Francisco

Jensen Clyde B 1997 *Common Paths in Medical Education, the training of allopaths, osteopaths and naturopaths.* Alternative and Complementary Therapies, August

Khalsa Sandesh Singh 2003 *The History of the National College of Naturopathic Medicine: 1956 to 1980.* National College of Naturopathic Medicine

Kirchfeld Friedhelm and Boyle Wade 1994 *Nature Doctors: Pioneers in Naturopathic Medicine.* NCNM Press, Portland Oregon

Kruger H. 1974 *Other healers, other cures: a guide to alternative medicine.* Bobbs-Merrill, New York

Kruzel Thomas A 1990 *History of Naturopathic Medicine*

Larson D 1968 *The Education and Regulation of Naturopaths in Ontario.* A study for the Ontario Committee on the Healing Art.

Levin Jeffrey S, Glass Thomas A, Kushi Lawrence H, et al. 1997 *Quantitative Methods in Research on Complementary and Alternative Medicine, a methodological manifesto.* Medical Care Vol35 No11, pg1079-1096.

Lindlahr H. *Philosophy of natural therapeutics.* Vol 1. Maidstronge, England

Lloyd, Iva 2005 *Messages from the Body, a guide to the energetics of health.* Naturopathic Publications, Ontario

Lloyd Iva 2009 *Energetics of Health, a naturopathic assessment,* Elsevier, England

Lust, Benedict 1918 *Universal Directory of Naturopathy.* Butler, Lust Publications, New Jersey

Lust, Benedict 1900 to 1940's various journals

MacDermot H.E. 1936 *History of the Canadian Medical Association 1867-1921.* The Canadian Medical Association Journal, March

Martin Marg 2004 *Naturopathic Philosophy: Time is of the Essence.* Journal of the Australian Traditional Medicine Society. Vol10, Issue2.

Micozzi Marc S. 1996 *Fundamentals of Complementary and Alternative Medicine* as taken from Pizzorno Joseph E 1996 *Natural Medicine.* Churchill Livingstone Inc., New York

Mills Donald 1966 *Royal Commission on Health Services: Study of Chiropractors, Osteopaths and Naturopaths in Canada.* Ottawa, Queen's Printer

Moor Fred B, Peterson Stella C, Manwell Ethel M, Noble Mary C, Muench Gertrude 1964 *Manual of Hydrotherapy and Massage.* Idaho, Pacific Press Publishing Association

Murray Michael T 1996 *Encyclopedia of Nutritional Supplements: the essential guide for improving your health naturally.* California, Prima Publishing

Murray Michael T and Pizzorno Joseph 1991 *Encyclopedia of Natural Medicine.* Prima Publishing, California

ONA / OAND minutes, records, journals and reports from 1950 to 2008

Pizzorno Joseph E 1996 *Natural Medicine.* Churchill Livingstone Inc., New York

Pizzorno Joseph E 1991 *Naturopathic medicine in the US 1990: review of a decade of challenge and accomplishment.* Complementary Medical Research, Vol5 No1.

Proby Jocelyn 2000 *Research Report on Naturopathy in Alberta and North America.* Edmonton

Washington State Naturopathic Association (WSNA) *Reader's Health Digest*, Public Relations Division, WSNA, Vol1

Ritchey Kris 2007 *US History of Physician Evolution*

Roy Leo 1984 *Health Freedoms Under Attack.* Medatic Research Inc. Toronto, Ontario

Schleich David John 2005 *From Nature-Cure to Naturopathic Medicine: The Institutionalizing of Naturopathic Medical Education in Ontario.* A thesis submitted to the Ontario Institute for Studies in Education of the University of Toronto

Shepherd Francis J *The First Medical School in Canada, its history and founders, with some personal reminiscences.* The Canadian Medical Association Journal. Pg 418-425.

Snider Pamela 1996 *The Future of Naturopathic Medical Education, primary care integrative natural medicine: the healing power of nature.* Bastyr University

Spaulding William B 1993 *Why Rockefeller Supported Medical Education in Canada.* The William Lyon Mackenzie King Connection. CBMH/BCHM. Vol10 pg 67-76.

Turner Christopher J 1986 *Naturopathy —What is it?* CNA

Turner Roger Newman 1990 *Naturopathic Medicine Treating the Whole Person, the principles and practice of naturopathy.* Great Britian, Health Advisory Lectures and Literature

Vanderhaeghe Lorna 1999 *The Evolution of Natural Medicine*

Vithoulkas George 1980 *The Science of Homeopathy.* Grove Press, New York

Vogel A. 1959 *The Nature Doctor, a kaleidoscopic collection of helpful hints from the Swiss folklore of healing.* Verlagsanstalt Merk & Co., Switzerland

Wright D. 2004 *Death, Disease and Degeneration: A History of Health and Health Care in Canada.* McMaster University, Waterloo

Yawney Carole 1983 *Naturopathic Medicine, a radical orthodoxy.* Health Sharing Spring.

Yawney Carole D 1986 *The Social Construction of Naturopathic Ideology in Ontario.* York University, Toronto

Zeff Jared L. 1997 *The Process of Healing: A Unifying Theory of Naturopathic Medicine.* Journal of Naturopathic Medicine, Vol7 Issue1, pg 122-126.